KV-086-893

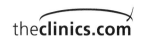
the**clinics.com**

CLINICS IN PERINATOLOGY

Iatrogenic Disease

GUEST EDITOR
Marcus C. Hermansen, MD

March 2008 • Volume 35 • Number 1

SAUNDERS

An Imprint of Elsevier, Inc.
PHILADELPHIA   LONDON   TORONTO   MONTREAL   SYDNEY   TOKYO

W.B. SAUNDERS COMPANY
A Division of Elsevier Inc.

Elsevier, Inc., 1600 John F. Kennedy Blvd., Suite 1800, Philadelphia, PA 19103-2899

http://www.theclinics.com

CLINICS IN PERINATOLOGY
March 2008
Editor: Carla Holloway

Volume 35, Number 1
ISSN 0095-5108
ISBN-10: 1-4160-5798-6
ISBN-13: 978-1-4160-5798-7

Clinics in Perinatology (ISSN 0095-5108) is published in quarterly by Elsevier Inc., 360 Park Avenue South, New York, NY 10010-1710. Months of issue are March, June, September, and December. Business and Editorial offices: 1600 John F. Kennedy Blvd., Suite 1800, Philadelphia, PA 19103-2899. Customer Service Office: 6277 Sea Harbor Drive, Orlando, FL 32887-4800. Periodicals postage paid at New York, NY and additional mailing offices. Subscription prices are $197.00 per year (US individuals), $297.00 per year (US institutions), $232.00 per year (Canadian individuals), $369.00 per year (Canadian institutions), $268.00 per year (foreign individuals), $369.00 per year (foreign institutions) $95.00 per year (US students), and $131.00 per year (Canadian and foreign students). Foreign air speed delivery is included in all Clinics subscription prices. All prices are subject to change without notice. **POSTMASTER:** Send address changes to *Clinics in Perinatology*; Elsevier Periodicals Customer Service, 6277 Sea Harbor Drive, Orlando, FL 32887-4800. Customer Service: 1-800-654-2452 (US). From outside the United States, call 1-407-563-6020. Fax: 1-407-363-9661. E-mail: JournalsCustomerService-usa@elsevier.com.

Clinics in Perinatology is also pubilshed in Spanish by McGraw-Hill Interamericana Editores S.A., P.O. Box 5-237, 06500 Mexico D.F., Mexico.

Clinics in Perinatology is covered in *Index Medicus, Current Contents, Excepta Medica, BIOSIS* and *ISI/BIOMED*.

Printed in the United States of America.

GUEST EDITOR

MARCUS C. HERMANSEN, MD, Associate Professor of Pediatrics; Adjunct Associate Professor of Obstetrics and Gynecology, Department of Pediatrics, Dartmouth Medical School, Lebanon; Neonatal Intensive Care Unit, Southern New Hampshire Medical Center, Nashua, New Hampshire

CONTRIBUTORS

CANDE V. ANANTH, PhD, MPH, Professor of Obstetrics and Gynecology; Director, Division of Epidemiology and Biostatistics, Department of Obstetrics, Gynecology, and Reproductive Sciences, UMDNJ-Robert Wood Johnson Medical School, New Brunswick, New Jersey

SABARATNAM ARULKUMARAN, MD, PhD, FRCOG, Professor, Department of Obstetrics and Gynaecology, St George's University of London, London, United Kingdom

STEPHEN BAUMGART, MD, Professor of Pediatrics, Children's National Medical Center, Department of Neonatology, George Washington University, School of Medicine, Washington, DC

CYNTHIA F. BEARER, MD, PhD, Professor of Pediatrics, Division of Neonatology, University Hospitals, Rainbow Babies and Childrens Hospital, Cleveland, Ohio

DAVID J. BIRNBACH, MD, MPH, Professor and Executive Vice Chair, Department of Anesthesiology; Director, UM-JMH Center for Patient Safety, Miller School of Medicine, Miami, Florida

MICHAEL D. BRANDLER, MD, Attending Neonatologist, Division of Neonatology, Department of Pediatrics, New York Hospital Queens, Affiliate Weill Medical College of Cornell University, Flushing, New York

ALISON J. CAREY, MD, Clinical Fellow, Division of Neonatology, Columbia University Medical Center, New York-Presbyterian Hospital, New York, New York

WALDEMAR A. CARLO, MD, Director, Division of Neonatology; Edwin M. Dixon Professor of Pediatrics, Department of Pediatrics, University of Alabama at Birmingham, Birmingham, Alabama

JOHN CHUO, MD, MS, Assistant Professor of Pediatrics; Director of Neonatal Intensive Care Unit and Neonatal Informatics, Robert Wood Johnson Medical School, University of Medicine and Dentistry of New Jersey, New Brunswick, New Jersey

STERGIOS K. DOUMOUCHTSIS, MD, PhD, MRCOG, Specialist Registrar, Department of Obstetrics and Gynaecology, St George's University of London, London, United Kingdom

ANTONI D'SOUZA, MD, Attending Neonatologist, Division of Neonatology, Department of Pediatrics, New York Hospital Queens, Affiliate Weill Medical College of Cornell University, Flushing, New York

RODNEY W. HICKS, PhD, RN, UMC Health System Endowed Chair for Patient Safety; Professor, Texas Tech University Health Sciences Center, Lubbock, Texas

LUCKY JAIN, MD, MBA, Professor, Division of Neonatology, Department of Pediatrics, Emory University School of Medicine, Atlanta, Georgia

TONI A. KFURI, MD, MPH, CMQ, FACOG, Research Analyst; Dr PH candidate, Department of Health Policy and Management, Johns Hopkins Bloomberg School of Public Health, Baltimore, Maryland

THOMAS T. LAI, MD, Division of Neonatology, University Hospitals, Rainbow Babies and Childrens Hospital, Cleveland, Ohio

CHRISTOPH U. LEHMANN, MD, Eudowood Neonatal Pulmonary Division, Department of Pediatrics; Department of Dermatology; Division of Health Sciences Informatics, Johns Hopkins University School of Medicine; School of Nursing, Johns Hopkins University, Baltimore, Maryland

DAVID C. MERRILL, MD, PhD, Professor; Chairman, Section on Maternal Fetal Medicine, Department of Obstetrics and Gynecology, Wake Forest University, Winston-Salem, North Carolina

HEATHER L. MERTZ, MD, Assistant Professor, Section on Maternal Fetal Medicine, Department of Obstetrics and Gynecology, Wake Forest University, Winston-Salem, North Carolina

J. DAVIN MILLER, MD, Fellow, Division of Neonatology, Department of Pediatrics, University of Alabama at Birmingham, Birmingham, Alabama

MARLENE R. MILLER, MD, MSc, Department of Pediatrics, Johns Hopkins University School of Medicine; Department of Health Policy and Management, Johns Hopkins University Bloomberg School of Public Health, Baltimore, Maryland; National Association of Children's Hospitals and Related Institutions, Alexandria, Virginia

LAURA MORLOCK, PhD, Professor and Deputy Chair, Department of Health Policy and Management, Johns Hopkins Bloomberg School of Public Health, Baltimore, Maryland

RICHARD A. POLIN, MD, Chief, Division of Neonatology, Columbia University Medical Center, New York-Presbyterian Hospital, New York, New York

ASHWIN RAMACHANDRAPPA, MD, MPH, Fellow, Division of Neonatology, Department of Pediatrics, Emory University School of Medicine, Atlanta, Georgia

JAYASHREE RAMASETHU, MD, FAAP, Associate Professor of Clinical Pediatrics; Associate Director, Neonatal Perinatal Medicine Fellowship Program, Division of Neonatology, Georgetown University Hospital, Washington, DC

J. SUDHARMA RANASINGHE, MD, FFARCSI, Associate Professor, Department of Anesthesiology, Miller School of Medicine, University of Miami, Miami, Florida

LISA SAIMAN, MD, MPH, Professor of Clinical Pediatrics, Division of Pediatric Infectious Disease, Columbia University Medical Center, New York-Presbyterian Hospital; Department of Hospital Epidemiology, Columbia University Medical Center, New York-Presbyterian Hospital, New York, New York

ANDREW D. SHORE, PhD, Assistant Scientist, Department of Health Policy and Management, Health Services Research and Development Center, The Johns Hopkins Bloomberg School of Public Health, Baltimore, Maryland

JENNIFER G. SMITH, MD, PhD, Instructor, Section on Maternal Fetal Medicine, Department of Obstetrics and Gynecology, Wake Forest University, Winston-Salem, North Carolina

PINCHI S. SRINIVASAN, MD, Associate Director; Assistant Professor of Clinical Pediatrics, Division of Neonatology, Department of Pediatrics, New York Hospital Queens, Affiliate Weill Medical College of Cornell University, Flushing, New York

THEODORA A. STAVROUDIS, MD, Eudowood Neonatal Pulmonary Division, Department of Pediatrics, Johns Hopkins University School of Medicine, Baltimore, Maryland

ANTHONY M. VINTZILEOS, MD, Professor and Chairman, Department of Obstetrics and Gynecology, Winthrop University Hospital, Mineola, New York

CONTENTS

during pregnancy. Furthermore, evidence of in-hospital medication errors from obstetric services has been provided by national medication error data voluntarily submitted from many hospitals. The data provide fresh insight into the nature of medication errors in obstetrics, especially regarding the medication use process, the most common types of errors reported, the most commonly reported products overall, as well as those that resulted in patient harm. Providers and staff working within health care organizations should be well aware that a substantial number of patients experience medication errors which can result in serious injuries.

Iatrogenic medication errors in the neonatal ICU (NICU) are reported to occur up to 2.6 times per 100 NICU days. It has been learned during the last decade that well-intended but faulty implementations of technology can increase the frequency of errors and also can give rise to new types. This article compares and discusses iatrogenic medication errors in the NICU that are related to computer entry and computerized physician order entry systems. The authors also propose a possible approach for evaluating technology that is intended to prevent iatrogenic mediation errors in the NICU.

Prevention of harm from medication errors has become a national priority. Medication errors in the neonatal intensive care unit are common, and most can be avoided. This article reviews the prevalence and types of medication errors affecting the care of the neonate and summarizes approaches that have been used to reduce these errors. Safety initiatives applicable to minimizing medication errors also are discussed.

Premature infants in the neonatal intensive care unit (NICU) face many illnesses and complications. Another potential source of iatrogenic disease is the NICU environment. Research in this area, however, is limited.

This article reviews the physiology of thermoregulation, hypothermia, and hyperthermia. The differential diagnosis of hypothermia and hyperthermia is discussed. The benefits of hypothermia following hypoxic-ischemic injury are discussed; however, both hypothermia and hyperthermia, in the extreme, are potentially harmful to the newborn. Recommendations for the prevention of these problems are discussed, as well as available treatments.

Insertion of an intravascular catheter is the most common invasive procedure in the neonatal ICU. With every passing decade, technological innovations in catheter materials and sizes have allowed vascular access in infants who are smaller and sicker for purposes of blood pressure monitoring, blood sampling, and infusion of intravenous fluids and medications. There is, however, growing recognition of potential risks to life and limb associated with the use of intravascular catheters. This article reviews complications of venous and arterial catheters in the neonatal ICU and discusses treatment approaches and methods to prevent such complications, based on current evidence.

Nosocomial infections are an important cause of morbidity and mortality in the preterm neonate. Extrinsic and intrinsic risk factors make the preterm neonate particularly susceptible to infection. This review focuses on two major pathogens that cause nosocomial infection, Candida and methicillin-resistant Staphylococcus aureus. The difficult diagnosis of meningitis in the neonate also is discussed.

In necrotizing enterocolitis (NEC) the small (most often distal) and/or large bowel becomes injured, develops intramural air, and may progress to frank necrosis with perforation. Even with early, aggressive treatment, the progression of necrosis, which is highly characteristic of NEC, can lead to sepsis and death. This article reviews the current scientific knowledge related to the etiology and patho-genesis of NEC and discusses some possible preventive measures.

Mechanical ventilation is necessary and life saving in many neonates. Most complications are inherent to this intervention and cannot be confused with iatrogenic errors in judgment or care practices by clinicians. Clinical data suggest that complications such as volutrauma and air leak syndromes can negatively affect long-term pulmonary and non-pulmonary outcomes. Careful attention to many aspects of neonatal care, such as delivery room resuscitation, ventilatory support, and routine care practices, is needed to decrease pulmonary complications of mechanical ventilation. Clinical research is needed to improve mechanical ventilator strategies to reduce pulmonary complications and improve long-term outcomes.

GOAL STATEMENT

The goal of *Clinics in Perinatology* is to keep practicing neonatologists and maternal-fetal medicine specialists up to date with current clinical practice in perinatology by providing timely articles reviewing the state of the art in patient care.

ACCREDITATION

The *Clinics in Perinatology* is planned and implemented in accordance with the Essential Areas and Policies of the Accreditation Council for Continuing Medical Education (ACCME) through the joint sponsorship of the University of Virginia School of Medicine and Elsevier. The University of Virginia School of Medicine is accredited by the ACCME to provide continuing medical education for physicians.

The University of Virginia School of Medicine designates this educational activity for a maximum of 60 *AMA PRA Category 1 Credits*™. Physicians should only claim credit commensurate with the extent of their participation in the activity.

The American Medical Association has determined that physicians not licensed in the US who participate in this CME activity are eligible for *AMA PRA Category 1 Credits*™.

Credit can be earned by reading the text material, taking the CME examination online at http://www.theclinics.com/home/cme, and completing the evaluation. After taking the test, you will be required to review any and all incorrect answers. Following completion of the test and evaluation, your credit will be awarded and you may print your certificate.

FACULTY DISCLOSURE/CONFLICT OF INTEREST

The University of Virginia School of Medicine, as an ACCME accredited provider, endorses and strives to comply with the Accreditation Council for Continuing Medical Education (ACCME) Standards of Commercial Support, Commonwealth of Virginia statutes, University of Virginia policies and procedures, and associated federal and private regulations and guidelines on the need for disclosure and monitoring of proprietary and financial interests that may affect the scientific integrity and balance of content delivered in continuing medical education activities under our auspices.

The University of Virginia School of Medicine requires that all CME activities accredited through this institution be developed independently and be scientifically rigorous, balanced and objective in the presentation/discussion of its content, theories and practices.

All authors/editors participating in an accredited CME activity are expected to disclose to the readers relevant financial relationships with commercial entities occurring within the past 12 months (such as grants or research support, employee, consultant, stock holder, member of speakers bureau, etc.).,The University of Virginia School of Medicine will employ appropriate mechanisms to resolve potential conflicts of interest to maintain the standards of fair and balanced education to the reader. Questions about specific strategies can be directed to the Office of Continuing Medical Education, University of Virginia School of Medicine, Charlottesville, Virginia.

The authors/editors listed below have identified no professional or financial affiliations for themselves or their spouse/partner:
Cande V. Ananth, PhD, MPH; Sabaratnam Arulkumaran, MD, PhD, FRCOG; Stephen Baumgart, MD; Cynthia F. Bearer, MD, PhD; David J. Birnbach, MD, MPH; Michael D. Brandler, MD; Alison J. Carey, MD; Waldemar A. Carlo, MD; John Chuo, MD, MS; Stergios K. Doumouchtsis, MD, PhD, MRCOG; Antoni D'Souza, MD; Marcus C. Hermansen, MD (Guest Editor); Carla Holloway (Acquisitions Editor); Toni A. Kfuri, MD, MPH, CMQ, FACOG; Thomas T. Lai, MD; Christoph U. Lehmann, MD; David C. Merrill, MD, PhD; Heather L. Mertz, MD; J. Davin Miller, MD; Marlene R. Miller, MD, MSc; Laura Morlock, PhD; Ashwin Ramachandrappa, MD, MPH; Jayashree Ramasethu, MD, FAAP; J. Sudharma Ranasinghe, MD, FFARCSI; Andrew D. Shore, PhD; Jennifer G. Smith, MD, PhD; Pinchi S. Srinivasan, MD; Theodora A. Stavroudis, MD; and Anthony M. Vintzileos, MD.

The authors/editors listed below identified the following professional or financial affiliations for themselves or their spouse/partner:
Rodney W. Hicks, PhD, RN employed by United States Pharmacopeia.
Lucky Jain, MD, MBA is a consultant for Schering Plough and serves on the speaker's bureau for iNO Therapeutics.
Richard A. Polin, MD serves on the Advisory Committee for Discovery Labs and is a consultant for Info Care.
Lisa Saiman, MD, MPH is a consultant for Transave, Inc. and serves on the Speaker's Bureau and the advisory board for Novartis.

Disclosure of Discussion of non-FDA approved uses for pharmaceutical products and/or medical devices:
The University of Virginia School of Medicine, as an ACCME provider, requires that all faculty presenters identify and disclose any "off label" uses for pharmaceutical and medical device products. The University of Virginia School of Medicine recommends that each physician fully review all the available data on new products or procedures prior to instituting them with patients.

TO ENROLL

To enroll in the Clinics in Perinatology Continuing Medical Education program, call customer service at 1-800-654-2452 or visit us online at www.theclinics.com/home/cme. The CME program is available to subscribers for an additional fee of $195.00.

FORTHCOMING ISSUES

RECENT ISSUES

CLINICS IN
PERINATOLOGY

Clin Perinatol 35 (2008) xv–xvi

Preface

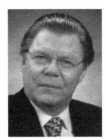

Marcus C. Hermansen, MD
Guest Editor

It is commonly believed that the phrase *primum non nocere* (above all [or first], do no harm) has its origin in the Hippocratic Oath. The Oath requires doctors to do what they consider beneficial for their patients and to "abstain from whatever is deleterious and mischievous." However, the Hippocratic Oath has no reference to doing no harm "first" or "above all" and should not be considered the source of the phrase.

Hippocrates (ca. 460–377 BC) did write in Greek in his *magnum opus, Epidemics*, Book 1, Section XI "Declare the past, diagnose the present, fore-tell the future; practice these acts. As to diseases, make a habit of two things – to help, or at least to do no harm." The prominent physician Galen (AD 129–ca. 200) is usually credited with translating Hippocrate's *Epidemics* from Greek to Latin and attaching "above all," producing *primum non nocere*. During the Middle Ages widespread use of Greek died out in Europe, and thereafter the phrase was passed down predominantly in Galen's Latin form. It was introduced into American and British medical cultures by Worthington Hooker in his 1847 book *Physician and Patient*. This was probably the first published translation of the phrase into English as "above all, do no harm." Hooker attributed the phrase to the oral teachings of Parisian pathologist and clinician Auguste François Chomel (1788–1858). In 1860, T. Inman credited the phrase not to Chomel but to Thomas Syndenham (1624–1689), sometimes referred to as the Father of English Medicine. Although the phrase was commonly spoken in the late 1800s, it rarely appeared in print early in the 20th century. Today the phrase is com-monly used. Medical students and physicians consider it to be a hallowed

0095-5108/08/$ - see front matter © 2008 Elsevier Inc. All rights reserved.
doi:10.1016/j.clp.2007.11.013   *perinatology.theclinics.com*

expression of hope, intention, humility, and recognition that human acts with good intentions may have unwanted consequences. The term, in both its English and Latin forms, has gained widespread use even outside the field of medicine, in fields as diverse as computer programming, religion, law enforcement, and criminal justice. *Primum non nocere*—above all, do no harm!

This issue of *Clinics in Perinatology* is my third, and presumably final, as guest editor. The common theme of the trilogy has been one of risk management with an emphasis on risk reduction. I have attempted to expose the reader to the intricacies of the medical malpractice system (*Clinics in Perinatology*, March 2005), to the various causes of cerebral palsy (*Clinics in Perinatology*, June 2006), and now to an analysis of the many complications of our care. A careful reading of this issue will provide the reader with countless strategies and tactics for risk reduction.

It has been an honor to have completed this project, and I thank all those who have participated, as well as Carla Holloway, Carin Davis, and the entire Elsevier staff for their professional efforts. I thank all the authors and contributors who shared their knowledge and wisdom with the readers. And most of all, I thank my wife Mary for her support, encouragement, and love throughout this endeavor.

Marcus C. Hermansen, MD
Neonatal Intensive Care Unit
Southern New Hampshire Medical Center
8 Prospect Street
Nashua, NH 03061

E-mail address: marcus.hermansen@snhmc.org

ELSEVIER
SAUNDERS

CLINICS IN
PERINATOLOGY

Clin Perinatol 35 (2008) 1–34

Iatrogenic Disorders in Modern Neonatology: A Focus on Safety and Quality of Care

Ashwin Ramachandrappa, MD, MPH*,
Lucky Jain, MD, MBA

*Division of Neonatology, Department of Pediatrics, Emory University
School of Medicine, 2015 Uppergate Drive NE, Atlanta, GA 30322, USA*

I am dying from the treatment of too many physicians.
Alexander the Great

Great strides have been made in the field of neonatal perinatal medicine since its birth in the 1950s. The neonatal mortality rate has declined 78%, from 20.5 per 1000 live births in the 1950s to 4.5 per 1000 live births in 2004 [1]. Rapid advances in the fields of physiology, chemistry, pharmacology, and diagnostics led to their adoption into this fledgling field to treat the less known diseases of newborns; the many successes have been intermingled with therapeutic misadventures. The introduction of these new modalities of treatment for the very premature infant and advanced life-support systems led to a decrease in the neonatal mortality rate, and a consequent increase in the population of the tiniest survivors.

Many of these premature infants that survive their neonatal intensive care unit (NICU) stay have permanent injury to their vital organs including eyes, lungs, brain, and gastrointestinal tract, causing them to have lifelong disabilities. Whether these injuries are a result of their prematurity, or are caused by the life-support systems and treatments is a subject of much dispute. As is often the case, hindsight reveals that the adoption of these new treatment modalities and drugs in neonatal medicine without adequate testing or trials has resulted in therapeutic misadventures, leading to new epidemics of iatrogenic disorders: neoiatroepidemics, as is vividly depicted in Fig. 1.

This article explains the process of iatrogenicity and separates the iatrogenic problems that are preventable from those that are currently

* Corresponding author.
  E-mail address: ashwin_ramachandrappa@oz.ped.emory.edu (A. Ramachandrappa).

0095-5108/08/$ - see front matter © 2008 Elsevier Inc. All rights reserved.
doi:10.1016/j.clp.2007.11.012   *perinatology.theclinics.com*

NEONATOLOGY

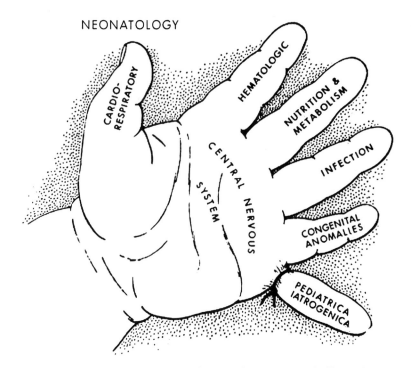

Fig. 1. Neonatology. (*Courtesy of* B.F. Andrews, MD, Louisville, KY.).

unpreventable. It is hoped that the reader's awareness will be raised particularly to those that are preventable; readers are also referred to a previous version of this article [2].

Definition

The word "iatrogenic" is derived from the Greek words "iatros," meaning physician and "genesis" for origin. As defined by Kassner [3], iatrogenic disorders include "all unintended adverse outcomes of diagnostic and/or therapeutic interventions, whether due to lack of physician skills, inherent hazard of intervention, susceptibility of the host, or extent of affliction being managed." Steel and colleagues [4] defined iatrogenic illness as "any illness that resulted from a diagnostic procedure, from any form of therapy, or from a harmful occurrence that was not a natural consequence of the patient's disease."

Historical background

Iatrogenic complications occurring in the course of perfectly well-intentioned therapy are not new to neonatal medicine. A historical review of the practice of neonatology over the last 60 years reveals interesting episodes of iatrogenic disorders (Table 1). For example, severe dehydration of preterm newborns was fairly common in the 1940s, when feeds were withheld for several days after birth for fear of death from aspiration [5]. Many dehydrated infants were then administered fluids subcutaneously, giving rise to a new set of complications. Incubator temperatures were held at 25°C since the early 1930s because the early incubators easily overheated at higher temperatures and bigger term babies did well at this temperature. The relative inexperience with premature babies led providers to believe that this was their normal physiologic temperature and they should not attempt artificially to increase their body temperature. It was not until Silverman's [6] study in 1954 on mortality at higher and lower temperature settings in the incubator did that practice start to change. Budin in the 1900s used oxygen in premature infants for apnea and cyanosis. A subsequent study by Wilson and colleagues in 1942 showed reduced apnea and periodic breathing with supplemental oxygen use; this, combined with a change in incubator technology designed to increase oxygen concentration in the incubator and its early adaptation without adequate testing, led to the retinopathy of prematurity (ROP) epidemic, blinding about 10,000 infants by the 1950s [5,7]. A randomized controlled trial conducted in 1954 clearly showed the association of oxygen with retrolental fibroplasia. The thalidomide disaster stunned the medical community and reminded of the extent of damage that can be caused by an iatroepidemic. Since then several new iatroepidemics in neonatal medicine have occurred.

Genesis

Several factors contribute to the genesis of an iatroepidemic. First, rapid technologic advances have revolutionized the practice of neonatal medicine. The influence of bioengineering in the present-day NICU can easily be seen when it is referred to as a "space station" [8]. A multitude of new therapeutic modalities have been introduced into the patient arena (Fig. 2). Some of them received critical evaluation and withstood the test of time; others managed to slip into use with less critical evaluation. Many of these therapeutic modalities are the major contributors to neoiatrogenesis; this can be easily seen in Table 1, which lists many interventions that although well intentioned, were never subjected to rigorous controlled trials. Research in basic sciences has predictably lagged behind. Most of the elemental problems in neonatology were tackled by an observational-authoritative approach. It is no wonder Silverman [6] stated that, "premature infants played the role of miners' canaries; they gave early warning about the danger of relying on the claims of recognized authorities who based their advice on inductive reasoning." In the absence of a sound knowledge of the physiologic effects of any given therapy, side effects cannot be predicted with accuracy and are likely to be missed.

Table 1
Major iatrogenic disorders during evolution of neonatology

Year	Problem	Treatment	Iatroepidemic
1930s	Temperature instability in premature infants, overheating incubators	Low incubator temperatures	Increased mortality and respiratory distress
	Enlarged thymus in infants with sudden infant death syndrome	Irradiation of thymus	Thyroid cancer
1940s	Aspiration of feed in preterm newborns	Withhold feed for 72 h	Dehydration, neurologic deficits
	Respiratory distress and periodic breathing in newborns	Liberal use of oxygen	Retinopathy of prematurity
	Blindness from retinopathy of prematurity	Restricted oxygen use	Increased mortality and neurologic sequelae
1950s	Vitamin K deficiency	Excessive synthetic vitamin K	Hemolysis, hyperbilirubinemia, and kernicterus
	Infections	Sulfisoxazole	Kernicterus
		Chramphenicol	"Gray baby" syndrome
	Nutrition	SMA (Wyeth Pharmaceuticals, Madison, New Jersey) formula	Seizures
1960s	Maternal sedation during pregnancy	Thalidomide	Limb defects in newborns
	Respiratory distress syndrome	Assisted ventilation	Air leak syndromes, bronchopulmonary dysplasia
	Invasive monitoring	Umbilical artery catheters	Aortic thrombus, gangrene
1970s	Persistent pulmonary hypertension	Tolazoline	Hypotension, bleed
	Nutrition	Hyperalimentation	Cholestasis, metabolic acidosis, essential fatty acid deficiency
		Premature infant formulas	Lactobezoars
1980s	Retinopathy of prematurity	Intravenous vitamin E	Multiorgan damage
	Solvent	Propylene glycol	Hyperosmolarity, seizures
	Persistent pulmonary hypertension	Hyperventilation	Air leak syndrome
		Extracorporeal membrane oxygenation	Intraventricular hemorrhage
1990s	Respiratory distress and bronchopulmonary dysplasia	Steroids	Cerebral palsy
	Extremely low birth weight infants	Advanced ventilation and equipment	Ethical problems: quality of life, financial burden

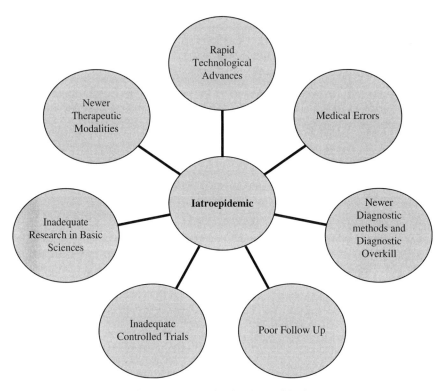

Fig. 2. Pathogenesis of an iatroepidemic.

Medical errors are an important part of iatrogenesis. An error is defined as the "failure of a planned action to be completed as intended (ie, error of execution) or the use of a wrong plan to achieve an aim (ie, error of planning)" [9]. Errors are not just pertinent to neonatology but are prevalent in the entire health care system. Brennan and colleagues in their landmark 1991 Harvard study [10] found adverse events to occur in 3.7% of all hospitalized patients, over half of which were preventable and 13.6% of which led to death. If this is extrapolated to the entire American health care system, over 180,000 die each year from preventable medical errors, the equivalent of three jumbo jet crashes every 2 days [11]. The Institutes of Medicine (IOM), in their landmark report "To Err is Human: Building a Safer Health System," attributed as many as 44,000 to 98,000 deaths annually to medical errors, higher than automobile accidents, AIDS, or breast cancer [9]. Other studies by Starfield [12] have estimated much higher number of deaths from errors, up to 250,000 per year. The IOM estimated that preventable adverse events (medical errors that result in injury) cost the United States economy between $17 and $29 billion, over half of which represents direct health care costs [9].

Overinterpretation of laboratory results and overdiagnosis similarly can contribute to iatrogenesis. Neonates undergo countless and sometimes unnecessary diagnostic tests; the habit of obtaining routine laboratory data is very prevalent in NICUs. Erroneous laboratory values can result in further blood draws and testing, which are not only worthless and time consuming but also may result in harm to the patient. The expanded newborn screening is a classic example; in states offering screening with tandem mass spectrometry, determination of inappropriate cutoff values for positive screens, especially in the premature neonates, have resulted in numerous abnormal results. Increased screening identifies more false-positive results, which triggers additional unnecessary and potentially harmful testing. A lack of accepted protocols and guidelines for work-up and poor availability of adequate educational materials describing disorders have also posed major challenges to parents [13].

It is generally agreed that the prospect of medicolegal liability has contributed to the practice of defensive medicine. This, in turn, contributes to iatrogenesis, although it is difficult to estimate the exact impact. A clear understanding among physicians as to the risk/benefit ratio of an intervention can minimize iatrogenic problems without the fear of medicolegal liability.

Types of iatrogenic disorders

It is quite difficult, and at times impossible, to categorize a given unfavorable outcome in a patient as a result of the underlying disease or from medical interventions. The IOM report defines an adverse event as "an injury caused by medical management rather than the underlying condition of the patient," and preventable adverse event as "an adverse event attributable to error" [9]. Adverse events can be preventable or unpreventable. Preventable disorders are usually caused by errors. Human error is the cause of most accidents in any industry, and medicine is no exception; it accounts for up to 60% to 80% of all accidents [9]. These errors can be defined as either slips or lapses (errors of execution, failure of a planned action to be completed as intended) and mistakes (errors of planning, the use of a wrong plan to achieve an aim) [9,11]. Errors can be active, occur at the level of the caregiver (physician or nurse), and its effects felt immediately; or errors can be latent, removed from the direct control of the caregiver (poor design or structure or system failures) [11,14]. Box 1 lists the classification of iatrogenic disorders.

The mechanism of errors are listed as follows:

1. Errors of execution: slips or lapses
2. Errors of planning: mistakes
3. Active errors: error at level of caregiver
4. Latent errors: errors of faulty design or system errors

In any rapidly changing specialty, medical progress may itself be a major cause of iatrogenesis. These problems are usually unanticipated complications of advancement. Some of the important problems in this category are discussed later. They usually continue to arise as long as one strives to improve their therapeutic abilities. It is unacceptable for one to retreat to

---

Box 1. Types of Iatrogenic disorders

1. Preventable
   a. Diagnostic
      - Error or delay in diagnosis
      - Failure to use indicated tests
      - Use of outmoded tests or therapy
      - Failure to act on results of monitoring or testing
   b. Treatment
      - Error in the performance of an operation, procedure, or test
      - Error in administering the treatment
      - Error in the dose or method of using a drug
      - Avoidable delay in treatment or in responding to an abnormal test
      - Inappropriate (not indicated) care
   c. Preventive
      - Failure to provide prophylactic treatment
      - Inadequate monitoring or follow-up of treatment
   d. Other
      - Failure of communication
      - Equipment failure
      - Other system failure
2. Potentially preventable
   - New or experimental modes of therapy
3. Currently unpreventable
   - Side effect of proved treatments or life-support systems

Modified from Kohn L, Corrigan J, Donaldson M. To err is human: building a safer health system. Washington: Institute of Medicine, National Academy Press; 2000; with permission.

---

the safer ground of therapeutic noninterference to reduce the present rate of iatrogenic complications. Instead, efforts should be focused at fostering research to establish maximal safety for new interventions and renew focus on safety and quality of care. This requires emphasis on well-designed animal studies followed by prospective, controlled, and blinded clinical trials. Long-term follow-up is essential to prevent problems that have a late onset. Several iatrogenic complications seen today result from the use of life-support systems with proved, albeit not perfect, efficacy. Without the use of these systems, mortality in sick newborns would have been extremely high. Infants who survive with the help of these therapeutic modalities will continue to manifest occasional signs of toxicity until better modalities are available.

Iatrogenic complications of therapy in modern neonatology

Reviews of iatrogenic disorders in newborns traditionally have included an exhaustive listing of birth injuries. These injuries have lessened considerably as a result of careful fetal monitoring and improved obstetric techniques. The following instead focuses on a few commonly used therapeutic modalities and their associated iatrogenic effects.

Medical and medication errors

The likelihood of an adverse event increases by 6% for each day spent in the hospital [15]. Patients that are sicker, have longer hospital stays, and are subjected to multiple interventions are more at risk for error [16,17]. Drug errors are seven times more likely to occur in the ICU than elsewhere [16]. It is no wonder that the sick premature neonate in the ICU is more prone to harm. Suresh and colleagues [18] reported that 47% of all adverse events in the NICU were from medication, blood products, and nutritional agents. Medication errors were the most common among errors to occur in the NICU; the recent report of three deaths of premature infants who received an overdose of heparin from an adult dose vial is a perfect example of the great harm medication errors can cause [19]. Chappel and Newman [20] found that more than one third of the doses prescribed in the NICU were for less than one tenth of the single drug vial and 8% of the errors were for a 10-fold drug overdose errors. Kaushal and colleagues [21] found medication errors occurred in 91 of 100 admissions and potential (intercepted) adverse drug events in 46 of 100 admissions, and they were significantly higher among neonates in the NICU than other wards. A total of 7.7% of these adverse drug events in this study were fatal or life threatening and 35% serious; 15.7% of the potential adverse drug events were fatal and 45% serious. In a review of 10 prospective and retrospective studies looking at medication errors and adverse events in the neonate, the incidence of adverse events and medication errors were 1 per 1000 to 157 per 1000 patient days [22]. Kanter and colleagues [23] looking at all neonatal discharges since 1997 from the Healthcare Cost and Use Project, which contains discharge data collected at community hospitals in more than 20 states in the United States, found medical error rates in premature neonates to be 1.2 per 100 discharges; there was a significant inverse relationship between birth weight and medical error rates (0.6% in 2000–2499 g birth weight to 5.2% in 500–749 g; $P < 0.001$) and there were more errors in the teaching hospitals than nonteaching hospitals. Two studies found that an increase in errors occurred when new doctors joined the rotation or when there was a change in the junior medical staff [16,24].

Suresh and colleagues [17] in their prospective study from 54 participating NICUs found that most errors were caused by failure to follow policy or protocol (47%); inattention (27%); and communication problems (22%). Other errors included documentation errors (13%); distraction (12%);

inexperience (10%); labeling error (10%); and poor teamwork (9%). Prescribing errors accounted for 71% to 74% of the medication errors in two studies [21,24], most of which were from incorrect doses [24]. Other studies found the most common cause to be administration error (27%–31%) [18,25]. Human error accounted for 63% to 88% of the errors in two studies [25,26]. These studies show that medical error is a serious problem and very prevalent in neonatology. Table 2 lists a review of articles and study results for medical errors in neonates [22].

Leape [11] and the IOM report [9] both concluded that most errors are caused by system errors; blaming an individual does not remove the risk of these errors recurring. Most health care workers are dedicated, intelligent, and conscientious; they do not intend to do harm. System deficiencies, such as poor design, inadequate staffing, incorrect installation, inadequate training, faulty maintenance, bad management decisions, and poorly structured organizations, allow for these errors to reach the patient [9]. For accidents to occur there has to be a combination of system and individual errors and breach of defenses, described as the "Swiss cheese" model where the holes all line up to allow the fault to pass from one end to the other, reaching the patient [11,27]. The recent example of the heparin overdose resulting in the death of three premature babies in an Indianapolis NICU comes to mind. These babies were given the 10,000 unit/mL dose of heparin instead of the 10 unit/mL dose of heparin. The failure in this case was at multiple levels; the nurse used the higher dose adult vial found in the drug cabinet without looking at the label, because the higher dose vials are usually never kept in the NICU and both vials look similar; the pharmacy technician stocked the wrong vial in the NICU; and the manufacturer uses the same kind of vial for both drugs and the labels are of similar color [19]. As can be seen from this example, multiple deficiencies went unchecked and reached the patient causing harm; no individual can be blamed in this case. If system deficiencies were identified earlier and proper protocols were in place, such as use of barcode technology to scan the medications, this accident could have been prevented.

A lot of injury and death can be prevented by identifying and reducing errors. Medication and medical errors have existed since time immemorial; it is only recently the effects of theses errors were quantified and their incidence estimated. Medical professionals are in the business of saving lives, and although they do not intend to cause harm, they should make every effort to reduce harm to patients. Mechanisms for error prevention are discussed later in this article.

Complications of parenteral nutrition

The early 1970s saw the beginning of the use of total parenteral nutrition (TPN) in very low birth weight (VLBW) infants with several studies being published by Driscoll [28], Benda [29] and others. Parenteral nutrition

Table 2
Review of studies on errors in neonatology

Reference	Total number of incidents included in study period	Incidents by type No. (%)	Etiology No. (%)	Degree of harm No. (%)	Preventability No. (%)
Folli et al [88] USA	281 (hospital 1) and 198 (hospital 2) errant medication orders (4.9/1000 and 4.5/1000 medication orders, respectively) Total error rate: 15.2/1000 patient days (PICU 32.6/1000, NICU 8.2/1000, ward 19.4/1000)	Overdose 264 (55.1) Underdose 129 (26.9) Wrong drug 27 (5.6) IV incompatibility 13 (2.7) Wrong route 9 (1.9) Drug interaction 9 (1.9) Drug allergy 2 (0.4) Other 26 (5.4)	Frequency of errant orders declined as physicians' training status increased ($P < 0.001$)	All areas: no actual harm NICU: No actual harm Potentially lethal 0.04/ 100 patient days Serious 0.23/100 patient days Significant 0.55/ 100 patient days	Pediatric pharmacists were able to detect errant medication orders and prevent medical errors

| Vincer et al [25] Canada | 313 medication incidents on 23 307 patient days (13.4/1000 patient days, approximately 13/100 admissions) | Human error 274 (87.5) Mechanical failures 8 (2.6) Other events 24 (7.7) Unknown 7 (2.2) | Administration 84 (27): neglecting to give a drug on scheduled time 52 (17) Failure to follow procedures 56 (18): intravenous infusion not properly regulated 32 (10) Physician's orders incorrect 51 (16) Faulty drug preparation 26 (8) Transcription of physician's order 26 (8) Interstitial intravenous line 18 (6) Other 52 (17) Relative risk of medication incidents increased with increasing level of care ($P<0.01$) Three serious errors were caused by verbal orders that differed from the subsequently written order | Errors in physician's orders resulted in more serious incidents (incidents with (potential for) patient morbidity), 20% compared with 6% of all other causes ($P<0.001$) | Not described |

(continued on next page)

Table 2 (*continued*)

Reference	Total number of incidents included in study period	Incidents by type No. (%)	Etiology No. (%)	Degree of harm No. (%)	Preventability No. (%)
Raju et al [72] USA	315 medication related errors among 2147 admissions (14.7/100 admissions, 8.8/1000 patient days)	Wrong time 68 (21.6) Wrong rate 43 (13.7) Wrong dose 43 (13.7) Unauthorized drug 42 (13.3) Wrong technique 41 (13) Omission 39 (12.4) Wrong preparation 26 (8.3) Wrong route 13 (4.1)	Improper placement of the decimal point was the commonest error in calculation	Substantial injury (long-term injury, toxic effects or death) 1 (0.3) Mild injury (no substantial treatment or intervention) 32 (10.2) No apparent injury 250 (79.4) Potentially serious (drug serum level in toxic range, or insufficient dose of a life-saving drug) 33 (10.5)	Not described
Frey et al [26] Switzerland	211 (45/100 neonatal admissions, 40/100 pediatric admissions)	Management/ environment 62 (29) Drugs 62 (29): wrong dose 37, wrong drug 11 Procedures 37 (18) Respiration 29 (14) Equipment dysfunction 15 (7) Nosocomial infections 6 (3)	Human error (63) Communication (14) Organizational problems (10) Equipment dysfunction (7) Milieu (3) No contributing factor identified (3)	Major: death (0), need for therapeutic intervention specific to the ICU (30) Moderate (requiring routine treatment available outside ICU) (25) Minor (no intervention required) (45) Most severe: incidents relating to respiration	Not described

| Ross et al [89] UK | Total hospital: 195 medication errors (0.15/100 admissions, 0.51/1000 patient days) NICU: 33 medication errors (0.83/100 admissions, 0.97/1000 patient days) PICU: 20 medication errors (0.61/100 admissions, 1.6/1000 patient days) | Parenteral medicines 109 (56): antibiotics 48 Oral medicines 66 (34) Other route 20 (10) Incorrect IV infusion rate 32 (15.8) Incorrect dose given 30 (14.8) Extra dose given 28 (13.8) Dose omitted 25 (12.3) Incorrect drug given 25 (12.3) Incorrect IV concentration 21 (10.3) Labelling error 20 (9.9) Incorrect route 9 (4.4) Incorrect patient 8 (3.9) Incorrect strength 1 (0.5) Other 4 (2) | Double check did not occur 58 (30) Unknown whether checking occurred 7 (3) Intravenous pump errors 23: many different types of syringe pump and volumetric pump in use Tenfold dosing errors 15 (8): 5 miscalculations of dose despite clear prescribing, 4 incorrect or unclear prescribing, 1 inaccurate verbal communication | Long-term morbidity or mortality 0 Serious (potential severe harm) 2 (1) Medium severity (clinical symptoms aggravated by error) 3 (2) Minor (no actual harm resulted) (96) Errors requiring active patient intervention 18 (9.2) | Errors involving morphine sulfate occurred when 10-mg, 15-mg, and 30-mg ampoules were available. In one case ampoules had been confused. |

(continued on next page)

Table 2 (*continued*)

Reference	Total number of incidents included in study period	Incidents by type No. (%)	Etiology No. (%)	Degree of harm No. (%)	Preventability No. (%)
Kaushal et al [21] USA	616 medication errors (5.7/100 orders, 55/100 admissions, 157/1000 patient days) 115 potential ADEs 26 ADEs neonates in the NICU: medication errors 91/100 admissions Potential ADEs 46/100 admissions Neonates in other wards: medication errors 50/100 admissions Potential ADEs 9/100 admissions	Dose 175 (28) Frequency 58 (9.4) Route 109 (18) Administration 85 (14) Wrong drug 8 (1.3) Wrong patient 1 (0.16) Known allergy 8 (1.3) Illegible order 14 (2.3) Missing or wrong weight 74 (12) No or wrong date 74 (12) Other 61 (9.9)	Prescription 454 (74) Transcription 62 (10) Administration 78 (13) Patient monitoring 4 (0.6) Missing 12 (1.9)	ADEs: fatal or life-threatening 2 (7.7), serious 9 (34.6), significant 15 (57.7) Potential ADEs: fatal or life threatening 18 (15.7), serious 52 (45.2), significant 45 (39.1)	Preventable ADEs: 5 (0.52/100 admissions) Nonpreventable ADEs: 21 (1.9/100 admissions)

| Frey et al [90] Switzerland | 284 drug-related incidents (including IV fluids and enteral and parenteral nutrition) | Catecholamines 31 (11) Anticoagulants 30 (11) Electrolytes 30 (11) Crystalloids 22 (8) Opiates 24 (9) Antibiotics 17 (6) Other 95 (34) | Prescription 102 (37) Preparation 162 (59) Administration 200 (73) | Major: death (0), need for therapeutic intervention specific to the ICU (5) Moderate (requiring routine treatment available outside ICU) (19) Minor (no intervention required) (76) Potentially life-threatening 24 (8) Most severe: sedative drugs, crystalloids, and enteral nutrition | 75 (27) incidents were caught before administration |
| Simpson et al [24] UK | 105 medication errors (14.7/1000 patient days): 24.1/1000 Patient days before intervention 5.1/1000 Patient days after intervention (pharmacist-led education program) 12.2/1000 Patient days after start of new junior medical staff | Parenteral medicines 63 (60): antibiotics 40, morphine 6 Oral medicines 41 (39) Topical medicines 1 (1) | Prescription 75 (71): 37 incorrect doses, 19 incorrect dose intervals, 14 incomplete prescriptions, 5 incorrect units Administration 30 (29): 16 poor documentation or communication | Most severe: two 10-fold dose miscalculations Serious (actual harm or very high risk of harm to the infant) 4 (4) Potentially serious (potential harm to the infant) 45 (43) Minor 56 (53) | A change over of junior medical staff was associated with an increase in medication errors |

(continued on next page)

Table 2 (*continued*)

Reference	Total number of incidents included in study period	Incidents by type No. (%)	Etiology No. (%)	Degree of harm No. (%)	Preventability No. (%)
Suresh et al [18] USA	1230 reports: 522 from phase 1 (free text reports) and 708 from phase 2 (structured reports)	Errors of diagnosis 137 (11.2) Errors of treatment 949 (77.2) Errors of prevention 0 Other errors 144 (11.7) Of all reported events, 581 (47%) were related to medication, nutritional agents, or blood products: administration (31), dispensing (25), ordering (16), transcribing (12), monitoring (1.4), wrong drug (8.4), uncertain (6)	In 584 (82.5) phase 2 reports at least one contributing factor was reported. In 52 (8.9) reports, 5–8 factors were selected for each report Most frequent contributing factors in these 584 reports: failure to follow policy/protocol 273 (47) Inattention 157 (27) Communication problem 131 (22) Charting or documentation error 78 (13) Distraction 69 (12) Inexperience 59 (10) Labelling error 56 (10) Poor teamwork 50 (9)	Outcome reported in 673 phase 2 reports: actual harm 181 (27): death 1 (0.2), serious (threat to life, impaired outcome) 13 (1.9), minor (increased monitoring, intervention) 167 (25) Potential harm, reached patient, no harm (34) Potential harm, did not reach patient (25) No potential for harm (14)	Not described

Kanter et al [23] USA	824 (1.2/100) premature neonates experienced a medical error	Procedural complications (60), including mechanical complications of device implants and grafts Medical care complications (25)	Significant inverse linear association between birth weight and medical error rates (birth weight 2000–2499 g, 0.6%, versus birth weight 500–749 g, 5.2%, $P<0.001$) More errors in urban teaching centers than in rural or urban nonteaching centers (OR = 1.69; 95% CI 1.18–2.43)	Not described	Not described

Abbreviations: ADE, adverse drug event; NICU, neonatal intensive care unit; PICU, pediatric intensive care unit.
Data from Snijders C, van Lingen RA, et al. Incidents and errors in neonatal intensive care: a review of the literature. Arch Dis Child Fetal Neonatal Ed 2007;92:F391–8.

(PN) was rapidly adopted over the existing glucose-only infusion as an alternate method for delivering nutrition to VLBW infants. Anderson [30] in the late 1970s demonstrated that addition of protein to the PN has several advantages in terms of positive nitrogen balance and enhanced protein stores. The widespread adoption and prolonged use of PN soon led to essential fatty acid deficiency. The availability of parenteral lipids in the 1980s solved the problem of limited energy intake and prevented fatty acid deficiency. Many centers advocated the early placement of central lines and high caloric intake to try and match the intrauterine growth; this in turn led to several complications of the central lines and the PN itself. Box 2 lists the types of complications from PN.

Inadequate supply of nutrients in TPN can result in symptomatic nutritional deficiencies. Metabolic bone disease continues to occur despite provision of large amounts of calcium, phosphorus, and vitamin D. Hypoalbuminemic edema can occur because of protein deficiency; essential fatty acid deficiency can lead to dermatitis, hair loss, and impaired wound healing, especially in infants with short-gut syndrome receiving prolonged PN. Although symptomatic deficiencies of essential fatty acids, vitamin E, trace elements, and carnitine have been described, micronutrient excess can cause several adverse effects, including liver disease from excess manganese, aluminum toxicity, and altered white cell function.

Box 2. Complications of total parenteral nutrition

Preventable
Metabolic complications
    Hypoglycemia and hyperglycemia
    Electrolyte imbalance
    Hypertriglyceridemia
    Fluid overload
    Trace element, mineral deficiency, excess
    Hypervitaminosis or hypovitaminosis
Complications of central lines
    Improper insertion, malposition, migration
    Cardiac tamponade
    Thrombus and occlusion
    Breakage
    Infection

Potentially preventable
Infection
Cholestasis, hepatocellular damage
Ricketts

Fluid overload can occur when more than the required volume of PN is given to improve caloric intake; this has been associated with a higher incidence of patent ductus arteriosus and bronchopulmonary dysplasia (BPD). Hyperglycemia commonly occurs in VLBW infants requiring glucose in excess of 4 to 6 mg/kg/min, which can in turn lead to osmotic diuresis, intraventricular hemorrhage, and cholestasis or hepatic steatosis. Lipid intolerance can lead to hyperlipidemia, kernicterus (displacement of the bilirubin from albumin binding sites by free fatty acids), and altered pulmonary diffusion capacity, resulting in exacerbation of chronic lung disease and increased risk of persistent pulmonary hypertension [31,32]. Lipids should be used cautiously in infants with documented sepsis and severe lung disease.

Cholestasis is a common problem in VLBW infants on prolonged PN (>2 weeks), but the underlying mechanisms remain to be completely elucidated. The incidence of cholestatic liver disease has decreased significantly over the last two decades; 40% to 60% percent of infants requiring long-term PN for intestinal failure develop cholestatic disease [33]. Cholestasis is inversely related to birth weight and gestational age [34]. Infants with PN-associated liver disease have increase in the direct bilirubin fraction greater than 2 mg/dL and accompanied increase in aminotransferases. The pathogenesis of cholestatic liver disease is best described by the "multiple hit" theory [35]; bile stasis secondary to delayed feeding, amino acid infusion, sepsis, hypoxia, hypotension, and hepatotoxic drugs all contribute toward the progressive liver disease. In most cases, cholestasis resolves once PN is discontinued and enteral feeds are initiated. Early or minimal enteral feeds stimulate bile flow, promote intestinal maturation, and stimulate enteric hormones. Studies have shown no increase in the risk of necrotizing enterocolitis and actually a decrease in TPN cholestasis with early feeds [36].

The availability of PN has provided an opportunity to support nutrition in the sickest and smallest infants, who are unable to receive enteral nutrition adequately. Amino acids should be started early to prevent negative nitrogen balance. Initial use of adult amino acid preparations in infants caused several complications from deficiency of certain amino acids to hyperammonemia and metabolic acidosis. Replacing hydrochloric salts of amino acids with acetate and addition of arginine in the newer pediatric formulations have decreased or eliminated the risk of metabolic acidosis and hyperammonemia [34,37]. Several nonessential amino acids are considered "conditionally essential" in neonates and reflect immature enzyme pathways or altered metabolism of parenterally administered amino acids. Cysteine is a conditionally essential amino acid in infants caused by low hepatic cystathionase activity; taurine, which is derived from cysteine, also needs to be added to the PN solution because it is essential for brain development [38]. Tyrosine levels are low in parenterally maintained infants despite adequate phenylalanine intake and needs to be added to PN. Since the availability of these safer formulations, all VLBW infants should be started on amino acid solution within 1 to 2 hours after birth; even the sickest infants can tolerate parenteral protein and have a positive nitrogen balance. It also leads to better glucose tolerance and prevents protein catabolism, hyperkalemia, and increased insulin production [33,36]. Other strategies to reduce the incidence of PN-associated liver disease including taurine, tauroursodeoxycholic acid, cholecystokinin-octreopeptide, phenobarbital, and removing copper and manganese from the PN have not been consistently successful [39]. The only way to resolve the cholestasis is discontinuing PN, which is not always feasible. Early initiation of feeds has helped reduce the duration of PN use and reduced the incidence of cholestasis. Further advances and research are required to identify the cause of PN-associated cholestasis and effective treatment and prevention.

Complications of invasive monitoring

The modern NICU takes pride in its ability to monitor precisely a variety of physiologic variables in sick newborns. Although the use of monitoring electrodes, catheters, and other devices has been shown to benefit the patient considerably, it also brings with it a significant amount of risk inherent to any invasive procedure. Iatrogenic disorders can result from malpositioning or malfunction of various catheters and instruments. Umbilical artery catheters and peripheral arterial lines are frequently used in the NICU for invasive monitoring. Umbilical artery catheters present an easy mode for monitoring blood pressure and blood sampling; it is easy to place and is invaluable especially in sick VLBW newborns. Most infants in the NICU, especially VLBW babies, have at least one catheter placed during their stay in the ICU. Despite their important role in monitoring vital signs of these sick infants, their use has several inherent risks. The most common visual symptom from umbilical or radial arterial lines is blanching or cyanosis of the distal extremity from vasospasm. This complication is more common in the low placement (L3-L4) umbilical artery catheter than the high placement umbilical artery catheter [40]. Management includes contralateral limb warming to produce reflex vasodilatation; if this does not work, the line must be removed to avoid the risk of gangrene in the affected extremity.

Thromboembolic events are common in infants with intravascular catheters. Their small vessel size, immature clotting mechanisms, and underlying disease puts them at a higher risk of forming a thrombus than adults and older children [41]. Tyson and colleagues [42] found thromboses in 59% of infants at autopsy who had an umbilical artery catheter, and another study found a thrombus in 30% of patients with an umbilical vein catheter [43]. Thrombus can form in different sites based on the catheter type and placement, including venous (renal, superior vena caval, portal-hepatic, and adrenal thrombus) and arterial (aorta, peripheral, cerebral, pulmonary, renal, and mesenteric). The duration of catheterization is usually not a determining factor in thrombus formation unlike infection [42], but the presence of the catheter itself predisposes the neonate to thrombus formation.

Treatment includes prompt removal of the catheter unless required for sustaining life; thrombolytic agents, such as heparin, streptokinase, or tissue plasminogen activator; and a surgical consult for clot removal. The recent availability of silicone catheters has shown decreased risk of thrombogenicity [44]. Long-term complications include hypertension, loss of limb or extremity, and short-gut syndrome. Less common complications include aortic aneurysms or coarctation, congestive heart failure, paraplegia, refractory hypoglycemia, peritoneal perforation, bladder injury, air embolism, and Wharton jelly embolus. The risk of infection is similar to other intravascular catheters and is discussed later. Complications can be reduced significantly by careful selection of patients for catheterization, limited duration of use, and prompt removal when no longer required. Adequate training of personnel involved in line placement and daily care is of paramount importance.

Complications of central venous lines

Central venous lines are widely used in the NICU, especially in LBW and VLBW infants. They provide easy access for giving medications, prolonged TPN use, exchange transfusions, and long-term intravenous access. Although very useful, they have inherent risks like infection; complications of malpositioning, including arrhythmia, cardiac tamponade, thromboembolic complications, hepatic abscess; and other rare complications, such as peritoneal perforation, necrotizing enterocolitis, and perforation of the colon. Schiff and Stonestreet [45] noted an increased risk of up to 85% for complications with central venous lines in VLBW infants.

Infection is a common complication of central lines. The latest annual national nosocomial infection surveillance report from the Centers for Disease Control and Prevention shows the current mean infection rate in the level III NICU for umbilical lines to range from 6.9 per 1000 catheter days for infants less than 750 g to 0.9 per 1000 catheter days for infants greater than 2500 g [46]. The risk of infection increases with lower gestation age, duration of catheter usage, number of breaks in the line for medication or blood product administration, and prolonged usage of TPN [47–49]. In several studies, an estimated 40% to 55% of umbilical artery catheters were colonized and 5% resulted in catheter-related bloodstream infections; umbilical vein catheters were associated with colonization in 22% to 59% of cases and with catheter-related bloodstream infections in 3% to 8% of cases [50].

The most common pathogens associated with central lines are coagulase-negative staphylococci, followed by gram-negative infections and fungal infections [41]. They present with apnea, bradycardia, feeding intolerance, respiratory distress, hypoxia, hypotension, and lethargy [49]. Diagnosis is confirmed by elevated or low white blood cell count with left shift, thrombocytopenia, elevated C-reactive protein, and positive blood culture. Some of these infections can be treated with the catheter in place, but they have to be removed if infection persists despite treatment and, in particular, for gram-negative infections and fungal infections. Vancomycin is commonly used to treat coagulase-negative staphylococci and gentamicin-cefotaxime is used to treat gram-negative infections. Infection can persist despite catheter removal and treatment with antibiotics in some cases; these infants should be evaluated for bacterial endocarditis.

Other rare complications are known to occur with umbilical vein catheters, such as hepatic abscess caused by direct infusion of PN or glucose into the liver. The Centers for Disease Control and Prevention recommends umbilical venous catheter removal within 14 days because of risk of complications and infection [50], but several institutions remove them earlier based on their hospital-specific infection rates.

Complications of peripherally inserted central catheter lines

Peripherally inserted central catheters have become very popular for prolonged intravenous access and TPN in sick preterm infants. They are long catheters made of silicone or polyurethane, inserted through a peripheral vein into a central vein, such as the inferior vena cava or the superior vena cava. They have similar complications as the other central venous catheters, such as thromboembolic events and infection, but they reduce the number of catheters required during the hospital stay [51]. Peripherally inserted central catheter lines have serious complications of arrhythmia, cardiac tamponade, and death associated with their use. Studies and case reports have suggested an incidence of 0.76% to 3% of cardiac tamponade and death [52,53]. The most common cause of tamponade includes improper positioning and more commonly migration into the heart from the superior vena cava or inferior vena cava. The catheter tip can easily perforate through the thin right atrial wall and cause pericardial effusion resulting in sudden cardiorespiratory compromise unresponsive to cardiopulmonary resuscitation. A survey of 390 NICUs in the country by Nadroo and colleagues [53] showed that myocardial perforation and pericardial effusion were reported by 29% and 43% of the units, respectively, and death from peripherally inserted central catheters was reported by 24% of the respondents. Mortality from tamponade is high at 34% to 45% [52].

Although not very common, in any infant with a peripherally inserted central catheter or umbilical venous line with sudden cardiorespiratory compromise unresponsive to cardiopulmonary resuscitation, tamponade must be considered and pericardiocentesis attempted if suspected. Mortality with pericardiocentesis is 8% and without is 75% [52]. Peripherally inserted central catheter lines must be positioned 1 cm outside the silhouette in preterm infants and 2 cm outside the silhouette in term infants to prevent this complication [52,54].

Complications of respiratory management

The introduction of assisted ventilation has played a major role in reducing mortality in infants with respiratory disease. Before its advent, neonates manifesting severe respiratory distress in the period usually died from intractable respiratory failure. With increasing survival of VLBW infants on assisted ventilation, a phenomenal increase in iatrogenic problems has been observed (Box 3). Although some of these complications are clearly iatrogenic, several others are an outcome of a complex situation with multifactorial etiology and may well have occurred spontaneously. Chronic lung disease in ventilated newborns is, in several ways, the most important neoiatroepidemic today.

Complications associated with endotracheal tube occur fairly commonly. Most acute complications are considered preventable and involve either trauma from or mechanical problems caused by the tube. Careful selection of patients and equipment for intubation, proper techniques, coupled with the close observation of the infant's condition can reduce a number of these complications. Newer equipment available today reduces movement of the endotracheal tubes, need for retaping, and number of accidental extubations. Avoiding malpositioning of the endotracheal tube is extremely important because it can lead to hypoxia and respiratory compromise. Such equipment as the end-tidal CO_2 detector, which is a durable colorimetric

---

Box 3. Complications of assisted ventilation

Preventable
Extensive air leaks
    Pneumothorax
    Pneumopericardium
    Pneumomediastinum
    Pneumoperitoneum
    Subcutaneous emphysema
    Air embolism
Complications of endotracheal intubation
    Malpositioning
    Trauma to vocal cords, pharynx, or esophagus
    Accidental extubation and obstruction

Potentially preventable
Pulmonary interstitial emphysema
Bronchopulmonary dysplasia
Subglottic stenosis
Palatal groves and defective dentition
Tracheomegaly

breath indicator for visualization of exhaled CO_2 to assist in verifying proper endotracheal tube placement, can be helpful in avoiding malpositioning [55]. Chronic complications can be reduced considerably by decreasing the number of reintubations and the total duration of assisted ventilation. Because suctioning has been associated with several complications, adequate attention must be paid to the suction pressure, catheter length, and prevention of hypoxemia during suctioning. Palatal implants have been used to reduce the risk of palatal groves and subsequent dentition problems [56,57].

Air leak syndrome is not an uncommon occurrence in infants on assisted ventilation and often is attributed to barotraumas. Despite a better understanding of pulmonary physiology and major technologic advances in respiratory support systems, air leaks contribute significantly to short- and long-term morbidity. The initiating event in all types of air leaks is alveolar rupture followed by the tracking of leaked air along any of the different routes available [58,59]. There are several excellent reviews on the subject to which the interested reader is referred [58–60].

Pneumothorax occurs when air in a subpleural hilar bleb ruptures into the pleural cavity. Alternatively, air from the anterior mediastinum can gain access to the pleural cavity. Occasionally, pneumothorax can result directly from either perforation of lung or bronchus by an endotracheal suction catheter [61] or secondary to needle aspiration of the chest for suspected pneumothorax. In infants on positive-pressure ventilation, tension pneumothorax can develop fairly quickly, seriously compromising cardiopulmonary function. Pneumopericardium occurs in a similar manner, and if under tension, can seriously compromise cardiac function. Air may sometimes track along the aorta or inferior vena cava into the retroperitoneum and lead to pneumoperitoneum.

Pulmonary interstitial emphysema is considered by some as the initiating event in all air leak syndromes. This complication is seen more frequently in preterm infants, in part because of an abundance of interstitial tissue [62]. Air arising from ruptured alveoli gets trapped in the interstitium.

In infants who have survived acute lung disease on assisted ventilation, BPD represents a formidable problem and a major contributor to prolonged hospitalization and late mortality [63]. Although the exact cause of BPD remains unclear, oxygen toxicity and barotrauma from assisted ventilation are important contributing factors [64]. The disease originally was described by Northway and coworkers [65] and is characterized by failure of infants in the healing phase of hyaline membrane disease to wean from assisted ventilation or oxygen. In infants weighing less than 1000 g, up to 30% have been reported to develop BPD [66]. How much of BPD is iatrogenic is difficult to assess. Several factors have been implicated as follows:

- Immaturity
- Barotrauma or volutrauma
- Oxygen toxicity

- Air leak syndrome
- Patent ductus arteriosus
- Inadequate nutrition
- Infections

Recent studies have shown that not all of BPD is unpreventable, and its occurrence may be related to individual practices [67]. Out of eight tertiary care nurseries reviewed for incidence of BPD, one center (Columbia) was shown to have a significantly lower incidence of chronic lung disease. This center was distinct from the rest for its nonaggressive approach in management of respiratory distress syndrome. Fewer infants were intubated and physicians accepted lower Po_2, pH, and higher Pco_2 values [67]. Since then, several studies have reported decreased incidence of BPD with noninvasive ventilation, such as nasal continuous positive airway pressure and bubble continuous positive airway pressure [68–70].

One of the biggest challenges today is prevention of acute and chronic iatrogenic problems in newborns with respiratory disease. Perelman [71] has recommended several areas that need to be explored. One cannot overemphasize the urgent need for reduction of preterm births. This involves a multipronged approach, including research in basic sciences to understand the causes and mechanism of preterm labor, and constitutional factors, with emphasis on antenatal care. The next step is to reduce the incidence and severity of neonatal respiratory disease. This requires adequate estimation and acceleration of fetal lung maturity, and early treatment with surfactant. Extensive research is being undertaken in these areas. The final step involves improving methods of artificial respiratory support to reduce the incidence of trauma to pulmonary tissue. Several new techniques, such as bubble continuous positive airway pressure and high-frequency ventilation, have been used but none has been consistently effective in reducing morbidity.

High-frequency oscillatory ventilation uses very small tidal volumes at extremely rapid rates to improve the efficacy of mechanical ventilation without causing excessive barotrauma. High-frequency oscillatory ventilation was introduced with great promise, because effective gas exchange could be achieved at relatively low mean airway pressures. The HIFI study group concluded that high-frequency oscillatory ventilation offers no significant advantage over conventional ventilation and was associated with several undesirable side effects, such as air leaks and intraventricular hemorrhage [72]. A Cochrane review by Henderson-Smart and colleagues [73] looked at 15 randomized controlled trials over 12 years and came to a similar conclusion. A recent review by Shah [74] looked at two more randomized controlled trials in addition to the trials from the Cochrane review and found a small statistically significant reduction in the incidence of chronic lung disease or death in the high-frequency oscillatory ventilation group (summary relative risk [RR] 0.90, 95% confidence interval [CI] 0.80–0.98; number needed to treat 20, 95% CI 11–100). There was no evidence of difference in the incidence of grade 3 or 4 intraventricular hemorrhage (summary RR 0.97, 95% CI 0.78–1.19) or pulmonary air leaks (summary RR 1.04, 95% CI 0.87–1.25). High-frequency oscillatory ventilation, although useful in certain cases, offers no advantage over conventional ventilation when it comes to BPD or death.

Retinopathy of prematurity

ROP is one of the biggest iatroepidemics witnessed in modern medicine. The study of its evolution teaches many important lessons. The disease was first reported from Boston in 1941, when Clifford identified infants with blindness that had been born prematurely [75]. Terry [76] in 1942 published a paper describing what he thought was an overgrowth of persistent vascular sheath behind the crystalline lens in preterm infants. Silverman coined the term "retrolental fibroplasias" for this condition in 1944 [77]. Soon thereafter the disease was recognized as a leading cause of blindness in the United States, blinding about 10,000 infants by 1953 [5]. Oxygen use was suggested to be the cause in 1951 by Campbell [78], and was later confirmed as the culprit in a trial conducted by 18 hospitals in the United States; however, as is often the case when the pendulum swings too far, severe restriction of oxygen use that followed led to increased mortality in infants with hyaline membrane disease [5].

Although frequently attributed to excessive oxygen use and medical progress, ROP is another disease with multifactorial etiology and is not entirely iatrogenic. Prematurity and oxygen exposure are now accepted as major contributing factors. Attempts to prevent the occurrence of this disease have failed in the past, mainly because sick premature infants continue to have oxygen requirements for prolonged periods. Use of antioxidants, like vitamin E, has produced mixed results [79]. Reports of toxic effects of vitamin E have prevented it from being used routinely for this purpose. The Supplemental Therapeutic Oxygen for Prethreshold ROP clinical trial showed that supplemental oxygen decreased the risk of reaching threshold in a small subset of infants, but the risks of pulmonary disease outweighed the benefits [80]. The Trial of Light Reduction for Reducing Frequency of ROP showed no increased risk of ROP from ambient lighting in the nursery [81]. The multicentered Trial of Cryotherapy for ROP found that cryoablative treatment of the avascular retina in eyes with advanced ROP decreases the chance of an unfavorable outcome (traction or detachment of the posterior retina) by 41% (21.8% in treated; 43% in untreated) [82]. Recent long-term follow-up from the Trial of Cryotherapy for ROP has shown that untreated eyes have a 30% increased risk of legal blindness [83]. With the development of lasers for retinal ablation, the risk of adverse effects from cryotherapy has been greatly reduced and this allows treatment of zone 1 disease more effectively; its use has now largely become the standard of care. Recent findings from the Early Treatment for ROP study showed a reduction in unfavorable visual acuity outcomes with earlier treatment from 19.8% to 14.3% and structural outcomes from 15.6% to 9% [84]. Advances in molecular biology have led to a greater understanding of angiogenesis, and newer therapies targeting vascular endothelial growth factor hold promise for better management of this condition. The incidence of ROP today is 70% for infants less than 1250 g birth weight and severe ROP occurs in less than 10% of these infants [85]. Although it looks like there has not been much progress in preventing ROP, the technologic and medical advances today allow a much greater population of the VLBW infants to survive, shifting the disease burden to these very premature and sick infants. Further research into newer novel therapies for preventing and treating ROP will go a long way in reducing the incidence of this disease.

Prevention

Given the complex and multifactorial causation of neoiatroepidemics, prevention has proved to be difficult and no one simple remedy exists. By reducing system faults, one can make it difficult for the individual to err. Attention needs to be paid to each stage of system development including design, construction, maintenance, training, and development of procedures and protocol so that there are fewer chances for accidents to occur. It is also important to monitor day-to-day processes and detect errors in a timely fashion. The recommendations of the IOM report include (1) creating a national focus to promote research and enhance the knowledge base about patient safety; (2) identifying errors from a combination of mandatory and voluntary reporting systems; and (3) raising standards and expectations through the action of oversight organizations and professional groups and creating safety systems inside health care organizations [9]. Box 4 lists the recommendations by the IOM committee.

Since the release of the IOM report in 1999, congress funded and entrusted the Agency for Healthcare Research and Quality to promote research in patient safety and support a variety of efforts targeted at reducing medical errors. Multiple research projects have been initiated and funded by Agency for Healthcare Research and Quality since then. Other organizations, such as the National Academy for State Health Policy, have been involved in developing state mandatory reporting protocols, standards, and enforcement of standards for health organizations. The Joint Commission on Accreditation of Healthcare Organizations has developed national patient safety goals, and works with hospitals to make system and infrastructure improvements to promote safety. Nonprofit and other voluntary agencies, such as the Leapfrog group, promote the use of computerized order entry systems to reduce medication errors and other agencies, such as National Patient Safety Foundation and Institute for Healthcare Improvement, have increased awareness on patient safety.

Box 4. Institute of Medicine committee recommendations

- Establishing a national focus to create leadership, research, tools, and protocols to enhance the knowledge base about safety
- Identify and learning from errors through immediate and strong mandatory reporting efforts, as well as the encouragement of voluntary efforts, both with the aim of making sure the system continues to be made safer for patients
- Raising standards and expectations for improvements in safety through the actions of oversight organizations, group purchasers, and professional groups
- Creating safety systems inside health care organizations through the implementation of safe practices at the delivery level. This level is the ultimate target of all the recommendations

---

From Kohn L, Corrigan J, Donaldson M. To err is human: building a safer health system. Washington: Institute of Medicine, National Academy Press; 2000; with permission.

Identifying the incidence of errors and the types of errors is crucial to develop safety systems. The IOM report recommended setting up of a national mandatory reporting system modeled after such systems as the Aviation Safety Reporting System in which all incidents pertaining to patient safety can be reported. The practicality and cost of setting up such a system are enormous, given how complex medicine is with its multiple specialties, so a specialty-specific or statewide system better serves the purpose. Twenty-five states have set up mandatory incident reporting systems with the help of the National Academy for State Health Policy. Such statewide and nationwide or specialty-specific systems can help in identifying the not so common or rare events.

Current incident reporting systems are used primarily to identify individual error and appropriate blame. Several studies have documented the advantages of using a nonpunitive, anonymous, voluntary reporting system [18,27,86,87]. The reporting rate is much higher than the mandatory system and the anonymous nature of the reporting reduces penalization of the reporters by their superiors and exposure to medicolegal liability. For an incident reporting system to be successful, it should not be used to penalize or appropriate blame on the worker by the health care worker. Rather, it should be used to identify the types of errors in the institution, perform a root cause analysis to find the cause of the error, provide feedback, and develop system changes to prevent further errors. Voluntary systems have proved very successful in anesthesia to identify and lower their adverse events; no such system exists in neonatology. Suresh and colleagues [18] conducted a study among 54 NICUs as a part of the Neonatal Intensive Care Quality Collaborative sponsored by the Vermont Oxford Network and found 1230 errors. The most frequent event categories were wrong medication, dose, schedule, or infusion rate including nutritional agents and blood products (47%); error in administration or method of using a treatment (14%); patient misidentification (11%); other system failure (9%); error or delay in diagnosis (7%); and error in the performance of an operation, procedure, or test (4%). The reporting system used in this study was Internet based, voluntary, anonymous, and nonpunitive; such systems can especially help in identifying the not so common, or rare events. Finally, there has to be collaboration between different agencies, such as hospital risk management, national and state reporting agencies, and relevant professional organizations, so that warnings about significant risks can be quickly disseminated among the health care workers and hospitals nationwide. Fig. 3 depicts the possible collaborations between different incident reporting systems.

There is an urgent need to set up a voluntary incident reporting system for neonatology; one can borrow from the experiences of available systems in other specialties (anesthesia) and industries (Aviation Safety Reporting

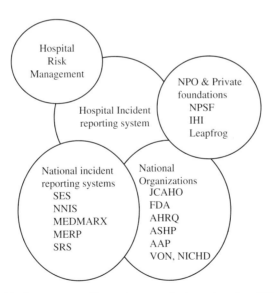

Fig. 3. Relationship between reporting systems, sentinel event system (SES), the national nosocomial infection surveillance system (NNIS), the national database for medication errors (MEDMARX), medication errors reporting program (MERP), state reporting systems (SRS), Joint commission on Accreditation of Healthcare Organizations (JCAHO), Food and Drug Administration (FDA), Agency for Healthcare Research and Quality (AHRQ), National Academy for State Health Policy (NASHP), American Academy of Pediatrics (AAP), Vermont Oxford Network (VON), National Institute for Child Health and Development (NICHD), National Patient Safety Foundation (NPSF), and Institute for Healthcare Improvement (IHI).

System). The reporting system set up by the Vermont Oxford Network is an important first step and needs to be made permanent, and expanded to all NICUs nationwide. Other methods, such as chart reviews, can help to identify errors that escaped reporting through the voluntary and mandatory reporting systems [86]. Individual case reviews through the departmental morbidity and mortality conferences, hospital quality assurance committees, and hospital risk management should help identify problem areas, perform root cause analysis to identify system deficiencies, and help develop protocols to enhance patient safety.

Several studies have shown that adoption of current technologies to reduce errors, such as electronic health records, computerized order entry systems, and use of allied health care professionals, such as pharmacists, physical therapists, and nutritionists, will help in reducing the number of adverse events [20,23,26]. Improving training for the nurses, residents, doctors, and health care workers and enhancing communication between them is also essential. Finally, collaboration between hospitals and national organizations is essential to facilitate data collection, analysis and research, and dissemination of information through their collaboratives, such as the Neonatal Intensive Care Quality Collaborative and the American Academy of Pediatrics.

The pursuit of basic sciences is an essential element in development of new technology and should precede and not follow the introduction of new modalities. Information obtained from research into basic sciences needs to be monitored constantly for accuracy and may need to be restructured. The resulting new technology and applied science need to be validated by appropriate prospective, randomized, controlled clinical trials before being applied to patient care. The statistical probability of a given outcome may be difficult to predict from small trials; premature publication of results before adequate confirmation of efficacy and safety should be avoided, because it can lead to widespread use of quasiscientific therapeutic modality with subsequent harmful effects in patients. The occurrence of such iatrogenic effects should be promptly reported, and therapy reappraised.

Neonatal medicine is passing through a very exciting phase of development. Although major advances in therapeutics continue to be made, clinicians must learn to be critical of shortcomings. It is not necessary to slow down the pace of technologic advancement. Instead, high priority should be given to establishing safety and efficacy of new therapeutic modalities.

References

[1] National Center for Health Statistics. Atlanta: Centers for Disease Control and Prevention; 2006.
[2] Jain L, Vidyasagar D. Iatrogenic disorders in modern neonatology. Clin Perinatol 1989; 16(1):255–73.
[3] Kassner EG. Iatrogenic disorders of the fetus, infant, and child. New York: Springer-Verlag; 1985.

[4] Steel K, Gertman PM, Crescenzi C, et al. Iatrogenic illness on a general medical service at a university hospital. N Engl J Med 1981;304(11):638–42.

[5] Robertson AF. Reflections on errors in neonatology: I. The "hands-off" years, 1920 to 1950. J Perinatol 2003;23(1):48–55.

[6] Silverman WA. The future of clinical experimentation in neonatal medicine. Pediatrics 1994; 94(6 Pt 1):932–8.

[7] Andrews BF. The importance of iatrogenesis in the founding of modern neonatology. J Perinatol 2004;24(11):671–3.

[8] Avery GB. Pathophysiology and management of the newborn. In: Neonatology: perspective in the mid 1980s. 3rd edition. Philadelphia: JB Lippincott; 1988. p. 7.

[9] Kohn L, Corrigan J, Donaldson M. To err is human: building a safer health system Institute of Medicine. Washington, DC: National Academy Press; 2000.

[10] Brennan TA, Leape LL, Laird N, et al. Incidence of adverse events and negligence in hospitalized patients: results of the Harvard Medical Practice Study I. N Engl J Med 1991;324: 370–6.

[11] Leape LL. Error in medicine. JAMA 1994;272(23):1851–7.

[12] Starfield B. Is US health really the best in the world? JAMA 2000;284(4):483–5.

[13] Tarini BA. The current revolution in newborn screening: new technology, old controversies. Arch Pediatr Adolesc Med 2007;161(8):767–72.

[14] Berwick DM, Leape LL. Reducing errors in medicine. BMJ 1999;319(7203):136–7.

[15] Andrews LB, Stocking C, Krizek T, et al. An alternative strategy for studying adverse events in medical care. Lancet 1997;349(9048):309–13.

[16] Wilson DG, McArtney RG, Newcombe RG, et al. Medication errors in paediatric practice: insights from a continuous quality improvement approach. Eur J Pediatr 1998;157(9): 769–74.

[17] Weingart SN, Wilson RM, Gibberd RW, et al. Epidemiology of medical error. BMJ 2000; 320(7237):774–7.

[18] Suresh G, Horbar JD, Plsek P, et al. Voluntary anonymous reporting of medical errors for neonatal intensive care. Pediatrics 2004;113(6):1609–18.

[19] Davies T. Fatal drug mix-up exposes hospital flaws. Available at: http://www.boston.com/news/nation/articles/2006/09/22/drug_mix_up_results_in_3_babies_deaths/, 2006. Accessed October 11, 2007.

[20] Chappell K, Newman C. Potential tenfold drug overdoses on a neonatal unit. Arch Dis Child Fetal Neonatal Ed 2004;89(6):F483–4.

[21] Kaushal R, Bates DW, Landrigan C, et al. Medication errors and adverse drug events in pediatric inpatients. JAMA 2001;285(16):2114–20.

[22] Snijders C, van Lingen RA, Molendijk A, et al. Incidents and errors in neonatal intensive care: a review of the literature. Arch Dis Child Fetal Neonatal Ed 2007;92(5):F391–8.

[23] Kanter DE, Turenne W, Slonim AD. Hospital-reported medical errors in premature neonates. Pediatr Crit Care Med 2004;5(2):119–23.

[24] Simpson JH, Lynch R, Grant J, et al. Reducing medication errors in the neonatal intensive care unit. Arch Dis Child Fetal Neonatal Ed 2004;89(6):F480–2.

[25] Vincer MJ, Murray JM, Yuill A, et al. Drug errors and incidents in a neonatal intensive care unit: a quality assurance activity. Am J Dis Child 1989;143(6):737–40.

[26] Frey B, Kehrer B, Losa M, et al. Comprehensive critical incident monitoring in a neonatal-pediatric intensive care unit: experience with the system approach. Intensive Care Med 2000; 26(1):69–74.

[27] Ahluwalia J, Marriott L. Critical incident reporting systems. Semin Fetal Neonatal Med 2005;10(1):31–7.

[28] Driscoll J. Total intravenous alimentation in low birth weight infants: a preliminary report. J Pediatr 1972;51:145–53.

[29] Benda GIM, Babson SG. Peripheral intravenous alimentation of small infants. J Pediatr 1971;79:494.

[30] Anderson TL, Muttart CR, Bieber MA, et al. A controlled trial of glucose versus glucose and amino acids in premature infants. J Pediatr 1979;94(6):947–51.

[31] Prasertsom W, Phillipos EZ, Van Aerde JE, et al. Pulmonary vascular resistance during lipid infusion in neonates. Arch Dis Child Fetal Neonatal Ed 1996;74(2):F95–8.

[32] Lloyd TR, Boucek MM. Effect of intralipid on the neonatal pulmonary bed: an echographic study. J Pediatr 1986;108(1):130–3.

[33] Heine RG, Bines JE. New approaches to parenteral nutrition in infants and children. J Paediatr Child Health 2002;38(5):433–7.

[34] Adamkin DH. Pragmatic approach to in-hospital nutrition in high-risk neonates. J Perinatol 2005;25(Suppl 2):S7–11.

[35] Pratt CA, Garcia MG, Kerner JA. Nutritional management of neonatal and infant liver disease. Neoreviews 2001;2(9):E215–21.

[36] Ehrenkranz RA. Early, aggressive nutritional management for very low birth weight infants: what is the evidence? Semin Perinatol 2007;31(2):48–55.

[37] Jadhav P, Parimi PS, Kalhan SC. Parenteral amino acid and metabolic acidosis in premature infants. JPEN J Parenter Enteral Nutr 2007;31(4):278–83.

[38] Sturman JA, Gaull GE. Taurine in the brain and liver of the developing human and monkey. J Neurochem 1975;25(6):831–5.

[39] Christensen RD, Henry E, Wiedmeier SE, et al. Identifying patients, on the first day of life, at high-risk of developing parenteral nutrition-associated liver disease. J Perinatol 2007;27(5): 284–90.

[40] Barrington KJ. Umbilical artery catheters in the newborn: effects of position of the catheter tip. Cochrane Database Syst Rev 2000;2:CD000505.

[41] Hermansen MC, Hermansen MG. Intravascular catheter complications in the neonatal intensive care unit. Clin Perinatol 2005;32(1):141–56, vii.

[42] Tyson JE, deSa DJ, Moore S. Thromboatheromatous complications of umbilical arterial catheterization in the newborn period: clinicopathological study. Arch Dis Child 1976; 51(10):744–54.

[43] Roy M, Turner-Gomes S, Gill G, et al. Accuracy of Doppler echocardiography for the diagnosis of thrombosis associated with umbilical venous catheters. J Pediatr 2002;140(1): 131–4.

[44] Martin R, Fanaroff A, Walsh M. Fanaroff and Martin's neonatal-perinatal medicine: diseases of the fetus and infant. 8th edition. Mosby; 2005. 1953.

[45] Schiff DE, Stonestreet BS. Central venous catheters in low birth weight infants: incidence of related complications. J Perinatol 1993;13(2):153–8.

[46] Edwards JR, Peterson KD, Andrus ML, et al. National Healthcare Safety Network (NHSN) Report, data summary for 2006 issued June 2007. Am J Infect Control 2007;35(5):290–301.

[47] Healy CM, Palazzi DL, Edwards MS, et al. Features of invasive staphylococcal disease in neonates. Pediatrics 2004;114(4):953–61.

[48] Gellert GA, Ewert DP, Bendana N, et al. A cluster of coagulase-negative staphylococcal bacteremias associated with peripheral vascular catheter colonization in a neonatal intensive care unit. Am J Infect Control 1993;21(1):16–20.

[49] Mireya UA, Marti PO, Xavier KV, et al. Nosocomial infections in paediatric and neonatal intensive care units. J Infect 2007;54(3):212–20.

[50] O'Grady NP, Alexander M, Dellinger EP, et al. Guidelines for the prevention of intravascular catheter-related infections. The Hospital Infection Control Practices Advisory Committee, Center for Disease Control and Prevention, U.S. Pediatrics 2002;110(5):E51.

[51] Ainsworth SB, Clerihew L, McGuire W. Percutaneous central venous catheters versus peripheral cannulae for delivery of parenteral nutrition in neonates. Cochrane Database Syst Rev 2007;3:CD004219.

[52] Nowlen TT, Rosenthal GL, Johnson GL, et al. Pericardial effusion and tamponade in infants with central catheters. Pediatrics 2002;110(1 Pt 1):137–42.

[53] Nadroo AM, Lin J, Green RS, et al. Death as a complication of peripherally inserted central catheters in neonates. J Pediatr 2001;138(4):599–601.

[54] Sehgal A, Cook V, Dunn M. Pericardial effusion associated with an appropriately placed umbilical venous catheter. J Perinatol 2007;27(5):317–9.

[55] The International Liaison Committee on Resuscitation. The International Liaison Committee on Resuscitation (ILCOR) consensus on science with treatment recommendations for pediatric and neonatal patients: neonatal resuscitation. Pediatrics 2006;117(5):E978–88.

[56] Erenberg A, Nowak AJ. Palatal groove formation in neonates and infants with orotracheal tubes. Am J Dis Child 1984;138(10):974–5.

[57] Macey-Dare LV, Moles DR, Evans RD, et al. Long-term effect of neonatal endotracheal intubation on palatal form and symmetry in 8-11-year-old children. Eur J Orthod 1999;21(6):703–10.

[58] Carey B. Neonatal air leaks: pneumothorax, pneumomediastinum, pulmonary interstitial emphysema, pneumopericardium. Neonatal Netw 1999;18(8):81–4.

[59] Plenat F, Vert P, Didier F, et al. Pulmonary interstitial emphysema. Clin Perinatol 1978;5(2):351–75.

[60] Morisot C, Kacet N, Bouchez MC, et al. Risk factors for fatal pulmonary interstitial emphysema in neonates. Eur J Pediatr 1990;149(7):493–5.

[61] Anderson KD, Chandra R. Pneumothorax secondary to perforation of sequential bronchi by suction catheters. J Pediatr Surg 1976;11(5):687–93.

[62] Reid L, Rubino L. The connective tissue septa in the fetal human being. Thorax 1959;14:3.

[63] Thompson T, Reynolds J. The results of intensive care therapy for neonates with respiratory distress syndrome: I. Neonatal mortality rates for neonates with RDS. II. Long-term prognosis for survivors with RDS. J Perinat Med 1977;5(4):149–71.

[64] Philip AG. Oxygen plus pressure plus time: the etiology of bronchopulmonary dysplasia. Pediatrics 1975;55(1):44–50.

[65] Northway WH Jr, Rosan RC, Porter DY. Pulmonary disease following respirator therapy of hyaline-membrane disease: bronchopulmonary dysplasia. N Engl J Med 1967;276(7):357–68.

[66] Walsh MC, Szefler S, Davis J, et al. Summary proceedings from the bronchopulmonary dysplasia group. Pediatrics 2006;117(3):S52–6.

[67] Avery ME, Tooley WH, Keller JB, et al. Is chronic lung disease in low birth weight infants preventable? A survey of eight centers. Pediatrics 1987;79(1):26–30.

[68] Aly H. Is there a strategy for preventing bronchopulmonary dysplasia? Absence of evidence is not evidence of absence. Pediatrics 2007;119(4):818–20.

[69] De Klerk AM, De Klerk RK. Nasal continuous positive airway pressure and outcomes of preterm infants. J Paediatr Child Health 2001;37(2):161–7.

[70] Lindner W, Vossbeck S, Hummler H, et al. Delivery room management of extremely low birth weight infants: spontaneous breathing or intubation? Pediatrics 1999;103(5):961–7.

[71] Perelman R. Reducing iatrogenic lung disease in the premature newborn. Semin Perinatol 1986;10(3):217–23.

[72] Raju TN, Kecskes S, Thornton JP, et al. Medication errors in neonatal and paediatric intensive-care units. Lancet 1989;2(8659):374–6.

[73] Henderson-Smart DJ, Cools F, Bhuta T, et al. Elective high frequency oscillatory ventilation versus conventional ventilation for acute pulmonary dysfunction in preterm infants. Cochrane Database Syst Rev 2007;3:CD000104.

[74] Shah S. Is elective high frequency oscillatory ventilation better than conventional mechanical ventilation in very low birth weight infants? Arch Dis Child 2003;88(9):833–4.

[75] Silverman WA. Retrolental fibroplasia: a modern parable. New York: Grune & Stratton; 1980.

[76] Terry TL. Extreme prematurity and fibroblastic overgrowth of persistent vascular sheath behind each crystalline lens. I. Preliminary report. Am J Ophthalmol 1942;25:203–4.

[77] Silverman WA. ROP–forme fruste. J Perinatol 2001;21(6):393–4.

[78] Campbell K. Intensive oxygen therapy as a possible cause of retrolental fibroplasias: a clinical approach. Med J Aust 1951;2:48–50.

[79] Raju TN, Langenberg P, Bhutani V, et al. Vitamin E prophylaxis to reduce retinopathy of prematurity: a reappraisal of published trials. J Pediatr 1997;131(6):844–50.

[80] Supplemental Therapeutic Oxygen for Prethreshold Retinopathy Of Prematurity (STOP-ROP), a randomized, controlled trial. I: primary outcomes. Pediatrics 2000;105(2):295–310.

[81] Reynolds JD, Hardy RJ, Kennedy KA, et al. Lack of efficacy of light reduction in preventing retinopathy of prematurity. Light Reduction in Retinopathy of Prematurity (LIGHT-ROP) Cooperative Group. N Engl J Med 1998;338(22):1572–6.

[82] Multicenter trial of cryotherapy for retinopathy of prematurity: preliminary results. Cryotherapy for Retinopathy of Prematurity Cooperative Group. Arch Ophthalmol 1988; 106(4):471–9.

[83] Multicenter trial of cryotherapy for retinopathy of prematurity: ophthalmological outcomes at 10 years. Arch Ophthalmol 2001;119(8):1110–8.

[84] Good WV. Final results of the Early Treatment for Retinopathy of Prematurity (ETROP) randomized trial. Trans Am Ophthalmol Soc 2004;102:233–48 [discussion: 248–50].

[85] Rosemary DH. 50 Years Ago in The Journal of Pediatrics: incidence of retrolental fibroplasias: Past and present. J pediatr 2006;148(6):778.

[86] Edwards WH. Patient safety in the neonatal intensive care unit. Clin Perinatol 2005;32(1): 97–106, vi.

[87] Papworth S, Cartlidge P. Learning from adverse events: the role of confidential enquiries. Semin Fetal Neonatal Med 2005;10(1):39–43.

[88] Folli HL, Poole RL, Benitz WE, et al. Medication error prevention by clinical pharmacists in two children's hospitals. Pediatrics 1987;79(5):718–22.

[89] Ross LM, Wallace J, Paton JY, et al. Medication errors in a paediatric teaching hospital in the UK: five years operational experience. Arch Dis Child 2000;83(6):492–7.

[90] Frey B, Buettiker V, Hug MI, et al. Does critical incident reporting contribute to medication error prevention? Eur J Pediatr 2002;161(11):594–9.

Anesthesia Complications in the Birthplace: Is the Neuraxial Block Always to Blame?

David J. Birnbach, MD, MPH[a],*,
J. Sudharma Ranasinghe, MD, FFARCSI[b]

[a]*Department of Anesthesiology, University of Miami–Jackson Memorial Hospital Center for Patient Safety, Miller School of Medicine, University of Miami, Room 300 JMH Central, 1611 NW 12th Ave., Miami, FL 33136, USA*
[b]*Department of Anesthesiology, Miller School of Medicine, University of Miami, Room 301 JMH Central, 1611 NW 12th Ave., Miami, FL 33136, USA*

Neurologic injuries may be associated with labor and delivery [1]; sometimes they are related to the use of a neuraxial technique (spinal, epidural, combined spinal-epidural), but often they are not. With the current worldwide increase in the use of neuraxial techniques to provide labor analgesia, many postpartum neurologic injuries, regardless of their true cause, are being attributed to the anesthetic. Although most neurologic complications are associated with pregnancy and delivery, some may be related to the anesthetic, and it often is difficult to determine the exact cause of a postpartum neuropathy. Although neuraxial analgesia is the safest and least depressant technique currently available to provide labor analgesia, the anesthetic indeed may be associated with complications, and these complications, if ignored, sometimes may produce devastating outcomes. This article highlights the common and some of the very serious complications that may occur following neuraxial analgesia for labor and delivery, including headache, backache, infection, hypotension, and hematoma. Total spinal block and failed block are discussed also, as are complications unique to epidural anesthesia, such as the intravascular injection of large volumes of local anesthetic (causing seizure or cardiac arrest) and accidental dural puncture.

No one is sure exactly how often neurologic complications occur after pregnancy or how many complications are caused by labor and delivery

---

* Corresponding author.
E-mail address: dbirnbach@miami.edu (D.J. Birnbach).

0095-5108/08/$ - see front matter © 2008 Elsevier Inc. All rights reserved.
doi:10.1016/j.clp.2007.11.011   *perinatology.theclinics.com*

rather than by neuraxial blocks. Complications following regional anesthesia probably are underreported, especially when the deficit is transient. Several factors may be responsible for this underreporting, including practitioner bias (written reports often come from institutions with high volumes of cases and expertise with these techniques), reporting bias (the quality of the data being reported is not always optimal, and many studies are underpowered or retrospective), timing bias (some complications become apparent several days after the block and thus may be missed), and publication bias (journals have a tendency to accept the first but not subsequent reports) [2].

Postpartum nerve palsies versus neuraxial anesthetic-related complications

In their classic 1954 paper, Vandam and Dripps [3] stated, "It is not scientific thinking always to attribute to the anesthetic a neurological complaint arising in a patient who has had a spinal anesthesia." These words remain true today and show the importance of remaining objective when attempting to determine the case of a postpartum neurologic dysfunction. Just because a neuraxial blockade was performed does not guarantee that it was the source. That said, it is important for anesthesiologists and obstetricians to have a clear understanding of these complications and knowledge of which ones need urgent attention.

Intrinsic obstetric palsies may occur following even routine and uncomplicated deliveries. Most often they are mononeuropathies of a lower extremity produced by an acute nerve injury. Several mechanisms have been proposed for this palsy, including transaction, stretch, vascular injury, and compression (Fig. 1) [4].

One of the more common postpartum neurologic deficits is foot drop, which commonly is caused by compression of the lumbosacral trunk at the pelvic brim during delivery. Katriji and colleagues [5] evaluated postpartum unilateral foot drop and reported that risk factors include short maternal stature, macrosomia, prolonged or arrested labor, and instrumental delivery. This list was increased further by Wong and colleagues [6], who added nulliparity and prolonged second stage of labor as risk factors. They also found that position might be involved; women pushing for extended periods in the semi-Fowler position had a much greater incidence of nerve injury. Of note, none of these authors have incriminated neuraxial analgesia techniques. Although in the past dense sensory and motor blockade were produced routinely in laboring patients receiving epidurals, current techniques are associated with little or no motor blockade and should not precipitate these traumatic events.

Another common postpartum nerve injury involves the lateral femoral cutaneous nerve, a condition termed "meralgia paresthetica." Entrapment of this nerve often occurs at the anterior superior iliac spine or during its

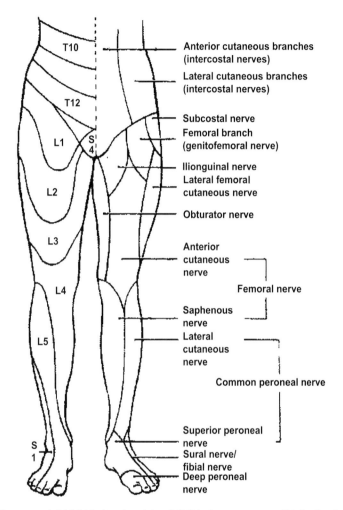

Fig. 1. The segmental (right leg) and peripheral (left leg) sensory nerve distribution is useful in distinguishing central from peripheral nerve injury. (*From* Redlick LF. Maternal perinatal nerve palsies. Postgrad Obstet Gynecol 1992;12:3; with permission.)

passage through the inguinal ligament [7] and is unrelated to neuraxial analgesia.

Neurologic injuries associated with pregnancy also include prolapsed disc, damage to the lumbosacral trunk, femoral nerve neuropathy, lateral femoral cutaneous neuropathy, sciatic neuropathy, obturator neuropathy, and common peroneal and saphenous nerve damage. Many of these injuries are caused by hyperacute hip flexion or the lithotomy position. In addition, compression of the fetal presenting part against the sacrum may produce neuropraxia, especially to the lumbosacral trunk (L4-5) (Fig. 2).

Table 1 illustrates the symptoms associated with various injuries.

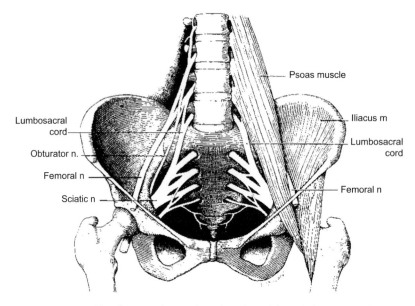

Fig. 2. The relationship of the lumbosacral cord to the pelvis and the psoas major muscle. (*From* Cole JT. Maternal obstetric paralysis. Am J Obstet Gynecol 1946;52:374; with permission.)

Neurologic complications associated with spinal or epidural anesthesia can result from the toxic effects of the injected agent, incorrect placement of a needle or catheter, infectious agents, or spinal cord compromise caused by ischemia or mass effect [8]. These complications, fortunately, are exceedingly rare in the obstetric population. According to one series, the incidence of neurologic complications has been reported as being between 0 and 36 per 10,000 epidural blocks and between 0 and 35 per 10,000 spinal blocks; these complications are predominantly reversible neuropathies [9]. Human error may also play a role; an assortment of agents have been accidentally injected epidurally

Table 1
Symptoms associated with various neurologic injuries during delivery

Damage	Symptoms
Infection	Pain, fever, leukocytosis, weakness
Lumbosacral nerve injury	Paralysis of dorsiflexors of ankle (foot drop)
	Numbness of lateral aspect of foot
	Weakness of quadriceps and hip adductors
Femoral nerve injury	Quadriceps paralysis
	Loss of patellar reflex
	Numbness of thigh
Peroneal nerve injury	Foot drop
Obturator nerve injury	Weakness of hip adduction
	Numbness of inner thigh

and intrathecally. For example, Balestrieri and colleagues [10] recently reported a case involving the accidental intrathecal injection of labetalol.

Complications associated with neuraxial blockade

Headache

Post–dural puncture headache (PDPH) develops in up to 50% of patients after accidental dural puncture with an epidural needle. These headaches also may occur following spinal techniques, especially when cutting edged spinal needles are chosen rather than the newer "atraumatic" needles. It is important to remember, however, that not all postpartum headaches occur as a result of dural puncture. A large analysis reported that headaches occurred in 15% of parturients who did not receive an epidural and in 12% of parturients who had an epidural but did not show evidence of dural puncture [11]. Other causes of headache in the postpartum period include nonspecific headache, migraine, hypertension, pneumocephalus, infection including sinusitis and meningitis, cortical vein thrombosis, and intracerebral pathology. In addition, because coffee intake is so prevalent today, caffeine withdrawal should be considered. PDPH typically presents as a postural headache that is worsened by standing and is relieved by lying down. If the headache is persistent and is accompanied by focal neurologic deficits, altered consciousness, or seizures, MRI is warranted to exclude subdural hematoma, which may result from rupture of bridge meningeal veins because of reduced cerebrospinal fluid (CSF) pressure. Cranial subdural hematoma has been reported even after puncture with a small-gauge atraumatic needle [12] and after an unintentional dural puncture that had been treated correctly by epidural blood patch [13]. MRI findings of a cranial subdural hematoma are illustrated in Fig. 3.

Generally, PDPH initially is treated conservatively with increased intake of both oral and intravenous caffeine and analgesics. Recently, the use of intravenous fluid has been questioned because no evidence has shown that even dramatically increasing fluid intake will cause a greater production of CSF. Drugs that have been used to treat PDPH include caffeine, vasopressin, theophylline, sumatriptan, and adrenocorticotropic hormone (ACTH). Caffeine, which is a cerebral vasoconstrictor, has been used successfully but may not produce permanent results [14] and seems to be more effective when headaches are the result of smaller spinal rather than larger epidural needles. Unfortunately, caffeine treatment may make the woman feel anxious and unable to sleep. In addition, seizures and cardiac arrhythmias have been reported after caffeine administration [15]. Sumatriptan, a serotonin agonist with cerebral vasoconstriction properties that is used to treat migraine headaches, also has been used in the treatment of PDPH [16], although not all studies support its effectiveness [17].

Epidural blood patch continues to be the most effective treatment of severe PDPH. Although early reports suggested immediate and permanent

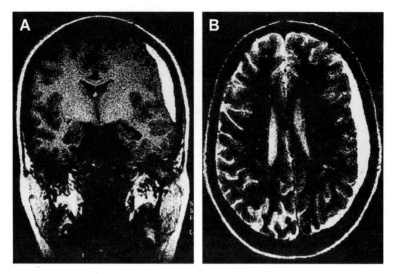

Fig. 3. MRI of cranial subdural hematoma. (*From* Davies JM, Murphy A, Smith M, et al. Subdural hematoma after dural puncture headache treated by epidural blood patch. Br J Anaesth 2001;86:721; with permission.)

cure of PDPH following epidural blood patch, it has been suggested recently that complete success rates are less than 75% and that the effectiveness of an epidural blood patch may be lower if the dural puncture was caused by a large-bore needle [18]. It has been reported that permanent cure after an epidural blood patch is achieved in approximately 60% of patients, not the results of better than 90% once described [19]. The mechanism of action of an epidural blood patch is probably not as simple as the clotted blood obstructing the dural tear. CSF volume replacement is not rapid, but the headache symptoms resolve almost immediately following injection of the blood. Other explanations for the rapid effectiveness of an epidural blood patch include an increase in CSF pressure and cerebral vasoconstriction [20].

Backache

Low back pain is common in pregnancy and also occurs commonly after labor and delivery. Many patients believe that back pain is linked in some way to epidural analgesia administered for labor, and several retrospective studies have suggested a relationship between labor epidurals and postpartum backache. One study reported new-onset long-term backache in 19% of women who delivered vaginally with labor epidural analgesia and in 10% of women who did not have an epidural in situ [21]. Another group of researchers reported an 18% incidence of new-onset postpartum back pain in women who delivered with an epidural versus a 12% incidence in those who delivered without an epidural [22]. More recently, however, several prospective studies evaluating labor epidural analgesia and postpartum back pain failed to find a significant link between epidural analgesia and back pain. In fact, it has been suggested that the incidence of postpartum backache in women who receive epidural anesthesia is equivalent to the incidence in those who did not. Further data analysis demonstrated an association of new-onset postpartum back pain with greater weight and shorter stature; postpartum back pain also was associated with a previous history of back pain, greater weight, and younger age [23]. Another recent study also found no difference in the incidence of long-term low back pain in patients receiving epidurals for labor and in controls who did not [24].

Hypotension

Hypotension is defined differently by different authors and in different settings. In obstetrics most anesthesiologists consider hypotension to be present when systolic blood pressure decreases to less than 90 to 100 mm Hg or to more than 20% to 30% less than baseline readings. The incidence and severity of hypotension depend on the height of the block and the position as well as the volume status of the parturient. In addition, the use of prophylactic measures, such as left uterine displacement, may play a major role, especially during neuraxial anesthesia for operative delivery. Fetal heart rate evaluation is helpful so that any adverse effects on the fetus can be corrected early. If recognized and treated promptly, transient maternal hypotension should not be associated with maternal or neonatal morbidity [25]. Many anesthesiologists still use intravenous ephedrine in 5- to 10-mg increments as a first-line treatment; however, recent evidence supports the use of phenylephrine as a safe and effective first-line drug to treat hypotension in the parturient [26]. Despite its continued use, the prophylactic administration of ephedrine does not seem to be of benefit and actually may pose risks [27]. A recent Cochrane database review has concluded that no interventions totally eliminate the need to treat hypotension [28].

Failed block

Failed block is defined as a neuraxial procedure (epidural, spinal, or combined spinal-epidural [CSE]) resulting in inadequate analgesia/anesthesia or no block after adequate dosing. The incidence and reasons for failure of obstetric neuraxial analgesia and anesthesia vary widely among reports. Most reports suggest that the failure rate is low in general surgical cases but is considerably higher in obstetric patients [28]. Pan and colleagues [29] performed a retrospective analysis of 19,259 deliveries that occurred in his institution during a 5-year period. The overall labor neuraxial analgesia failure rate was 12%, including initial failures from intravenous or subarachnoid catheter placement, unanticipated puncture of the dura, or no CSF or analgesia during the spinal portion of CSE. Excluding these initial failures and problems, only 6.8% of the labor epidural catheters provided inadequate analgesia and required replacement. The rate of epidural catheter replacement reported in this study was higher than the 4.7% rate of epidural reinsertion reported by Peach and colleagues [30] but was less than the 13.1% rate reported by Eappen and colleagues [31] or the 15.4% rate reported by Crawford [32]. Pan and colleagues reported a 7.1% failure rate of labor epidural catheters when used for cesarean sections. Riley and Papasin [33] reported a higher failure rate of labor epidural catheters for cesarean sections if more frequent redosing was required during labor analgesia or nonobstetric anesthesia specialists were involved.

The differences in reported failure rates for neuraxial block probably are related to several factors, including technique factors, catheter-related factors, and patient factors.

Technique factors.

1. Specialists versus trainees or nonobstetric specialists performing the block: Nearly all neuraxial blocks in Pan and colleagues' [29] study were performed by residents, possibly accounting for the higher failure rate in this study compared with that reported by Peach and colleagues [30].
2. The length of catheter inserted inside the epidural space: It has been suggested that no more than 3 to 4 cm of catheter should be inserted into the epidural space. A radiologic study by Bridenbaugh and colleagues [34] reported a 4.5% incidence of transforaminal escape when more than 5 cm of catheter was inserted into the epidural space. The transforaminal escape (clinically or radiologically) has been detected only in obstetric patients, however, not in general surgical patients. The distension of the epidural venous system in pregnancy is thought to be a causative factor for the escape [35]. It was estimated that only about half of these cases were treated successfully by withdrawing the catheter to a more suitable length and further local anesthetic injection; the proposed mechanism was that although the catheter tips were repositioned correctly, the subsequent doses of local anesthetic followed the path opened by the errant catheter and previous solutions out of the epidural space [35].
3. The loss-of-resistance technique used (to air or to saline): Beilin and colleagues [36] found that the frequency of adequate analgesia was higher when a saline-filled syringe was used for the loss-of-resistance technique than when air was used. They found that women in air group requested additional medication more often (36%) than women in the saline group (19%). Anesthesiologists who preferentially use saline suggest that air is detrimental because it is more likely to cause pneumocephalus with resultant headache and that epidural air bubbles may cause incomplete block by preventing spread of local anesthetic.
4. The relative percentage of CSEs versus epidurals used: The incidence of overall failure is significantly lower with the CSE than with the epidural technique. When either epidural or spinal anesthesia is used alone, an

alternative technique is required in approximately 4% of cases [37]. If the two techniques are used together (as in CSE), in theory, the expected failures rates would be 0.16%. In the authors' institution, a retrospective analysis of 525 cases in which CSE was used for cesarean delivery revealed a failure rate of 0.6% (6:1000) requiring rescue with general anesthesia [38].

Catheter-related factors. Inadequate or failed blocks may be caused by blockage of the catheter or uneven delivery of local anesthetic. Two types of epidural catheters are used commonly: single-orifice (open ended) catheters and multiorifice, closed-tip catheters with three lateral holes. Studies have compared the success rates and complication rates of the two types of catheters. Magides and colleagues [39] performed lumbar epidurography with multiorifice and single-orifice epidural catheters. They randomly chose 20 patients presenting for hysterectomy to receive postoperative epidural anesthesia using either multiorifice catheters or single-orifice catheters and studied the spread of iohexol dye in the epidural space when injected through these catheters. The total number of vertebral segments covered by dye was comparable in the two groups, but the sacral extension of dye was observed only in the single-orifice catheter group. The investigators thought this difference was related to the larger diameter of the single orifice and the resultant higher epidural pressure on injection.

Morrison and colleagues [40] showed that, although multiorifice catheters may be less safe because they can be sited partially subdurally and allow multicompartmental spread of local anesthetic, they are less likely to occlude and require re-siting.

Michael and colleagues [41] found that differences in the type of complication that occurred with the two types of epidural catheters, although the complication rate was similar. Bloody taps were more common with multiorifice catheters, and missed segments were more common when single-orifice catheters were used.

Patient factors.

1. Spinal deformity, disease, or previous spinal surgery: Unilateral blocks have been described in the presence of asymptomatic, fairly minor degrees of scoliosis. Epidural spread of solution, and in one case the catheter itself, was directed away from the primary scoliosis. This misdirection may cause uneven distribution of solutions, leading to unilateral block [35]. More severe deformities, therefore, may be associated with failed or patchy blocks. Similarly, inadequate blocks are seen following spinal surgery such as scoliosis corrections because scar tissue, adhesions, or bone grafts may disrupt the spread of local anesthetic. Lumbar disc disease also has been shown to interfere with the spread of contrast material and, presumably, local anesthetic in the lumbar

epidural space. In their series of 600 epidurograms, Luyendyk and Van Voorthusien [42] found that contrast material failed to reach the affected nerve roots in 33% of patients who had uncomplicated disc prolapse.

2. The midline barrier: A unilateral block seems to result from maldistribution of local anesthetic by a midline barrier in the epidural space. These patients have reported identical unilateral blocks in successive pregnancies [35]. Blomberg [43] summarized his findings following epiduroscopy of 48 autopsy subjects aged between 20 and 88 years: "In every case there was a dorsal connective tissue band in the midline (referred to as plica mediana dorsalis) of the epidural space. The appearance of the band varied from strands of connective tissue to a complete membrane (in 2% of cadavers). The membranes were found to extend vertically over at least two lumbar segments, which was as far as could be visualized with the epiduroscope." The septal barriers that have been demonstrated are incomplete in most patients [35], and increased volume of local anesthetic eventually can reach the unblocked side via either the cephalad or caudad end of the septum. Therefore, management of a unilateral block may include partial withdrawal of the epidural catheter, additional fractionated doses of local anesthetic (perhaps combined with an opioid) to cross the barrier, and possibly change of posture.

3. Differences in patient demographics and expectations: One study showed that younger parturients with higher body mass indices and longer periods of gestation are at increased risk of being unable to extend labor epidural analgesia to epidural anesthesia for cesarean delivery [44]. Bishton and colleagues [45] found a statistically significant relationship between the migration of epidural catheters and the patient's body mass index. They postulated that in obese patients a large amount of subcutaneous fat may allow greater relative movement between the skin exit site and the point of entry into the supraspinous ligament, causing the epidural catheter to migrate out of the epidural space and coil up in the subcutaneous tissue.

Infection, abscess, and meningitis

Infectious complications, although rare, may occur following neuraxial techniques and range from minimal risk (colonization of the catheter in an asymptomatic patient) to major risk (meningitis, abscess). The risk of epidural-related infection is extremely low. Scott and Hibbard [46] reviewed more than 500,000 labor epidurals in the United Kingdom and reported only a single epidural abscess. When discussing infection, an important question is whether there is a need (or a way) to decrease the risk of infection. Reduction of risk would need to involve all facets of aseptic technique as well as use of different techniques and agents for antisepsis. Although there is much literature surrounding the risks associated with intravascular (central venous) catheters, there is conflicting evidence regarding the risk of infection following neuraxial block. Unfortunately, neither the numerator nor the denominator is known for complications following neuraxial blocks, and these complications are so rare that prospective studies become problematic. Although numerous anecdotal and case reports about infection following epidurals exist, there is little hard evidence on which to base guidelines or standards. There currently are no standards or guidelines in the United States for antisepsis as related to initiating epidurals or spinals; some other countries, however, do require that cap and mask be worn, or that hands be washed, or in the most extreme case, that anesthesiologists wear surgical gowns. The Centers for Disease Control and the World Health Organization both have advocated the requirement for hand hygiene before placing sterile gloves for techniques that require aseptic technique. Although anesthesiologists performing neuraxial blocks for surgery must wear a cap and mask because they are in the operating room, the requirement is not always in force for labor and delivery suites, where these blocks typically are performed in an environment with less stringent antiseptic conditions. Surveys of anesthesiologists in the United Kingdom and Australia have reported that many do not wear masks or wash their hands before the procedure [47].

There also seems to be no standard for disinfecting the skin of the back. Most anesthesiologists in the United States use povidone iodine (PI), and most of those using PI prefer single-use bottles or packets rather than multiuse bottles. Some use two swabs, and some use three; some let the PI dry, and others wipe it off; and some continue to use multiuse bottles of PI (which occasionally have been shown to support bacterial growth) [48]. Some anesthesiologists use alcohol alone, some use alcohol plus PI, and some use an iodinated solution plus alcohol. Still others (and most Europeans) use chlorhexidine. The Food and Drug Administration, however, still warns about a potential neurotoxicity risk with chlorhexidine despite a lack of clinical evidence to support such a risk.

The number of reports in the non-anesthesia literature of infections related to inappropriate or suboptimal disinfection practices or sterile techniques associated with neuraxial analgesia/anesthesia are disquieting. Many of these reports incriminate lack of sterile technique, and most have not been reported in the anesthesia literature [49–51].

In addition, physicians do not seem to be very good at picking up the signs of postepidural or spinal meningitis, and several bad outcomes have occurred because of major delays in diagnosis. For example a study that identified 42 catheter-related epidural abscesses reported that the correct diagnosis was considered originally in only 15 cases, and that the time from symptoms to treatment was as long as 108 days [52].

Total spinal block

A total spinal block is a rare and potentially life-threatening complication that occurs after excessive cephalad spread of spinally or epidurally administered anesthetic. It can occur during single-shot spinal anesthesia or, more commonly, as a result of unanticipated intrathecal spread of epidural medication after unintentional dural puncture or unsuspected catheter migration from the epidural to either subdural or spinal space. Subdural spread of the local anesthetic also can cause a high block characterized by a high sensory level, sacral sparing, and incomplete or absent motor block [53].

Bleeding/epidural hematoma

Spinal hematoma is caused by bleeding within the spinal neuraxis and may produce permanent paralysis from spinal cord compression. Hematoma following neuraxial blockade is extremely rare but is not a new phenomenon. Less than 10 years after the first spinal anesthetic was performed by Bier, a spinal hematoma was reported [54]. That patient did have spinal pathology (spina bifida), but no coagulopathy was seen. Today much emphasis is placed on the coagulation status of the parturient who is to receive a neuraxial block. Risk factors for coagulopathy (eg, pre-eclampsia, the hemolysis, elevated liver enzymes, and low platelet count syndrome, and intrauterine fetal demise) should cause concern. Recently, as low molecular weight heparin therapy has gained popularity for the prevention of perioperative thromboembolism, these concerns have been renewed and amplified. If cord compression is suspected, prompt diagnosis and intervention is necessary to prevent permanent neurologic insult, including paralysis.

The volume of blood required to cause ischemia of the cord is variable, depending on the site of bleeding and the speed with which blood accumulates. Adding to the confusion, several cases of hematoma have been associated with volumes of blood less than those routinely administered for epidural blood patch [55].

Accidental dural puncture

A relatively common complication of epidural block placement is the unanticipated puncture of the dura, which has an incidence of up to 3% [56]. This complication can lead to the development of PDPH in up to 70% of cases. The traditional management of accidental dural puncture was to reposition the epidural at a different interspace, but many anesthesiologists currently advocate passing the epidural catheter into the spinal space (converting to a "macrocatheter" continuous spinal technique) [57]. This technique establishes rapid and effective pain relief and probably decreases the incidence of headache. Analysis of aggregate data from limited retrospective trials demonstrates a significant reduction in the incidence of PDPH and the need for an epidural blood patch in patients who receive continuous spinal analgesia after unintentional dural puncture [58]. In addition, the catheter provides excellent labor analgesia and an immediate onset of blockade for cesarean section. A recent review of cases in which epidural anesthesia was complicated by an unintentional dural puncture suggested that spinal headache could be reduced if five steps were followed: (1) injection of CSF from the epidural syringe back into the subarachnoid space through the epidural needle, (2) insertion of an epidural catheter into the subarachnoid space, (3) injection of preservative-free normal saline through the intrathecal catheter before its removal, (4) administration of continuous intrathecal labor analgesia, and (5) leaving the intrathecal catheter in situ for a total of 12 to 20 hours [59].

Pneumocephalus

Pneumocephalus, the introduction of air into the cranial cavity, is a rare complication typically associated with placement of an epidural anesthetic using the loss-of-resistance-to-air technique. The neurologic findings associated with pneumocephalus can be impressive but usually resolve spontaneously following resorption of collection of air [60,61]. Seizure associated with pneumocephalus also has been reported [62].

The use of a hyperbaric chamber has been advocated for severe neurologic symptoms associated with pneumocephalus [63].

Because of the risk of pneumocephalus, many authors now advocate the use of a loss-of-resistance-to-saline technique. An added advantage to using loss of resistance to saline is that it also may decrease the incidence of failed blocks and decrease the risk of accidental dural puncture by the epidural needle [64].

Spinal cord injury

Direct injury to the spinal cord following epidural block is exceedingly rare, because the epidural space generally is entered at the L3-4 ($\pm$ 1) interspace, well below the end of the spinal cord. Nonetheless, spinal cord injury associated with epidural analgesia for labor has been reported [65]. How does this injury occur? Broadbent and colleagues [65] have shown that anesthesiologists often place neuraxial blocks at spaces remote from the presumed interspace. The actual level of markers ranged from one space below to four spaces above the level at which the anesthesiologist believed it to be.

Another reason for this error is the variation in the vertebral level of termination of the cord, which varies between the bodies of T12 and L3 and is lower in women than in men.

Reynolds [66] also reported damage to the spinal cord during placement of spinal anesthesia and has suggested that lower spaces be used (Fig. 4).

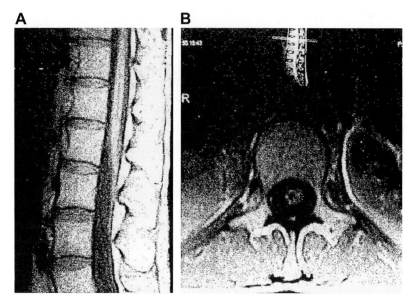

Fig. 4. MRI of conus lesion. (*From* Reynolds F. Damage to the conus medullaris following spinal anesthesia. Anesthesia 2001;56:240; with permission.)

Horner's syndrome and trigeminal nerve palsy

Horner's syndrome is a very rare complication of epidural analgesia for labor, as is trigeminal nerve palsy. Both were reported as having occurred in one patient following placement of epidural analgesia for labor, presumably resulting from a subdural block [67].

Changes in fetal heart rate

Changes in fetal heart rate have been reported following initiation of neuraxial analgesia but are more common with intrathecal opioids, especially when high doses are used [68]. This phenomenon was reported first in 1989 by Clarke and colleagues [69].

Complications associated with epidural catheters

Transient paresthesias frequently occur during epidural needle or catheter placement; one study found the rate of paresthesias associated with catheter insertion to be greater than 40% [70]. An analysis of prospective data was collected on all epidural blocks performed at a single institution. Minor complications included failed or abandoned insertion of the catheter (5%) and inadequate anesthesia (1.7%) or analgesia (0.9%). In addition, 3% of insertions were associated with venous puncture [30].

Summary

Neuraxial blockade offers the most effective and least depressant option for labor analgesia. It may be associated with complications, as discussed in this article, but all too often any postpartum neurologic abnormality is attributed to the neuraxial anesthetic. Lord Justice Denning, in his opinion in the Wooley and Roe case, wrote, "We must insist on due care for the patient at every point, but we must not condemn as negligence that which is only a misadventure" [71]. These words are just as true today. Misadventures occur during labor and delivery; they seldom are the result of neuraxial blocks and should not automatically be assumed to result from negligence on the part of the anesthesiologist.

References

[1] Sahai-Srivastava S, Amezcua L. Compressive neuropathies complicating normal childbirth: case report and literature review. Birth 2007;34:173–5.

[2] Benhamou D, Auroy Y. Overview of regional anesthesia complications. In: Neal JM, Rathmell JP, editors. Complications in regional anesthesia and pain medicine. Philadelphia: Elsevier; 2007.

[3] Vandam LD, Dripps RD. Long term follow-up of patients who received 10,098 spinal anesthetics. IV. Neurologic disease incident to traumatic lumbar puncture during spinal anesthesia. JAMA 1960;172:1483–7.

[4] Birnbach DJ, Hernandez M, Van Zundert AJ. Neurologic complications of neuraxial analgesia for labor. Curr Opin Anaesthesiol 2005;18:513–7.

[5] Katriji B, Wilbourn AJ, Scarberry SL, et al. Intrapartum maternal lumbosacral plexopathy. Muscle Nerve 2002;26:340–7.

[6] Wong CA, Scavone BM, Dugan S, et al. Incidence of postpartum lumbosacral spine and lower extremity nerve injuries. Obstet Gynecol 2003;101:279–88.

[7] Ferra Verdera M, Ribera L. Two cases of paresthetic meralgia of the femoral cutaneous nerve. Rev Esp Anestesiol Reanim 2003;50:154–6.

[8] Horlocker TT, Wedel DJ. Neurologic complications of spinal and epidural anesthesia. Reg Anesth Pain Med 2000;25:83–98.

[9] Kerr S, O'Sullivan G. Neurologic complications in obstetric regional anesthesia. Anaesth Intensive Care 2004;5:271–3.

[10] Balestrieri PJ, Hamza MS, Ting PH, et al. Inadvertent intrathecal injection of labetalol in a patient undergoing post-partum tubal ligation. Int J Obstet Anesth 2005;14:340–2.

[11] Benhamou D, Hamza J, Ducot B. Postpartum headache after epidural analgesia without dural puncture. Int J Obstet Anesth 1995;4:17–20.

[12] Cantais E, Benhamou D, Pete D, et al. Acute subdural hematoma following spinal anesthesia with a very small spinal needle. Anesthesiology 2000;93:1354–5.

[13] Davies JM, Murphy A, Smith M, et al. Subdural hematoma after dural puncture headache treated by epidural blood patch. Br J Anaesth 2001;86:720–3.

[14] Camann WR, Murray RS, Mushlin PS, et al. Effects of oral caffeine on postdural puncture headache: a double-blind placebo-controlled trial. Anesth Analg 1990;70: 181–4.

[15] Bolton VE, Leicht CH, Scanlon TS. Postpartum seizure after epidural blood patch and intravenous caffeine sodium benzoate. Anesthesiology 1989;70:146–9.

[16] Hodgson C, Roitberg HA. The use of sumatriptan in the treatment of postdural puncture headache. Anaesthesia 1997;52:808.

[17] Paech M, Banks S, Gurrin L, et al. An audit of accidental dural puncture during epidural insertion of a Tuohy needle in obstetric patients. Int J Obstet Anesth 2001;10:162–7.

[18] Safa-Tisseront V, Thormann F, Malassine P, et al. Effectiveness of epidural blood patch in the management of post–dural puncture headache. Anesthesiology 2001;95: 334–9.

[19] Taivaninen T, Pitkanen M, Touminen M, et al. Efficacy of epidural blood patch for post-dural puncture headache. Acta Anaesthesiol Scand 1993;37:702–5.

[20] Coombs DW, Hooper D. Subarachnoid pressure with epidural blood patch. Reg Anesth 1979;4:3–6.

[21] Macarthur C, Lewis M, Knox FG, et al. Epidural anaesthesia and longterm backache after childbirth. BMJ 1990;301:9–12.

[22] Russell R, Groves P, Taub N, et al. Assessing longterm backache after childbirth. BMJ 1993; 306:1299–303.

[23] Breen TW, Ransil BJ, Groves PA, et al. Factors associated with back pain after childbirth. Anesthesiology 1994;81:29–34.

[24] Howell CJ, Dean T, Lucking L, et al. Randomised study of longterm outcome after epidural versus non-epidural analgesia during labour. BMJ 2002;325:357–61.

[25] Corke BC, Datta S, Ostheimer GW, et al. Spinal anaesthesia for caesarean section. The influence of hypotension on neonatal outcomes. Anaesthesia 1982;37:658–62.

[26] Ngan Kee WD, Khaw KS. Vasopressors in obstetrics: what should we be using? Curr Opin Anaesthesiol 2006;19:238–43.

[27] Ngan Kee WD, Khaw K, Lee BB, et al. A dose-response study of prophylactic intravenous ephedrine for the prevention of hypotension during spinal anesthesia for cesarean delivery. Anesth Analg 2000;90:1390–5.

[28] Cyna AM, Emmett RS, Middleton P, et al. Techniques for preventing hypotension during spinal anaesthesia for caesarean section. Cochrane Database Syst Rev 2006;4:CD002251.

[29] Pan PH, Bogard TD, Owen MD. Incidence and characteristics of failures in obstetrical neuraxial analgesia and anesthesia: a retrospective analysis of 19,259 deliveries. Int J Obstet Anesth 2004;13:227–33.

[30] Peach MJ, Godkin R, Webster S. Complications of obstetric epidural analgesia and anesthesia: a prospective analysis of 10995 cases. Int J Obstet Anesth 1998;7:5–11.

[31] Eappen S, Blinn A, Segal S. Incidence of epidural catheter replacement in parturients: a retrospective chart review. Int J Obstet Anesth 1998;7:220–5.

[32] Crawford JS. The second thousand epidural blocks in an obstetric hospital practice. Br J Anaesth 1972;44:1277–86.

[33] Riley ET, Papasin J. Epidural catheter function during labor predicts anesthetic efficacy for subsequent cesarean delivery. Int J Obstet Anesth 2002;11:81–4.

[34] Bridenbaugh LD, Moore DC, Bagdi P, et al. The position of plastic tubing in continuous block technique: an X-ray study of 552 patients. Anesthesiology 1968;29:1047–9.

[35] Collier CB. Why obstetric epidurals fail: a study of epidurograms. Int J Obstet Anesth 1996; 5:19–31.

[36] Beilin Y, Arnold I, Telfeyan C, et al. Quality of analgesia when air versus saline is used for identification of the epidural space in the parturient. Reg Anesth Pain Med 2000;25(6):596–9.

[37] Milne MK, Lawson J. Epidural analgesia for cesarean section. A review of 182 cases. Br J Anaesth 1973;45:1206–10.

[38] Ranasinghe JS, Steadman J, Toyama T, et al. Combined spinal epidural anesthesia is better than spinal or epidural alone for caesarean delivery. Br J Anaesth 2003;91:299–300.

[39] Magides AD, Sprigg A, Richmond MN. Lumbar epidurography with multi-orifice and single orifice and epidural catheters. Anaesthesia 1996;51:757–63.

[40] Morrison LMM, Buchan AS. Comparison of complications associated with single-holed and multiholed extradural catheters. Br J Anaesth 1990;64:183–5.

[41] Michael S, Richmond MN, Birks RJS. A comparison between open end (single hole) and closed end (three lateral holes) epidural catheters. Anaesthesia 1989;44:78–80.

[42] Luyendyk W, Van Voorthuisen AE. Contrast examination of the spinal epidural space. Acta Radiol Diagn 1966;5:1051–66.

[43] Blomberg R. The dorsomedian connective tissue band in the lumbar epidural space of humans. An anatomical study using epiduroscopy in autoscopy cases. Anesth Analg 1986;65:747–52.

[44] Orbach-Zinger S, Avramovich A, Ilgiaeva N, et al. Risk factors for failure to extend labor epidural analgesia to epidural anesthesia for cesarean section. Acta Anaesthesiol Scand 2006;50:1014–8.

[45] Bishton IM, Martin PH, Vernon JM, et al. Factors influencing epidural catheter migration. Anaesthesia 1992;47:610–2.

[46] Scott DB, Hibbard BM. Serious non-fatal complications associated with extradural block in obstetric practice. Br J Anaesth 1990;64:537–41.

[47] Sellors JE, Cyna AM, Simmons SW, et al. Aseptic precautions for inserting an epidural catheter: a survey of obstetric anaesthetists. Anaesthesia 2002;57:593–6.

[48] Birnbach DJ, Stein DJ, Murray O, et al. Povidone iodine and skin disinfection before initiation of epidural anesthesia. Anesthesiology 1998;88:668–72.

[49] Rodrigo N, Perera KN, Ranwala R, et al. Aspergillus meningitis following spinal aneaesthesia for caesarean section in Colmbo, Sri Lanka. Int J Obstet Anesth 2007;16:256–60.

[50] Moen V. Meningitis is a rare complication of spinal anesthesia. Good hygiene and face masks are simple preventive measures. Lakartidningen 1998;95:631–2.

[51] Schneeberger PM, Janssen M, Voss A. Alpha-hemolytic streptococci: a major pathogen of iatrogenic meningitis following lumbar puncture. Infection 1996;24:29–33.

[52] Kindler CH, Seeberger MD, Staender SE. Epidural abscess complicating epidural anesthesia and analgesia. An analysis of the literature. Acta Anaesthesiol Scand 1998;42:614–20.

[53] Reynolds F, Speedy HM. The subdural space: the third place to go astray. Anaesthesia 1990; 45:120–3.

[54] Usubiaga JE. Neurologic complications following epidural anesthesia. Int Anesthesiol Clin 1975;13:1–153.

[55] Horlocker TT, Wedel DJ. Neuraxial block and low molecular weight heparin: balancing perioperative analgesia and thromboprophylaxis. Reg Anesth Pain Med 1998;23:164–77.

[56] Norris MC, Leighton BL, DeSimone CA. Needle bevel orientation and headache after inadvertent dural puncture. Anesthesiology 1989;70:729–31.

[57] Hall JM, Hinchliffe D, Levy DM. Prolonged intrathecal catheterisation after inadvertent dural taps in labour. Anaesthesia 1999;54:611–2.

[58] Russell I. In the event of accidental dural puncture by an epidural needle in labour, the catheter should be passed into the subarachnoid space. Int J Obstet Anesth 2002;11:23–7.

[59] Kuczkowski KM, Benumof JL. Decrease in the incidence of post–dural puncture headache: maintaining CSF volume. Acta Anaesthesiol Scand 2003;47:98–100.

[60] Smarkusky L, DeCarvalho M, Bermudez A, et al. Acute onset headache complicating labor epidural caused by intrapartum pneumocephalus. Obstet Gynecol 2006;108:795–8.

[61] Velickovic IA, Pavlik R. Pneumocephalus complicated by postdural puncture headache after unintentional dural puncture. Anesth Analg 2007;104:747–8.

[62] van den Berg AA, Nguyen L, von-Maszewski M, et al. Unexplained fitting in patients with post dural puncture headache. Risk of iatrogenic pneumocephalus with air rationalizes use of loss of resistance to saline. Br J Anaesth 2003;90:810–1.

[63] Panni MK, Camann W, Bhavani Shankar K. Hyperbaric therapy for a postpartum patient with prolonged epidural blockade and tomographic evidence of epidural air. Anesth Analg 2003;97:1810–1.

[64] Gleeson CM, Reynolds F. Accidental dural puncture rates in UK obstetric practice. Int J Obstet Anesth 1998;7:242–6.

[65] Broadbent CR, Maxwell WB, Ferrie R, et al. Ability of anaesthetists to identify a marked lumbar interspace. Anaesthesia 2000;55(11):1122–6.

[66] Reynolds F. Damage to conus medullaris following spinal anaesthesia. Anaesthesia 2001;56:238–47.

[67] De la Gala F, Reyes A, Avellard M, et al. Trigeminal nerve palsy and Horner's syndrome following epidural analgesia for labor: a subdural block? Int J Obstet Anesth 2007;16:180–2.
[68] van de Velde M. Neuraxial analgesia and fetal bradycardia. Curr Opin Anaesthesiol 2005;18: 253–6.
[69] Clarke VT, Smiley RM, Finster M. Uterine hyperactivity after intrathecal injection of fentanyl for analgesia during labor: a cause of fetal bradycardia. Anesthesiology 1994;81:1083.
[70] Rolbin SH, Hew E, Ogilvie G. A comparison of two types of epidural catheter. Can J Anaesth 1987;34:459–61.
[71] Cope RW. The Wooley and Roe case. Anaesthesia 1995;50:162–73.

Clin Perinatol 35 (2008) 53–67

Medically Indicated Preterm Birth: Recognizing the Importance of the Problem

Cande V. Ananth, PhD, MPH[a],*,
Anthony M. Vintzileos, MD[b]

[a]*Division of Epidemiology and Biostatistics, Department of Obstetrics, Gynecology,
and Reproductive Sciences, UMDNJ-Robert Wood Johnson Medical School,
125 Paterson Street, New Brunswick, NJ 08901-1977, USA*
[b]*Department of Obstetrics and Gynecology, Winthrop University Hospital, 259 First Street,
Mineola, NY, USA*

Preterm birth—delivery before 37 completed weeks—complicates over 500,000 births annually, affecting 12.5% of pregnancies in the United States [1]. It is one of the leading causes of perinatal morbidity and mortality [2–4] in industrialized countries. Although prevention of preterm birth remains a perinatal priority [5,6], clinical and community-based interventions have clearly fallen short of reducing preterm birth [7]. In fact, the rate of preterm birth has been increasing in the United States [8–11] and in several other Western societies in recent decades [12–14]. The temporal increase in preterm births in the United States has occurred following a concurrent increase in medically indicated preterm birth [9]. In spite of the dramatic improvements and advances in neonatal care, therapeutic interventions have had limited effects on adverse outcomes attributable to preterm birth [15]. The therapies, themselves, are expensive and can lead to important morbidity; hence, it is important to consider primary prevention. However, it is almost impossible to target prevention programs without an understanding of the etiologies and preventable causes of preterm birth.

Preterm birth is arguably the most studied problem in contemporary obstetrics. Despite extensive research, the problem has continued to be elusive in regards to etiology and prevention. While efforts to reduce perinatal and infant mortality rates and morbidity in the newborn in general, and as

* Corresponding author.
E-mail address: cande.ananth@umdnj.edu (C.V. Ananth).

0095-5108/08/$ - see front matter © 2008 Elsevier Inc. All rights reserved.
doi:10.1016/j.clp.2007.11.001   *perinatology.theclinics.com*

a consequence of preterm birth in particular, have been successful, primary prevention of preterm birth has been disappointing [16–18]. Several issues of importance have been overlooked in recent efforts aimed at preterm birth prevention, including the failure to distinguish preterm birth as a heterogeneous clinical end point with varied clinical pathways of spontaneous and medically indicated preterm birth [2,19–23]. In fact, most preterm birth prevention programs have been largely restricted to women with spontaneous preterm birth. However, medically indicated preterm births constitute roughly 35% to 40% of all preterm births [9,16,24], and efforts to understand this group have largely been ignored.

The remainder of this article will largely focus on medically indicated preterm birth, including its incidence rate, temporal trends, recurrence, and a focused discussion of the underlying maternal and fetal indications leading to medical interventions at preterm gestational ages.

Impact of ischemic placental disease on medically indicated preterm birth

Preterm birth affects more than one in eight births in the United States. The pathways to preterm birth can be broadly classified into two clinical subtypes: medically indicated and spontaneous preterm birth (composed of both preterm premature rupture of membranes and spontaneous onset of labor at preterm gestations) [21]. Although this stratification facilitates epidemiologic research, the considerable heterogeneity in etiologic profiles within these two broad distinctions has been largely neglected, and is necessary to advance the field.

Preterm birth shows considerable race disparity [9,17,25–27], with African American women at 1.8- to 2.0-fold higher risk (17%) than white women (9%) [9]. The preterm birth rate among white women in the United States has increased over the recent decade by 14% (from 8.3% in 1989 to 9.4% in 2000). In contrast, the rate among African American women over the same period has declined by 15% (from 18.5% in 1989 to 16.2% in 2000).

The race-disparity in preterm birth trends also persists within clinical subtypes of preterm birth. The overall increase in preterm birth among white is accompanied by a concurrent temporal increase in medically indicated preterm birth (55%). This is a stark contrast to the temporal decline in preterm births among African American women following a decline in spontaneous preterm birth. Of note is that the medically indicated preterm birth among African American women increased by 32% [9].

The frequency and extent to which common maternal and fetal indications warranting either a labor induction and/or a prelabor cesarean at preterm gestational ages was reported by our group [28]. The common indications that were analyzed in a cohort of roughly 650,000 singleton live births included medical and obstetrical complications of pregnancy (Table 1). These data suggest that preeclampsia, fetal distress, small for

Table 1

Associations of maternal and fetal conditions with all and medically indicated preterm birth at <35 weeks

Maternal-fetal conditions	Near-term/term birth ≥35 weeks (n = 653,473)	Medically indicated preterm birth (n = 7347)		
		Rate (per 100)	RR (95% CI)	PAF (%)
Ischemic placental disease				
Preeclampsia	3.9	23.3	5.5 (5.1, 5.9)	19.1
Fetal distress	5.9	23.0	1.4 (1.3, 1.5)	6.6
Small for gestational age	9.6	18.9	1.3 (1.2, 1.4)	4.4
Placental abruption	0.5	11.9	8.4 (7.7, 9.2)	10.5
At least 1 ischemic cause	17.7	53.2	4.9 (4.7, 5.2)	43.1
Miscellaneous causes				
Chronic hypertension	0.8	4.3	3.0 (2.6, 3.4)	2.9
Placenta previa	0.3	5.6	6.7 (5.9, 7.7)	4.8
Unexplained vaginal bleeding	0.5	3.1	3.3 (2.8, 4.0)	2.2
Diabetes (all types)	2.4	4.6	1.3 (1.1, 1.4)	1.1
Renal disease	0.2	1.1	2.7 (2.2, 3.8)	0.7
Rh sensitization	0.4	0.9	2.7 (2.1, 3.5)	0.6
Congenital malformation[a]	3.7	12.7	3.4 (3.2, 3.6)	9.0
At least 1 miscellaneous cause	7.6	25.9	4.0 (3.8, 4.2)	19.4

Relative risks are adjusted for the confounding effects of period of birth, maternal age, parity, maternal race/ethnicity, marital status, maternal education, smoking and alcohol use during pregnancy, and prepregnancy body-mass index.

Abbreviations: RR, relative risk; CI, confidence interval; PAF, population attributable fraction percent.

[a] Excludes any chromosomal abnormalities.

Data from Ananth CV, Vintzileos AM. Maternal-fetal conditions necessitating a medical intervention resulting in preterm birth. Am J Obstet Gynecol 2006;195(6):1557–63.

gestational age (birth weight below the 10th percentile for gestational age), and placental abruption were the most common conditions present among medically indicated preterm births. In other words, one or more of these conditions were present in more than 1 of 2 indicated preterm births (53.2%) and were almost five-fold more common (relative risk 4.9, 95% confidence interval 4.7, 5.2), compared with 17.7% of singleton births at near-term or term gestations. The frequency of other medical conditions in indicated preterm births and term births are also contrasted in Table 1.

Recurrence of medically indicated preterm birth

The strongest risk factor for preterm birth is a history of preterm birth (Fig. 1) [25,29–36]. Studies more recently have demonstrated patterns of recurrence of preterm birth within the two clinical subtypes, namely,

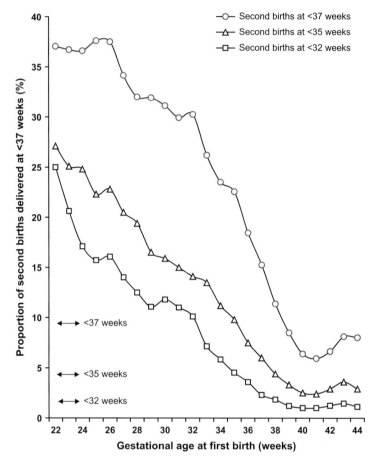

Fig. 1. Proportion of second births that were delivered at <37, <35 and <32 weeks, conditional on gestational age at delivery of the first birth. The horizontal lines denote preterm birth rates at <37, <35, and <32 weeks in the first pregnancy. (*From* Ananth CV, Getahun D, Peltier MR, et al. Recurrence of spontaneous versus medically indicated preterm birth. Am J Obstet Gynecol 2006;195(3):643–50; with permission).

medically indicated and spontaneous preterm births. While women with a prior preterm birth have a 2.9-fold (95% confidence interval 2.8, 3.0) increased risk of delivering preterm in the subsequent pregnancy, there is considerable heterogeneity in recurrence risks across clinical subtypes [29]. In other words, women with an indicated preterm birth in the first pregnancy are not only more likely to deliver preterm for medical indications in the second pregnancy (Fig. 2), but are also at increased risk of spontaneously delivering preterm, and vice versa [29]. A population-based cohort study from the Maternal-Fetal Medicine network also showed women with a prior spontaneous preterm birth at less than 35 weeks were at an increased risk

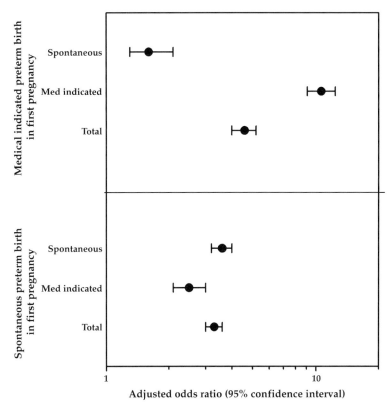

Fig. 2. Recurrence of medically indicated and spontaneous preterm birth (<35 weeks) in a population-based cohort of 154,809 women with the first two consecutive singleton pregnancies resulting in live births.

of delivering a spontaneous preterm birth in the following pregnancy [37]. However, whether such increased recurrence risk persisted for medically indicated preterm births was not explored in this study. These findings, in general, suggest that the two clinical subtypes of preterm birth are likely to share common etiologies—a notion also strongly supported by epidemiologic observations [2,3,19,22,23,38].

Main indications for medically indicated preterm births

Labor induction and/or cesarean section at preterm gestational ages are usually performed for maternal and/or fetal indications. The goal of such interventions is to balance maternal and fetal risks of untoward outcomes and benefits with carefully planned and appropriately timed interventions during gestation [39]. These medical indications for delivery have consequently led to increases in rates of preterm birth. In fact, such interventions have also led to a considerable "left shift" in the distribution of gestational age, thereby increasing the proportion of births at term (37 to 41 weeks) and postterm (42 weeks and beyond) gestations. This phenomenon has been documented to occur in the United States [8,9,24,40], Canada [12,13,41], France [42–44], and other developed countries [14,45], as well as between singleton [9,12,13,40–42] and multiple [9,24,46] gestations.

The clinical manifestations of preeclampsia, intrauterine growth restriction, and placental abruption are disorders that may involve the placenta. These disorders, while heterogeneous in their clinical manifestations, may be causally associated with some common biologic underpinnings [47,48]. These include uteroplacental underperfusion, chronic hypoxia, and uteroplacental ischemia [49–51]. Given the similarities in the pathophysiologic mechanisms of these clinical conditions, we hypothesized that these disease states can be classified as "ischemic placental disease" to facilitate etiologic research [28]. Compelling arguments in support of ischemic placental disease being a common pathophysiologic mechanism for preeclampsia, IUGR, and placental abruption are provided by several Doppler studies of uterine and umbilical arteries, placental histology, and biochemical factors.

Epidemiology of ischemic placental disease

Several epidemiologic, clinical, uterine and umbilical artery Doppler findings, biochemical markers, as well as placental histologic data provide evidence to support the concept that ischemic placental disease may provide an acceptable etiologic underpinning common to preterm preeclampsia, intrauterine growth restriction (IUGR) and placental abruption (Table 2) [52–66]. Numerous studies have also shown that both preeclampsia and

Table 2
Distribution of ischemic placental disease among medically indicated preterm birth at <35 weeks and among term/near term births

Ischemic placental disease	Near term/term birth ≥35 weeks rate, %	Medically indicated preterm birth	
		Rate, %	RR (95% CI)
PE only	3.2	13.4	5.2 (4.9, 5.5)
PE + SGA	0.7	8.3	14.7 (13.6, 15.9)
PE + Placental abruption	0.03	1.1	41.0 (31.5, 53.4)
PE + SGA + Placental abruption	0.02	0.5	49.8 (34.9, 71.2)
Small for gestational age only	8.8	8.3	1.3 (1.2, 1.4)
SGA + Placental abruption	0.1	1.9	18.7 (15.9, 21.9)
Placental abruption only	0.4	8.5	26.5 (24.4, 28.8)

Relative risks (RR) are adjusted for the confounding effects of period of birth, maternal age, parity, maternal race/ethnicity, marital status, maternal education, smoking and alcohol use during pregnancy, and prepregnancy body mass index.

Abbreviations: CI, confidence interval; PE, preeclampsia; RR, relative risk; SGA, small for gestational age.

IUGR, especially at preterm gestational ages, are associated with failure of trophoblast invasion and abnormal Doppler findings in both the uterine and umbilical arteries [61,67,68]. It has been postulated that the degree of trophoblast invasion will dictate what the clinical manifestation(s) may be including preeclampsia, preterm birth, and/or IUGR or their combination [60]. Finally, placental histologic studies have revealed remarkable similarity between preterm preeclampsia and early-onset IUGR [55,59].

Biochemical angiogenic factors, ischemic placental disease, and indicated preterm births

Although there are no accepted reliable biomarkers for predicting preeclampsia, IUGR, or placental abruption, recent and accumulating data suggest that these conditions may be associated with functional changes in circulating proteins involved in angiogenesis [69–76]. These proteins include vascular endothelial growth factor (VEGF), placental growth factor (PlGF), soluble fms-like tyrosine kinase-1 receptors (sFlt-1 also referred to as sVEGFR-1), and soluble Endoglin. One potential mechanism for the development of ischemic placental disease is inadequate or aberrant production of factors responsible for angiogenesis at the maternal-fetal interface (Fig. 3). This aberration can lead to reduced vascular development and/or fetal-placental hypoxia. Although many proteins with angiogenic factors have previously been described, VEGF, PlGF, sFlt-1, and Endoglin are best studied at the maternal-fetal interface and have already been studied extensively for some subtypes of ischemic placental disease, notably preeclampsia [70,74,77–79] and, to a lesser extent, for IUGR and placental abruption [75].

VEGF is produced by trophoblasts, placental macrophages, and decidua under the influence of macrophage colony-stimulating factor (M-CSF) and tissue hypoxia [80]. It regulates branching types of angiogenesis and also stimulates the growth and proliferation of stem villi [81]. As pregnancy advances and the vasculature becomes established, VEGF gene expression in the placenta decreases [82]. In placentas isolated from women with preeclampsia, there was evidence of decreased production of VEGF (mRNA). Although some studies have reported decreased production of this growth factor in maternal circulation [83–86], others have reported that maternal concentrations of VEGF may be increased [87–89]. Increased production of VEGF is associated with vascular resistance and may reflect a compensatory mechanism [90,91].

PlGF is a growth factor that induces nonbranching angiogenesis and stimulates the development of the trunks of the vascular trees during pregnancy. Unlike VEGF, PlGF is negatively regulated by hypoxia [80,92] and maternal levels dramatically augmented by increased placental perfusion [93]. Decreased levels of this factor have been associated with IUGR,

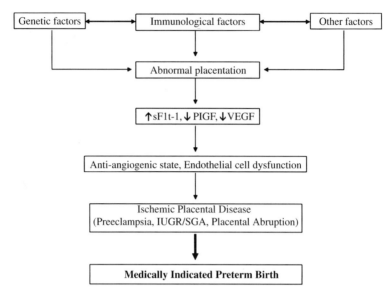

Fig. 3. The role of angiogenic factors in the pathogenesis of ischemic placental disease and medically indicated preterm birth. (*Adapted from* Karumanchi SA, Bdolah Y. Hypoxia and sFlt-1 in preeclampsia: the "chicken-and-egg" question. Endocrinology 2004;145(11):4835–7; with permission).

preeclampsia [86], and preeclampsia accompanied with IUGR [83,94]. However, some studies have reported increased production of PlGF in IUGR [92].

The sFlt-1 protein acts by adhering to the receptor-binding domains of VEGF and PlGF, preventing their ability to interact with endothelial receptors on the cell surface, and thereby inducing endothelial cell dysfunction [70,74]. sFlt-1 was significantly elevated in the plasma of women with preeclampsia [95] and increased levels of this factor precede the development of clinical disease [70]. Administration of adenoviral vectors expressing this molecule to pregnant rats caused the animals to develop hypertension, proteinuria, and glomerular endotheliosis [96], classic signs of preeclampsia. Therefore, decreased bioavailability of VEGF and PlGF because of inadequate production or excessive neutralization by sFlt-1 and Endoglin may be a significant cause of preeclampsia.

Disentangling the associations between these angiogenic proteins and risks of ischemic placental disease at preterm and term gestations is essential, and most previous studies have failed to accomplish this. Taken together, ischemic placental disease at preterm gestations is etiologically different from those that occur at term gestations, and this observation is supported by epidemiologic studies, placental histologic data, and Doppler velocimetry findings.

Recurrence of ischemic placental disease

The last piece of evidence in support of our previous hypothesis [16,28] that preeclampsia, IUGR, and placental abruption have a common pathophysiologic mechanism, ie, ischemic placental disease, is provided by the data on recurrence of ischemic placental disease [97]. We recently reported that if women developed preeclampsia in the first pregnancy, then they were at increased risk of not only a recurrent preeclampsia in the subsequent

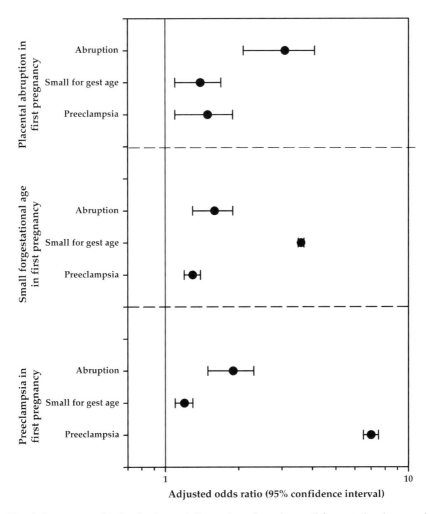

Fig. 4. Recurrence of ischemic placental disease (preeclampsia, small for gestational age, and placental abruption) between the first and second pregnancies. (*From* Ananth CV, Peltier MR, Chavez MR, et al. Recurrence of ischemic placental disease. Obstet Gynecol 2007;110:128–33; with permission).

pregnancy, but also at increased risk of developing placental abruption or delivering a small for gestational age birth in the second pregnancy. This finding also persisted for situations when women delivered a small for gestational age infant or developed placental abruption in the first pregnancy to be at increased risk of any of the three conditions of ischemic placental disease (Fig. 4). These findings also partially supported in other studies that showed increased risk for placental abruption in the second pregnancy among women with a prior small for gestational age birth or preeclampsia [51].

Summary

The recent temporal increase in medically indicated births at preterm gestational ages is accompanied by a concurrent substantial and impressive decline in perinatal mortality rates. Preeclampsia, fetal growth restriction, and placental abruption—conditions that constitute ischemic placental disease—are implicated in more than *one of every two medically indicated preterm births*, one of four spontaneous preterm births, and one of five births at term [28]. Ischemic placental disease at preterm gestations is etiologically different from those that occur at term gestations. This observation is further supported by epidemiologic studies, placental histologic findings, and Doppler velocimetry of the umbilical artery.

Most research to date on preterm births has focused on spontaneous preterm birth, and consequently clinical and community-based interventions to reduce the preterm birth rate have been largely unsuccessful. The heterogeneity in indicated preterm birth may not be as high as once thought, and targeted interventions designed to prevent medically indicated preterm births following preeclampsia, IUGR, and placental abruption may help reduce the overall preterm birth rate and costs associated with it. The decline in perinatal mortality following indicated preterm births may have inadvertently increased the burden of newborn morbidity and long-term neurodevelopmental and cognitive impairments. Other mechanisms that underlie medically indicated preterm births, including the role of infection and inflammation [98–101] and genetic underpinning [102–104], need to be carefully examined. Comprehensive evaluation risk factors, with careful consideration of heterogeneity in the syndrome of medically indicated preterm birth and ischemic placental disease will provide important clues to predict and subsequently prevent preterm birth and associated adverse outcomes.

Acknowledgments

The authors thank Morgan R. Peltier, PhD, for comments on an earlier version of the manuscript that helped improve the manuscript.

References

[1] Martin JA, Hamilton BE, Menacker F, et al. Preliminary births for 2004: infant and maternal health. Health e-stats Released November 15, 205 2005. Available at: http://www.cdc.gov/nchs/products/pubs/hestats/prelimbirths04/prelimbirths04health.htm. Accessed May 9, 2006.

[2] Berkowitz GS, Blackmore-Prince C, Lapinski RH, et al. Risk factors for preterm birth subtypes. Epidemiology 1998;9(3):279–85.

[3] Berkowitz GS, Papiernik E. Epidemiology of preterm birth. Epidemiol Rev 1993;15(2):414–43.

[4] Kramer MS, Demissie K, Yang H, et al. The contribution of mild and moderate preterm birth to infant mortality. Fetal and Infant Health Study Group of the Canadian Perinatal Surveillance System. JAMA 2000;284(7):843–9.

[5] Buekens P, Klebanoff M. Preterm birth research: from disillusion to the search for new mechanisms. Paediatr Perinat Epidemiol 2001;15(Suppl 2):159–61.

[6] Slattery MM, Morrison JJ. Preterm delivery. Lancet 2002;360(9344):1489–97.

[7] Goldenberg RL, Jobe AH. Prospects for research in reproductive health and birth outcomes. JAMA 2001;285(5):633–9.

[8] Ananth CV, Joseph KS, Kinzler WL. The influence of obstetric intervention on trends in twin stillbirths: United States, 1989–99. J Matern Fetal Neonatal Med 2004;15(6):380–7.

[9] Ananth CV, Joseph KS, Oyelese Y, et al. Trends in preterm birth and perinatal mortality among singletons: United States, 1989 through 2000. Obstet Gynecol 2005;105(5 Pt 1):1084–91.

[10] Branum AM, Schoendorf KC. Changing patterns of low birthweight and preterm birth in the United States, 1981–98. Paediatr Perinat Epidemiol 2002;16(1):8–15.

[11] Demissie K, Rhoads GG, Ananth CV, et al. Trends in preterm birth and neonatal mortality among blacks and whites in the United States from 1989 to 1997. Am J Epidemiol 2001;154(4):307–15.

[12] Joseph KS, Kramer MS, Marcoux S, et al. Determinants of preterm birth rates in Canada from 1981 through 1983 and from 1992 through 1994. N Engl J Med 1998;339(20):1434–9.

[13] Kramer MS, Platt R, Yang H, et al. Secular trends in preterm birth: a hospital-based cohort study. JAMA 1998;280(21):1849–54.

[14] Roberts CL, Algert CS, Raynes-Greenow C, et al. Delivery of singleton preterm infants in New South Wales, 1990–1997. Aust N Z J Obstet Gynaecol 2003;43(1):32–7.

[15] Wisborg K, Henriksen TB, Hedegaard M, et al. Smoking during pregnancy and preterm birth. Br J Obstet Gynaecol 1996;103(8):800–5.

[16] Ananth CV, Vintzileos AM. Epidemiology of preterm birth and its clinical subtypes. J Matern Fetal Neonatal Med 2006;19(12):773–82.

[17] Goldenberg RL, Rouse DJ. Prevention of premature birth. N Engl J Med 1998;339(5):313–20.

[18] Holzman C, Paneth N. Preterm birth: from prediction to prevention. Am J Public Health 1998;88(2):183–4.

[19] Meis PJ, Michielutte R, Peters TJ, et al. Factors associated with preterm birth in Cardiff, Wales. II. Indicated and spontaneous preterm birth. Am J Obstet Gynecol 1995;173(2):597–602.

[20] Pickett KE, Abrams B, Selvin S. Defining preterm delivery—the epidemiology of clinical presentation. Paediatr Perinat Epidemiol 2000;14(4):305–8.

[21] Savitz DA, Blackmore CA, Thorp JM. Epidemiologic characteristics of preterm delivery: etiologic heterogeneity. Am J Obstet Gynecol 1991;164(2):467–71.

[22] Savitz DA, Dole N, Herring AH, et al. Should spontaneous and medically indicated preterm births be separated for studying aetiology? Paediatr Perinat Epidemiol 2005;19(2):97–105.

[23] Zhang J, Savitz DA. Preterm birth subtypes among blacks and whites. Epidemiology 1992; 3(5):428–33.

[24] Ananth CV, Joseph KS, Demissie K, et al. Trends in twin preterm birth subtypes in the United States, 1989 through 2000: impact on perinatal mortality. Am J Obstet Gynecol 2005;193(3 Pt 2):1076–82.

[25] Kistka ZA, Palomar L, Lee KA, et al. Racial disparity in the frequency of recurrence of preterm birth. Am J Obstet Gynecol 2007;196(2):131 e1–6.

[26] Kramer MS, Goulet L, Lydon J, et al. Socio-economic disparities in preterm birth: causal pathways and mechanisms. Paediatr Perinat Epidemiol 2001;15(Suppl 2):104–23.

[27] Schieve LA, Handler A. Preterm delivery and perinatal death among black and white infants in a Chicago-area perinatal registry. Obstet Gynecol 1996;88(3):356–63.

[28] Ananth CV, Vintzileos AM. Maternal-fetal conditions necessitating a medical intervention resulting in preterm birth. Am J Obstet Gynecol 2006;195(6):1557–63.

[29] Ananth CV, Getahun D, Peltier MR, et al. Recurrence of spontaneous versus medically indicated preterm birth. Am J Obstet Gynecol 2006;195(3):643–50.

[30] Bakewell JM, Stockbauer JW, Schramm WF. Factors associated with repetition of low birthweight: Missouri longitudinal study. Paediatr Perinat Epidemiol 1997;11(Suppl 1):119–29.

[31] Bloom SL, Yost NP, McIntire DD, et al. Recurrence of preterm birth in singleton and twin pregnancies. Obstet Gynecol 2001;98(3):379–85.

[32] Carr-Hill RA, Hall MH. The repetition of spontaneous preterm labour. Br J Obstet Gynaecol 1985;92(9):921–8.

[33] Cnattingius S, Granath F, Petersson G, et al. The influence of gestational age and smoking habits on the risk of subsequent preterm deliveries. N Engl J Med 1999;341(13):943–8.

[34] Mazaki-Tovi S, Romero R, Kusanovic JP, et al. Recurrent preterm birth. Semin Perinatol 2007;31(3):142–58.

[35] Adams MM, Elam-Evans LD, Wilson HG, et al. Rates of and factors associated with recurrence of preterm delivery. JAMA 2000;283(12):1591–6.

[36] Melve KK, Skjaerven R, Gjessing HK, et al. Recurrence of gestational age in sibships: implications for perinatal mortality. Am J Epidemiol 1999;150(7):756–62.

[37] Mercer BM, Goldenberg RL, Moawad AH, et al. The preterm prediction study: effect of gestational age and cause of preterm birth on subsequent obstetric outcome. National Institute of Child Health and Human Development Maternal-Fetal Medicine Units Network. Am J Obstet Gynecol 1999;181(5 Pt 1):1216–21.

[38] Meis PJ, Goldenberg RL, Mercer BM, et al. The preterm prediction study: risk factors for indicated preterm births. Maternal-Fetal Medicine Units Network of the National Institute of Child Health and Human Development. Am J Obstet Gynecol 1998;178(3):562–7.

[39] Joseph KS. Theory of obstetrics: an epidemiologic framework for justifying medically indicated early delivery. BMC Pregnancy Childbirth 2007;7(1):4.

[40] Joseph KS, Huang L, Liu S, et al. Reconciling the high rates of preterm and postterm birth in the United States. Obstet Gynecol 2007;109(4):813–22.

[41] Joseph KS, Demissie K, Kramer MS. Obstetric intervention, stillbirth, and preterm birth. Semin Perinatol 2002;26(4):250–9.

[42] Papiernik E, Zeitlin J, Rivera L, et al. Preterm birth in a French population: the importance of births by medical decision. BJOG 2003;110(4):430–2.

[43] Breart G, Blondel B, Tuppin P, et al. Did preterm deliveries continue to decrease in France in the 1980s? Paediatr Perinat Epidemiol 1995;9(3):296–306.

[44] Foix-L'Helias L, Blondel B. Changes in risk factors of preterm delivery in France between 1981 and 1995. Paediatr Perinat Epidemiol 2000;14(4):314–23.

[45] Olsen P, Laara E, Rantakallio P, et al. Epidemiology of preterm delivery in two birth cohorts with an interval of 20 years. Am J Epidemiol 1995;142(11):1184–93.

[46] Blondel B, Kogan MD, Alexander GR, et al. The impact of the increasing number of multiple births on the rates of preterm birth and low birthweight: an international study. Am J Public Health 2002;92(8):1323–30.

[47] Villar J, Abalos E, Carroli G, et al. Heterogeneity of perinatal outcomes in the preterm delivery syndrome. Obstet Gynecol 2004;104(1):78–87.

[48] Moutquin JM. Classification and heterogeneity of preterm birth. Br J Obstet Gynaecol 2003;110(Suppl 20):30–3.

[49] Naeye RL. Pregnancy hypertension, placental evidences of low uteroplacental blood flow, and spontaneous premature delivery. Hum Pathol 1989;20(5):441–4.

[50] Ananth CV, Oyelese Y, Prasad V, et al. Evidence of placental abruption as a chronic process: associations with vaginal bleeding early in pregnancy and placental lesions. Eur J Obstet Gynecol Reprod Biol 2006;128(1–2):15–21.

[51] Rasmussen S, Irgens LM, Dalaker K. A history of placental dysfunction and risk of placental abruption. Paediatr Perinat Epidemiol 1999;13(1):9–21.

[52] Aardema MW, Saro MC, Lander M, et al. Second trimester Doppler ultrasound screening of the uterine arteries differentiates between subsequent normal and poor outcomes of hypertensive pregnancy: two different pathophysiological entities? Clin Sci (Lond) 2004; 106(4):377–82.

[53] Audibert F, Benchimol Y, Benattar C, et al. Prediction of preeclampsia or intrauterine growth restriction by second trimester serum screening and uterine Doppler velocimetry. Fetal Diagn Ther 2005;20(1):48–53.

[54] Crispi F, Dominguez C, Llurba E, et al. Placental angiogenic growth factors and uterine artery Doppler findings for characterization of different subsets in preeclampsia and in isolated intrauterine growth restriction. Am J Obstet Gynecol 2006;195(1):201–7.

[55] Egbor M, Ansari T, Morris N, et al. Morphometric placental villous and vascular abnormalities in early- and late-onset pre-eclampsia with and without fetal growth restriction. BJOG 2006;113(5):580–9.

[56] Egbor M, Ansari T, Morris N, et al. Pre-eclampsia and fetal growth restriction: how morphometrically different is the placenta? Placenta 2006;27(6–7):727–34.

[57] El-Hamedi A, Shillito J, Simpson NA, et al. A prospective analysis of the role of uterine artery Doppler waveform notching in the assessment of at-risk pregnancies. Hypertens Pregnancy 2005;24(2):137–45.

[58] Lau WL, Lam HS, Leung WC. Reversed diastolic flow in the uterine artery—a new Doppler finding related to placental insufficiency? Ultrasound Obstet Gynecol 2007;29(2):232–5.

[59] Mayhew TM, Manwani R, Ohadike C, et al. The placenta in pre-eclampsia and intrauterine growth restriction: studies on exchange surface areas, diffusion distances and villous membrane diffusive conductances. Placenta 2007;28(2–3):233–8.

[60] Norwitz ER. Defective implantation and placentation: laying the blueprint for pregnancy complications. Reprod Biomed Online 2006;13(4):591–9.

[61] Papageorghiou AT, Yu CK, Cicero S, et al. Second-trimester uterine artery Doppler screening in unselected populations: a review. J Matern Fetal Neonatal Med 2002;12(2):78–88.

[62] Phupong V, Dejthevaporn T, Tanawattanacharoen S, et al. Predicting the risk of preeclampsia and small for gestational age infants by uterine artery Doppler in low-risk women. Arch Gynecol Obstet 2003;268(3):158–61.

[63] Pilalis A, Souka AP, Antsaklis P, et al. Screening for pre-eclampsia and fetal growth restriction by uterine artery Doppler and PAPP-A at 11-14 weeks' gestation. Ultrasound Obstet Gynecol 2007;29(2):135–40.

[64] Schiessl B, Kainer F, Oberhoffer R, et al. Doppler sonography of the uterine and the cubital arteries in normal pregnancies, preeclampsia and intrauterine growth restriction: evidence for a systemic vessel involvement. J Perinat Med 2006;34(2):139–44.

[65] Stepan H, Kramer T, Faber R. Maternal plasma concentrations of soluble endoglin in pregnancies with intrauterine growth restriction. J Clin Endocrinol Metab 2007;92(7): 2831–4.

[66] Stepan H, Unversucht A, Wessel N, et al. Predictive value of maternal angiogenic factors in second trimester pregnancies with abnormal uterine perfusion. Hypertension 2007;49(4): 818–24.

[67] Papageorghiou AT, Yu CK, Nicolaides KH. The role of uterine artery Doppler in predicting adverse pregnancy outcome. Best Pract Res Clin Obstet Gynaecol 2004;18(3): 383–96.

[68] Espinoza J, Romero R, Nien JK, et al. Identification of patients at risk for early onset and/or severe preeclampsia with the use of uterine artery Doppler velocimetry and placental growth factor. Am J Obstet Gynecol 2007;196(4):326. e1–13.

[69] Levine RJ, Lam C, Qian C, et al. Soluble endoglin and other circulating antiangiogenic factors in preeclampsia. N Engl J Med 2006;355(10):992–1005.

[70] Levine RJ, Maynard SE, Qian C, et al. Circulating angiogenic factors and the risk of preeclampsia. N Engl J Med 2004;350(7):672–83.

[71] Lockwood CJ, Toti P, Arcuri F, et al. Thrombin regulates soluble fms-like tyrosine kinase-1 (sFlt-1) expression in first trimester decidua: implications for preeclampsia. Am J Pathol 2007;170(4):1398–405.

[72] Papazoglou D, Galazios G, Koukourakis MI, et al. Vascular endothelial growth factor gene polymorphisms and pre-eclampsia. Mol Hum Reprod 2004;10(5):321–4.

[73] Powers RW, Roberts JM, Cooper KM, et al. Maternal serum soluble fms-like tyrosine kinase 1 concentrations are not increased in early pregnancy and decrease more slowly postpartum in women who develop preeclampsia. Am J Obstet Gynecol 2005;193(1): 185–91.

[74] Shibata E, Rajakumar A, Powers RW, et al. Soluble fms-like tyrosine kinase 1 is increased in preeclampsia but not in normotensive pregnancies with small-for-gestational-age neonates: relationship to circulating placental growth factor. J Clin Endocrinol Metab 2005; 90(8):4895–903.

[75] Signore C, Mills JL, Qian C, et al. Circulating angiogenic factors and placental abruption. Obstet Gynecol 2006;108(2):338–44.

[76] Karumanchi SA, Bdolah Y. Hypoxia and sFlt-1 in preeclampsia: the "chicken-and-egg" question. Endocrinology 2004;145(11):4835–7.

[77] Levine RJ, Karumanchi SA. Circulating angiogenic factors in preeclampsia. Clin Obstet Gynecol 2005;48(2):372–86.

[78] Rana S, Karumanchi SA, Levine RJ, et al. Sequential changes in antiangiogenic factors in early pregnancy and risk of developing preeclampsia. Hypertension 2007;50(1):137–42.

[79] Tjoa ML, Levine RJ, Karumanchi SA. Angiogenic factors and preeclampsia. Front Biosci 2007;12:2395–402.

[80] Lash GE, Taylor CM, Trew AJ, et al. Vascular endothelial growth factor and placental growth factor release in cultured trophoblast cells under different oxygen tensions. Growth Factors 2002;20(4):189–96.

[81] Kingdom JC, Kaufmann P. Oxygen and placental vascular development. Adv Exp Med Biol 1999;474:259–75.

[82] Cooper JC, Sharkey AM, Charnock-Jones DS, et al. VEGF mRNA levels in placentae from pregnancies complicated by pre-eclampsia. Br J Obstet Gynaecol 1996;103(12):1191–6.

[83] Reuvekamp A, Velsing-Aarts FV, Poulina IE, et al. Selective deficit of angiogenic growth factors characterises pregnancies complicated by pre-eclampsia. Br J Obstet Gynaecol 1999;106(10):1019–22.

[84] Lyall F, Greer IA, Boswell F, et al. Suppression of serum vascular endothelial growth factor immunoreactivity in normal pregnancy and in pre-eclampsia. Br J Obstet Gynaecol 1997; 104(2):223–8.

[85] Hunter A, Aitkenhead M, Caldwell C, et al. Serum levels of vascular endothelial growth factor in preeclamptic and normotensive pregnancy. Hypertension 2000;36(6):965–9.

[86] Polliotti BM, Fry AG, Saller DN, et al. Second-trimester maternal serum placental growth factor and vascular endothelial growth factor for predicting severe, early-onset preeclampsia. Obstet Gynecol 2003;101(6):1266–74.

[87] Kuperminc MJ, Daniel Y, Englender T, et al. Vascular endothelial growth factor is increased in patients with preeclampsia. Am J Reprod Immunol 1997;38(4):302–6.

[88] Sharkey AM, Cooper JC, Balmforth JR, et al. Maternal plasma levels of vascular endothelial growth factor in normotensive pregnancies and in pregnancies complicated by preeclampsia. Eur J Clin Invest 1996;26(12):1182–5.

[89] Levin ED, Torry D. Acute and chronic nicotine effects on working memory in aged rats. Psychopharmacology (Berl) 1996;123(1):88–97.

[90] Simmons LA, Hennessy A, Gillin AG, et al. Uteroplacental blood flow and placental vascular endothelial growth factor in normotensive and pre-eclamptic pregnancy. Bjog 2000; 107(5):678–85.

[91] Bosio PM, Wheeler T, Anthony F, et al. Maternal plasma vascular endothelial growth factor concentrations in normal and hypertensive pregnancies and their relationship to peripheral vascular resistance. Am J Obstet Gynecol 2001;184(2):146–52.

[92] Khaliq A, Dunk C, Jiang J, et al. Hypoxia down-regulates placenta growth factor, whereas fetal growth restriction up-regulates placenta growth factor expression: molecular evidence for "placental hyperoxia" in intrauterine growth restriction. Lab Invest 1999;79(2):151–70.

[93] Welch PC, Amankwah KS, Miller P, et al. Correlations of placental perfusion and PlGF protein expression in early human pregnancy. Am J Obstet Gynecol 2006;194(6):1625–9 [discussion: 1629–31].

[94] Taylor RN, Grimwood J, Taylor RS, et al. Longitudinal serum concentrations of placental growth factor: evidence for abnormal placental angiogenesis in pathologic pregnancies. Am J Obstet Gynecol 2003;188(1):177–82.

[95] Koga K, Osuga Y, Yoshino O, et al. Elevated serum soluble vascular endothelial growth factor receptor 1 (sVEGFR-1) levels in women with preeclampsia. J Clin Endocrinol Metab 2003;88(5):2348–51.

[96] Maynard SE, Min JY, Merchan J, et al. Excess placental soluble fms-like tyrosine kinase 1 (sFlt1) may contribute to endothelial dysfunction, hypertension, and proteinuria in preeclampsia. J Clin Invest 2003;111(5):649–58.

[97] Ananth CV, Peltier MR, Chavez MR, et al. Recurrence of ischemic placental disease. Obstet Gynecol 2007;110(1):128–33.

[98] Peltier MR. Immunology of term and preterm labor. Reprod Biol Endocrinol 2003;1:122.

[99] Goldenberg RL, Hauth JC, Andrews WW. Intrauterine infection and preterm delivery. N Engl J Med 2000;342(20):1500–7.

[100] Romero R, Erez O, Espinoza J. Intrauterine infection, preterm labor, and cytokines. J Soc Gynecol Investig 2005;12(7):463–5.

[101] Romero R, Espinoza J, Goncalves LF, et al. The role of inflammation and infection in preterm birth. Semin Reprod Med 2007;25(1):21–39.

[102] Adams KM, Eschenbach DA. The genetic contribution towards preterm delivery. Semin Fetal Neonatal Med 2004;9(6):445–52.

[103] Hao K, Wang X, Niu T, et al. A candidate gene association study on preterm delivery: application of high-throughput genotyping technology and advanced statistical methods. Hum Mol Genet 2004;13(7):683–91.

[104] Romero R, Kuivaniemi H, Tromp G. Functional genomics and proteomics in term and preterm parturition. J Clin Endocrinol Metab 2002;87(6):2431–4.

CLINICS IN
PERINATOLOGY

Clin Perinatol 35 (2008) 69–83

Head Trauma After Instrumental Births

Stergios K. Doumouchtsis, MD, PhD, MRCOG*,
Sabaratnam Arulkumaran, MD, PhD, FRCOG

*Department of Obstetrics and Gynaecology, St. George's
University of London, Cranmer Terrace, London SW17 0RE, UK*

Instrumental delivery may be performed for fetal or maternal indications. The most common indication is a prolonged second stage of labor when it is caused by malposition of the fetal head, and fetal distress or presumed fetal compromise, where any delay may result in hypoxic brain damage or fetal death if no intervention is undertaken. Maternal indications include severe heart disease or cerebral vascular malformations [1]. The rate of instrumental vaginal delivery in different countries varies between 10% and 15% [1–6]. Over the past two decades, in the United Kingdom, the use of forceps has decreased by 50% in favor of vacuum extraction or caesarean section [7].

Types of head trauma

Extracranial trauma

Scalp bruises and lacerations
Infants delivered by vacuum extraction may sustain minor scalp injuries. Most of them are of no clinical significance. Bruising and vacuum marks resolve quickly without sequelae [8]. Most of the scalp abrasions and lacerations are superficial and minor in degree [9]. Scalp and face injuries occur on average in 16% of vacuum deliveries and 17% of forceps deliveries [10]. Alopecia due to vacuum-associated scalp trauma has been reported [11]. The incidence of scalp abrasions is higher in infants delivered by Omnicup vacuum (Clinical Innovations Inc, Murray, Utah) or metal cup devices compared with those delivered by silastic cup [12]. Bruising and lacerations are more frequent in vacuum deliveries by metal cup, but there is no difference between deliveries by Omnicup and the standard silastic cup [13].

---

* Corresponding author.
E-mail address: sdoum@yahoo.com (S.K. Doumouchtsis).

0095-5108/08/$ - see front matter © 2008 Elsevier Inc. All rights reserved.
doi:10.1016/j.clp.2007.11.006
perinatology.theclinics.com

Facial nerve palsy

Forceps are associated with facial nerve injury due to pressure on the sty-lomastoid foramen or compression of the bone overlying the vertical segment of the facial canal. However, 33% of facial nerve injuries occur in spontane-ous delivery, probably due to compression against the maternal sacral prom-ontory [14]. The injury is rare with an incidence rate of 2.9 to 5 per 1000 forceps deliveries. The prognosis is good with recovery within 2 weeks [15].

Caput succedaneum

Caput succedaneum is a serosanguinous, extraperiosteal collection which extends across the midline and over suture lines. It is caused by mechanical compression of the presenting part of the fetal head pushing through a dilat-ing cervix [16].

Chignon

During application of the vacuum cup on the fetal head a collection of interstitial fluid and micro-hemorrhages, or chignon, fill the internal diame-ter of the vacuum cup in a key-in-lock fashion [9]. This is created by the pressure gradient between the vacuum and the mean arterial pressure of the fetus and is less pronounced when using soft cups. The chignon is most pronounced immediately after the removal of the cup, but typically re-solves within 12 to 18 hours. [9]. No treatment is required.

Cephalhematoma

Cephalhematoma is a subperiosteal collection secondary to rupture of the bridging blood vessels between the skull and the periosteum. It is delineated by the suture lines and thus can be differentiated from subgaleal hemor-rhage. Because a limited volume can accumulate in the subperiosteal space, these hematomas are limited in size, and anemia and hypotension are rare sequelae.

Cephalhematoma occurs in 1% to 2% of spontaneous vaginal deliveries, in 6% to 10% of vacuum extractions (range 1%–26%) [8,10,17,18] and in 4% of forceps deliveries [10]. Vacuum extraction has therefore a stronger as-sociation with cephalhematoma compared with forceps (odds ratio [OR] 2.38) [10]. Metal cups are more likely to cause cephalhematoma than silastic cups or the Omnicup [13]. Vacuum extractions at mid- or low station are as-sociated with a higher incidence of cephalhematoma (13.11% and 13.56%) when compared with vacuum applied at the outlet (6.81%; relative risk [RR] 1.92, 1.99) [17]. Following a failed vacuum delivery there is no difference in the incidence of cephalhematoma between a sequential instrumental vaginal delivery and caesarean section [19].

Uncomplicated cephalhematomas usually resolve within a few weeks and do not require treatment [20]. Underlying skull fractures may also be pres-ent. Suspected depressed skull fractures and neurologic symptoms should be investigated by a skull radiograph and cranial CT. Infection is a rare complication which may lead to meningitis or osteomyelitis and can be diagnosed by aspiration [21].

Subgaleal hemorrhage

Subgaleal hemorrhage develops by an accumulation of blood in the subaponeurotic space between the periosteum of the skull and the galea aponeurotica. The galea aponeurotica covers the vault of the cranium and is attached to the overlying skin and the subcutaneous tissues [22]. Beneath the galea aponeurotica, the loose subaponeurotic layer contains large emissary veins which connect the dural sinuses and the scalp veins. This space extends to the orbital margins anteriorly, the nuchal ridge posteriorly, and the temporal fascia laterally, and has a capacity of up to 260 mL in term infants [23].

The traction force applied during instrumental delivery pulls the aponeurosis from the cranium, thus avulsing the subgaleal space and causing hemorrhage. The pathogenesis also includes skull fracture or rupture of an interosseous synchondrosis. Subgaleal hemorrhage with a loss of 20% to 40% of the circulating blood volume will result in hypovolemic shock [22,23], disseminated intravascular coagulation, multiorgan failure and neonatal death in up to 25% of cases [22,24,25].

Vacuum extraction (OR 7.17; 95% CI: 5.43–10.25) and forceps delivery (OR 2.66; 95% CI: 1.78–5.18) are risk factors associated with subgaleal hemorrhage [25]. The reported incidence rate after spontaneous vaginal deliveries is 4 per 10,000 [22] and ranges between 0% and 21% following vacuum extractions [17,22,26]. Maternal nulliparity, placement of vacuum extraction cup over the sagittal suture close to the infant's anterior fontanel, and failed vacuum extraction predispose infants to subgaleal hemorrhage [26]. Other risk factors include prolonged second stage of labor, fetal distress, and macrosomia [24,25]. The potential role of a coagulopathy is controversial, as it is not clear whether the hemostatic disturbance is the cause or the effect of the bleeding [22]. There is no difference between rigid and soft vacuum extractor cups in the incidence of subgaleal hemorrhage [8].

Management consists of blood and blood-products transfusion. In severe cases, surgery may be required to cauterize the bleeding vessels. Depending on the severity of subgaleal hemorrhage, the mortality can be as high as 25% [27]. A decrease in hematocrit that is greater than 25% of the baseline value at birth and an associated significant birth asphyxia are the most important risk factors for mortality [28].

Cranial trauma

The incidence rate of skull fractures after vacuum extractions is higher in newborns from nulliparous (6.58%) than multiparous mothers (2.35%; RR 2.79). Among the latter, older age (>35 years) is associated with an incidence rate of 7.94%, compared with no fracture among younger multiparous women (<35 years) [17]. Skull fractures are usually linear, affecting the parietal bones, or depressed, forming the so-called "ping-pong ball-type" fracture [14,20]. A skull fracture must be suspected in any cephalhematoma or subarachnoid hemorrhage [14]. In a study of neonatal complications following vacuum extractions, cephalhematoma was associated with a higher incidence of skull fracture (10.10%; RR 2.05) [17]. Nevertheless, the authors of this study found a higher incidence of skull fracture (5.04% compared with 0%–0.5%) than generally estimated [29,30] and attributed this finding to the systematic radiologic screening during the postpartum period [17]. O'Mahony and colleagues [31] reviewed a national UK database to ascertain the causes of intrapartum-related fetal and neonatal deaths and found that cranial and intracranial injury was almost always associated with physical difficulty at delivery and instrumentation. Moreover, in 24 of 37 cases, at least two separate attempts with a different instrument were made. Skull fractures are caused by compression from forceps blades or by compression of the skull against the maternal bony pelvis.

Linear fractures are usually of no clinical significance and require no specific treatment. The management of depressed fractures remains controversial [32,33]. Nonsurgical techniques, such as digital pressure, a breast pump, and an obstetric vacuum extractor, have been used [34]. Neurosurgical management is indicated when there are bone fragments in the cerebrum, neurologic deficits, signs of intracranial injury, or signs of cerebrospinal fluid beneath the galea, and in cases of failed closed manipulation [20].

Intracranial trauma

Intracranial hemorrhage

Intracranial hemorrhage may occur in the subdural, subarachnoid, intraparenchymal, and intraventricular spaces [17]. It occurs in approximately 5 to 6 live births per 10,000 and can be potentially fatal or cause lifelong disability. Forceps and vacuum delivery, precipitous delivery, prolonged second stage of labor, and macrosomia are recognized risk factors [35,36]. Following vacuum extraction the incidence of intracranial hemorrhage is 0.87% [17]. Simonson and colleagues observed more intracranial hemorrhages than generally reported (0.87% compared with 0.11%–0.34%) [29,37–40]. It remains unclear whether this is due to the use of transfontanellar ultrasonography and skull radiography used in this study [17].

Other causes of intracranial hemorrhage may include birth asphyxia, prematurity, hemorrhagic diathesis, infection, and vascular abnormalities [17]. The higher rates of intracranial hemorrhage among infants delivered by instrumental or cesarean delivery during labor than among infants delivered by uncomplicated vaginal delivery or elective cesarean delivery suggest that abnormal labor rather than the mode of delivery may be the major risk factor of intracranial hemorrhage [38]. Towner and colleagues [38] showed that the rate of subdural or cerebral hemorrhage did not differ significantly between forceps delivery and vacuum extraction. Wen and colleagues [39] on the other hand, found a higher incidence of subarachnoid hemorrhages after vacuum extractions (0.06%) than after forceps application (0.01%) or after spontaneous vaginal deliveries (0.01%). Jhawar and colleagues [41] found that among full term infants forceps delivery was six times more likely to be complicated by subarachnoid or subdural hemorrhage than spontaneous vaginal delivery.

These differences may reflect a number of confounders among observational studies [38–40,42]. Nevertheless, the incidence of intracranial hemorrhage is consistently increased for forceps and vacuum-assisted deliveries [15]. Cesarean section after a failed attempt of operative vaginal delivery and the sequential use of vacuum and forceps are additional risk factors [38,40,42].

The types of intracranial hemorrhage associated with instrumental deliveries are subdural and subarachnoid hemorrhages rather than intraventricular [38,39,41].

Epidural hemorrhage

Epidural hemorrhage is a blood collection between a calvarial bone and its inner periosteum or between the periosteal membrane and the underlying outer dura fibrous stratum [16]. It is associated with difficult parturition and instrumental delivery in nulliparous women, and breech delivery [43]. It typically results from the mechanical forces exerted on the fetal head during birth, with or without instrumental interference [44]. During labor, overriding of the vault's bones (moulding) can occur. An increased degree of moulding leading to excessive displacement of the skull bones may cause considerable injury to the dura matter [45]. Epidural hemorrhage is usually a result of injury to the middle meningeal artery, and is frequently associated with a cephalhematoma or skull fracture [43]. In neonates, the meningeal arteries are not embedded in the cranial bones and therefore less susceptible to injury [20]. This probably explains the rarity of epidural hemorrhage in neonates, which accounts for approximately 2% of all cases of intracranial hemorrhage [46].

The association between epidural hemorrhage and cephalhematoma is a consequence of a communication of two distinctive hematomas, bleeding from one area to another through a skull fracture or intracranial extension of an underlying cephalhematoma [44].

Epidural hemorrhage may present with diffuse neurologic symptoms, increased intracranial pressure, and bulging fontanel or localized symptoms, such as lateralizing seizures and eye deviation [20]. Diagnosis is established by cranial CT. Large hemorrhages require surgical decompression and ligation of bleeding points. Smaller, epidural hematomas in a stable infant may resolve without surgery [43].

Subdural hemorrhage

Subdural hemorrhage can be supratentorial or infratentorial. Pollina and colleagues [35] found that 73% of cranial birth injuries in term neonates were subdural hemorrhages. In this study, the number of vacuum and forceps deliveries was significantly higher in the group of neonates who had cranial injuries compared with a group of neonates who did not.

The incidence rate of subdural or cerebral hemorrhage, per 10,000 in each case, is 2.9 after spontaneous delivery, 4.1 after caesarean section without labor, 8.0 after vacuum delivery, 9.8 after forceps delivery, 25.7 after casarean section following failed instrumental vaginal delivery, and 21.3 after combined vacuum and forceps delivery [38].

Subdural hematomas have been diagnosed antenatally in utero [47,48] and in asymptomatic newborns after uncomplicated vaginal deliveries [49–51]. Whitby and colleagues [51] examined 111 newborn infants using MRI and showed that, of the nine infants who had asymptomatic subdural hemorrhages, three were normal vaginal deliveries, five were delivered by forceps after an attempted vacuum delivery, and one had a traumatic vacuum delivery. Their findings agreed with those of earlier studies showing that subdural hemorrhage is not necessarily indicative of excessive birth trauma [52]. Subdural hematomas have also been associated with coagulation disturbances [53].

The pathophysiology of a subdural hematoma involves mechanical compression and distortion of the fetal cranium during labor, tearing of veins and venous sinuses, and bleeding into the subdural space. Another possible mechanism, called *occipital osteodiastasis*, is the separation of the squamous and lateral parts of the occipital bone, leading to rupture of the occipital sinus, direct cerebellar trauma, and brain-stem compression [54].

Subdural hemorrhages present with apnea, unequal pupils, eye deviation, irritability, tense fontanel, seizures, and coma [20,54]. Diagnosis is established by cranial CT or MRI. Treatment is usually conservative as most subdural hemorrhages are small and resolve without sequelae [51–53, 55,56], or surgical, depending on the extent of the lesion and the presence of acute hydrocephalus or signs of brainstem compression [53,55].

The long-term outcome depends on the size of the lesion and the presence of intraparenchymal lesions [20]. Perrin and colleagues [53] reviewed a series of 15 neonates who had posterior fossa subdural hemorrhages with a mean follow-up of 4.5 years. Of the 15, 7 had normal neurologic development, 3 were mildly delayed, 2 were moderately delayed, and 3 were profoundly delayed.

Subarachnoid hemorrhage

Subarachnoid hemorrhage is most frequently caused by rupture of the small bridging vessels of the leptomeninges [46]. It is the second most common intracranial hemorrhage after instrumental deliveries [38,39].

Towner and colleagues [38] showed that the incidence rate of subarachnoid hemorrhage was 1.3 per 10,000 after spontaneous vaginal delivery, 2.2 per 10,000 after vacuum extraction, 3.3 per 10,000 after forceps delivery, and 10.7 per 10,000 after combined vacuum and forceps delivery was. In contrast, Wen and colleagues [39] found an incidence rate of subarachnoid hemorrhage of 0.6 per 1,000 after vacuum extraction, 0.1 per 1,000 after forceps delivery, and 0.1 per 1,000 after spontaneous vaginal delivery. Vacuum was therefore more likely to cause subarachnoid hemorrhage compared with forceps delivery (OR 5.4; 95% CI: 1.3–23.4). However, these large retrospective studies are based on databases and lack clinical data.

Clinical manifestations include seizures, irritability, recurrent apnea, depressed level of consciousness and focal neurologic signs. The diagnosis is made by cranial CT. Investigations include lumbar puncture and examination of cerebral spinal fluid for red blood cells. No specific treatment is available, though close observation for signs of hydrocephalus is recommended [46].

Reducing fetal head trauma

Before instrumental delivery is attempted, a number of parameters should be ascertained, including fetal and maternal condition, cervical dilatation, uterine contractions, progress of labor, station, position and molding of the fetal head, adequate analgesia, and experience of the operator.

Reducing the rates of instrumental deliveries

Avoidance of unnecessary instrumental deliveries is an important measure in reducing fetal head trauma. Nonoperative interventions, such as one-to-one support, partogram use, oxytocin use, and delayed pushing in women using epidurals, will decrease the need for instrumental delivery [1].

The diagnosis of prolonged second stage of labor and resort to instrumental delivery should not be based only on time limits when there is progressive descent and the fetal heart rate is normal [4]. In cases of prolonged second stage of labor, cephalopelvic disproportion should be excluded and, unless contraindicated, oxytocin should be used before instrumental delivery [57]. Delaying directed pushing (by 1–3 hours, or less if the woman has an involuntary urge to push), compared with directed pushing at diagnosis of second stage, reduces the risk of a midpelvic or rotational instrumental birth [58]. Continuous electronic fetal monitoring increases the risks of instrumental vaginal delivery especially among women who have low-risk pregnancies [58], and should be used only when indicated.

Contraindications of instrumental vaginal delivery

Absolute contraindications include malpresentation (eg, brow, face, mento-posterior), unengaged fetal head, cephalopelvic disproportion, and fetal clotting disorder (eg, alloimmune thrombocytopenia) [4]. In cases of cephalopelvic disproportion, excessive molding of the fetal head can lead to distortion of the tentorium and falx structures and subdural hemorrhage. Significant resistance and repetitive pushing against the birth canal tissues can generate shear forces leading to scalp trauma and cephalhematomas. Vacuum traction adds a shear force that can cause tears in the subperiosteal space [15].

The most common relative contraindications are unfavourable position and attitude of fetal head, presenting part at midstation and fetal prematurity. Among premature newborns delivered by vacuum extraction, 14.29% exhibit scalp edema, 21.43% bone fracture, and 21.43% cephalhematoma [17]. The Royal College of Obstetricians and Gynecologists (RCOG) recommends avoiding the use of ventouse below 34 weeks because of the susceptibility of the preterm infant to cephalhematoma, intracranial hemorrhage, and neonatal jaundice [2].

Instrumental delivery should not be attempted with an incompletely dilated cervix. Possible exceptions include cord prolapse at 9 cm in a multiparous woman or a second twin [2] and situations where the benefits significantly outweigh the risks and there is no viable alternative [1].

When there is significant caput and molding, vaginal examination may be misleading and clinical assessment should always include abdominal palpation. Vaginal examination during instrumental delivery fails to identify the correct fetal head position in 25% [59] to 65% [60] of cases. Therefore, intrapartum translabial ultrasound may provide objective information on the fetal head station, position, and progress of labor [61]. Some authors recommend the routine performance of abdominal and translabial ultrasound scanning in the labor room [62].

Forceps may only be applied in vertex presentation, face presentation if mento-anterior, and breech presentation for the delivery of the aftercoming head. Application of a vacuum cup when the position is uncertain may result in failed vacuum and increase the risks of fetal trauma [4].

Analgesia

Epidural analgesia is associated with a longer second stage of labor and an increase in instrumental birth [58]. Moreover, high concentrations of local anesthetic to maintain regional epidural analgesia result in increased instrumental delivery rates, whereas the addition of opioids to low-concentration local anesthetics provides effective analgesia with less motor block and less instrumental birth [58]. On the other hand, the absence of adequate analgesia during instrumental delivery may lead to lower success rates because of significant pain and lack of patient cooperation, which can affect the decision of the obstetrician to continue with instrumental delivery or to use forceps after a vacuum failure [63].

Choice of instrument

Although the incidence of instrumental delivery has remained essentially unchanged, ventouse has become more popular than forceps. Over the past two decades, in the United Kingdom, the use of forceps has decreased by 50% in favor of vacuum extraction or caesarean section [7]. In the United States, the rate of vacuum delivery surpassed the rate of forceps delivery in 1992 [3,64]. In Canada, forceps delivery has decreased in the last decade from 11.2% in 1991 to 6.8% in 2001 [1].

The use of vacuum extractor is associated with a significant reduction of maternal morbidity compared with the use of forceps [65]. However, it is associated with higher failure rates (RR 1.7) [10,63], which is a concern in light of the risks of sequential instrumentation for delivery [38]. Compared with forceps, vacuum delivery is more likely to cause cephalhematoma or retinal hemorrhage, but less likely to be associated with significant maternal perineal and vaginal trauma [10].

The RCOG recommends that operators choose the instrument most appropriate to the clinical circumstances and their level of skill [2].

Appropriate use of instruments

The instruments should be checked before applications to ensure that the vacuum device is working and that the forceps blades match. Correct placement of the vacuum cup is a major determinant of the outcome. The 'flexion point' is the site on the fetal scalp over which the center of the vacuum cup should be placed to achieve a flexing median application. This point is on the sagittal suture, 3 cm anteriorly to the posterior fontanel. Application of the vacuum cup on this point promotes synclitism and flexion of the fetal head, presenting the optimal diameters of the fetal head to the maternal pelvis. The more significant vacuum associated scalp injuries are related to wrong placement of the cup, excessive or poorly directed traction, or cephalopelvic disproportion [9]. By misplacing the vacuum cup, the fetal head will present with a larger diameter, which will increase the difficulty and risk of injury [8]. Deflexing and paramedial placement of the vacuum increases the risk of subgaleal hemorrhage [26]. A registry of neonatal deaths attributable to intrapartum trauma revealed that cranial injury was almost always associated with physical difficulty at delivery, the use of instruments, and poorly judged persistence in the presence of failure to progress or signs of fetal compromise [31]. Detachment of the cup is associated with increased incidence of cranial fractures (9.58%, RR 2.11) cephalhematoma (18.56%; RR 1.86) and scalp edema (26.34%; RR 1.41) [17].

Whitlow and colleagues [66] showed that the traction force indicators of the vacuum devices are reliable and recommended that attention to the force and duration may help to reduce the incidence of cephalhematomas and subgaleal hemorrhages. It has been suggested that in vacuum extractions the traction force should not exceed 11.5 kg, the duration of the procedure should be restricted to 15 minutes and the number of pulls limited to three for the descent phase and three for the perineal phase [67]. A traction force exceeding 13.5 kg is associated with an increased risk of fetal scalp injury [67]. Higher levels of traction force and a greater number of pulls, however, may be required during the outlet phase of the vacuum delivery, as resistance is greatest at this stage. For this reason, additional time and pulls should be allowed for the perineum to stretch over the head, especially if the birth is managed without episiotomy [67]. The traction force is less when the head descends with the cup during traction compared with a situation where the head does not descend with traction. Hence, additional pulls with descent are less likely to be harmful compared with traction on a head that does not descend with three pulls.

Application of the forceps to the fetal head is extremely important for a safe procedure and a successful outcome. The exact location of the sagittal suture and posterior fontanel should be ascertained. The forceps blades should be applied gently between contractions. The blades are correctly placed when they are situated in the spaces between the fetal orbits and ears. When the blades are locked, the sagittal suture should be perpendicular to the shanks, the occiput should be 3 to 4 cm above the shanks (so that the traction line is along the flexion point to cause flexion and expose the minimal diameter) and the space between the heel of the blade and the head does not admit more than a finger's breadth (reassures synclitism). Checking these points confirms correct application. No force should be required to apply the blades. If there is resistance, the blades should be removed and reapplied. The use of protective covers over forceps reduces rates of facial abrasions and skin bruises [68]. Leslie and colleagues [69] studied the maximum traction residents could apply to forceps during simulations with the use of visual feedback. They found that residents of both sexes, but especially men, can generate traction forces exceeding the recommended limit, and forces generated from the sitting position can often exceed the preferred range.

An instrumental delivery should be abandoned if there is difficulty in applying the instrument, if there is no appreciable descent with each pull, or if descent is not significant following three pulls of a correctly applied instrument and the baby has not been delivered after 15 to 20 minutes [4].

Conditions where difficulty or failure are anticipated include situations in which: one-fifth of the head is palpable abdominally; the presenting part is at the level of the spines; the fetus is in occiput posterior position; there is excessive molding of the fetal head or fetal macrosomia; the mother is undergoing dysfunctional or prolonged labor and has a body mass index >30 [70]. In those cases of a trial of instrumental vaginal delivery, a back-up plan should always be in place [2] and it should be performed in an operating theater equipped for cesarean section [4].

When one instrument has failed to effect delivery, sequential use of instruments offers the advantage of avoiding the complications of cesarean section at full dilatation with a low head, but increases the risks of fetal trauma [19,42]. Appropriate case selection with careful decision-making is of paramount importance [4]. If the head has descended to the introitus, a sequential delivery is rational and less likely to cause harm compared with the use of a second instrument when there is no or minimal descent.

Diagnosis of head injuries

All infants delivered by vacuum or forceps should be clinically examined. Systematic radiographic and ultrasonographic examination may lead to the discovery of asymptomatic complications that are not clinically significant and require no therapeutic intervention, such as nondepressed fracture, cephalhematoma, and scalp edema. For this reason they are not recommended as routine screening tools. Nevertheless, in cases of suspected depressed skull fracture or neurologic symptoms, skull radiography and cranial CT are indicated [17].

Training

Adequate clinical experience and training of the operator are essential to the safe performance of instrumental deliveries [1]. Lack of experience may lead to inappropriate use of instruments [71]. Experienced obstetricians have been shown to demonstrate a higher level of repeatability of the forceps maneuvers than junior doctors [72].

The obstetrician must be confident in the assessment of any signs of cephalopelvic disproportion, determine the cervical dilatation, and assess the engagement of the fetal vertex and fetal position and station. It is also essential to determine flexion, asynclitism, caput and molding. The decrease in the number of forceps deliveries and increase in litigation has an impact on the residents' training opportunities. Vacuum delivery is perceived to be easier to learn than forceps; however, incorrect use of this device may result in increased failure rates and complications. Cheong and colleagues [73] showed that formal training results in a significant decrease in maternal as well as neonatal morbidity associated with admission to Special Care Baby Unit, severe neonatal scalp injury and facial injuries. Thus, formal education and training can result in improved safety for mother and baby. Obstetric simulators and forceps with spatial location sensors have been designed to facilitate training and assessment of the quality of the maneuvers [72]. Traction-force training using computer-assisted visual feedback can be useful in training practitioners to produce appropriate traction forces during obstetric forceps deliveries. [69]. The RCOG recommends that only practitioners who are adequately trained, or who are under the supervision of trained practitioners, should undertake instrumental delivery [2].

Summary

Instrumental vaginal deliveries have risks of failure and complications. The obstetrician should critically appraise the indications for the procedure and the risk factors to provide a safe delivery for fetus and mother. Knowledge of the injuries that can be caused by improper use of vacuum and forceps is of paramount importance in the decision-making process.

The most appropriate intervention needs to be decided after consideration of the clinical circumstances as well as the operator's skills and experience. An alternative plan that will result in a safe delivery should always be in place.

References

[1] Society of Obstetricians and Gynaecologists of Canada. Guidelines for operative vaginal birth. SOGC. Number 148, May 2004. Int J Gynaecol Obstet 2005;88:229–36.
[2] Operative vaginal delivery. Guideline No. 26. Clinical green top guidelines. Royal College of Obstetricians and Gynaecologists; 2005.
[3] Kozak LJ, Weeks JD. U.S. trends in obstetric procedures, 1990–2000. Birth 2002;29:157–61.
[4] Edozien LC. Towards safe practice in instrumental vaginal delivery. Best Pract Res Clin Obstet Gynaecol 2007;21:639–55.
[5] Dupuis O, Silveira R, Redarce T, et al. [Instrumental extraction in 2002 in the "AURORE" hospital network: incidence and serious neonatal complications]. Gynecol Obstet Fertil 2003;31:920–6 [in French].
[6] American College of Obstetrics and Gynecology. Operative vaginal delivery. Clinical management guidelines for obstetrician-gynecologists. American College of Obstetrics and Gynecology. Int J Gynaecol Obstet 2001;74:69–76.
[7] Patel RR, Murphy DJ. Forceps delivery in modern obstetric practice. BMJ 2004;328:1302–5.
[8] Vacca A. Vacuum-assisted delivery. Best Pract Res Clin Obstet Gynaecol 2002;16:17–30.
[9] McQuivey RW. Vacuum-assisted delivery: a review. J Matern Fetal Neonatal Med 2004;16: 171–80.
[10] Johanson RB, Menon BK. Vacuum extraction versus forceps for assisted vaginal delivery. Cochrane Database Syst Rev 2000:CD000224.
[11] Lykoudis EG, Spyropoulou GA, Lavasidis LG, et al. Alopecia associated with birth injury. Obstet Gynecol 2007;110:487–90.
[12] Hayman R, Gilby J, Arulkumaran S. Clinical evaluation of a "hand pump" vacuum delivery device. Obstet Gynecol 2002;100:1190–5.
[13] Attilakos G, Sibanda T, Winter C, et al. A randomised controlled trial of a new handheld vacuum extraction device. BJOG 2005;112:1510–5.
[14] Hughes CA, Harley EH, Milmoe G, et al. Birth trauma in the head and neck. Arch Otolaryngol Head Neck Surg 1999;125:193–9.
[15] Towner DR, Ciotti MC. Operative vaginal delivery: a cause of birth injury or is it? Clin Obstet Gynecol 2007;50:563–81.
[16] Doumouchtsis SK, Arulkumaran S. Head injuries after instrumental vaginal deliveries. Curr Opin Obstet Gynecol 2006;18:129–34.
[17] Simonson C, Barlow P, Dehennin N, et al. Neonatal complications of vacuum-assisted delivery. Obstet Gynecol 2007;109:626–33.
[18] Johanson R, Menon V. Soft versus rigid vacuum extractor cups for assisted vaginal delivery. Cochrane Database Syst Rev 2000:CD000446.
[19] Sadan O, Ginath S, Gomel A, et al. What to do after a failed attempt of vacuum delivery? Eur J Obstet Gynecol Reprod Biol 2003;107:151–5.

[20] Uhing MR. Management of birth injuries. Clin Perinatol 2005;32:19–38.

[21] LeBlanc CM, Allen UD, Ventureyra E. Cephalhematomas revisited. When should a diagnostic tap be performed? Clin Pediatr (Phila) 1995;34:86–9.

[22] Uchil D, Arulkumaran S. Neonatal subgaleal hemorrhage and its relationship to delivery by vacuum extraction. Obstet Gynecol Surv 2003;58:687–93.

[23] Davis DJ. Neonatal subgaleal hemorrhage: diagnosis and management. CMAJ 2001;164: 1452–3.

[24] Plauche WC. Subgaleal hematoma. A complication of instrumental delivery. JAMA 1980; 244:1597–8.

[25] Gebremariam A. Subgaleal haemorrhage: risk factors and neurological and developmental outcome in survivors. Ann Trop Paediatr 1999;19:45–50.

[26] Boo NY, Foong KW, Mahdy ZA, et al. Risk factors associated with subaponeurotic haemorrhage in full-term infants exposed to vacuum extraction. BJOG 2005;112:1516–21.

[27] Amar AP, Aryan HE, Meltzer HS, et al. Neonatal subgaleal hematoma causing brain compression: report of two cases and review of the literature. Neurosurgery 2003;52: 1470–4 [discussion: 1474].

[28] Ng PC, Siu YK, Lewindon PJ. Subaponeurotic haemorrhage in the 1990s: a 3-year surveillance. Acta Paediatr 1995;84:1065–9.

[29] Maryniak GM, Frank JB. Clinical assessment of the Kobayashi vacuum extractor. Obstet Gynecol 1984;64:431–5.

[30] Berkus MD, Ramamurthy RS, O'Connor PS, et al. Cohort study of silastic obstetric vacuum cup deliveries: I. Safety of the instrument. Obstet Gynecol 1985;66:503–9.

[31] O'Mahony F, Settatree R, Platt C, et al. Review of singleton fetal and neonatal deaths associated with cranial trauma and cephalic delivery during a national intrapartum-related confidential enquiry. BJOG 2005;112:619–26.

[32] Nakahara T, Sakoda K, Uozumi T, et al. Intrauterine depressed skull fracture. A report of two cases. Pediatr Neurosci 1989;15:121–4.

[33] Garza-Mercado R. Intrauterine depressed skull fractures of the newborn. Neurosurgery 1982;10:694–7.

[34] Pollak L, Raziel A, Ariely S, et al. Revival of non-surgical management of neonatal depressed skull fractures. J Paediatr Child Health 1999;35:96–7.

[35] Pollina J, Dias MS, Li V, et al. Cranial birth injuries in term newborn infants. Pediatr Neurosurg 2001;35:113–9.

[36] Sachs BP, Acker D, Tuomala R, et al. The incidence of symptomatic intracranial hemorrhage in term appropriate-for-gestation-age infants. Clin Pediatr (Phila) 1987;26: 355–8.

[37] Plauche WC. Fetal cranial injuries related to delivery with the Malmstrom vacuum extractor. Obstet Gynecol 1979;53:750–7.

[38] Towner D, Castro MA, Eby-Wilkens E, et al. Effect of mode of delivery in nulliparous women on neonatal intracranial injury. N Engl J Med 1999;341:1709–14.

[39] Wen SW, Liu S, Kramer MS, et al. Comparison of maternal and infant outcomes between vacuum extraction and forceps deliveries. Am J Epidemiol 2001;153:103–7.

[40] Demissie K, Rhoads GG, Smulian JC, et al. Operative vaginal delivery and neonatal and infant adverse outcomes: population based retrospective analysis. BMJ 2004;329:24–9.

[41] Jhawar BS, Ranger A, Steven D, et al. Risk factors for intracranial hemorrhage among full-term infants: a case-control study. Neurosurgery 2003;52:581–90 [discussion: 588–90].

[42] Gardella C, Taylor M, Benedetti T, et al. The effect of sequential use of vacuum and forceps for assisted vaginal delivery on neonatal and maternal outcomes. Am J Obstet Gynecol 2001; 185:896–902.

[43] Negishi H, Lee Y, Itoh K, et al. Nonsurgical management of epidural hematoma in neonates. Pediatr Neurol 1989;5:253–6.

[44] Hamlat A, Heckly A, Adn M, et al. Pathophysiology of intracranial epidural haematoma following birth. Medical Hypotheses 2006;66:371–4.

[45] Lapeer RJ, Prager RW. Fetal head moulding: finite element analysis of a fetal skull subjected to uterine pressures during the first stage of labour. J Biomech 2001;34:1125–33.

[46] Perlman JM. Brain injury in the term infant. Semin Perinatol 2004;28:415–24.

[47] Mateos F, Esteban J, Ramos JT, et al. Fetal subdural hematoma: diagnosis in utero. Case report. Pediatr Neurosci 1987;13:125–8.

[48] Hanigan WC, Ali MB, Cusack TJ, et al. Diagnosis of subdural hemorrhage in utero. Case report. J Neurosurg 1985;63:977–9.

[49] Holden KR, Titus MO, Van Tassel P. Cranial magnetic resonance imaging examination of normal term neonates: a pilot study. J Child Neurol 1999;14:708–10.

[50] Tavani F, Zimmerman RA, Clancy RR, et al. Incidental intracranial hemorrhage after uncomplicated birth: MRI before and after neonatal heart surgery. Neuroradiology 2003;45: 253–8.

[51] Whitby EH, Griffiths PD, Rutter S, et al. Frequency and natural history of subdural haemorrhages in babies and relation to obstetric factors. Lancet 2004;363:846–51.

[52] Chamnanvanakij S, Rollins N, Perlman JM. Subdural hematoma in term infants. Pediatr Neurol 2002;26:301–4.

[53] Perrin RG, Rutka JT, Drake JM, et al. Management and outcomes of posterior fossa subdural hematomas in neonates. Neurosurgery 1997;40:1190–9 [discussion: 1199–200].

[54] Haase R, Kursawe I, Nagel F, et al. Acute subdural hematoma after caesarean section: a case report. Pediatr Crit Care Med 2003;4:246–8.

[55] Huang CC, Shen EY. Tentorial subdural hemorrhage in term newborns: ultrasonographic diagnosis and clinical correlates. Pediatr Neurol 1991;7:171–7.

[56] Odita JC, Hebi S. CT and MRI characteristics of intracranial hemorrhage complicating breech and vacuum delivery. Pediatr Radiol 1996;26:782–5.

[57] Saunders NJ, Spiby H, Gilbert L, et al. Oxytocin infusion during second stage of labour in primiparous women using epidural analgesia: a randomised double blind placebo controlled trial. BMJ 1989;299:1423–6.

[58] Intrapartum care. care of healthy women and their babies during childbirth. Clinical guideline. NICE (National Institute for Health and Clinical Excellence). 2007.

[59] Akmal S, Kametas N, Tsoi E, et al. Comparison of transvaginal digital examination with intrapartum sonography to determine fetal head position before instrumental delivery. Ultrasound Obstet Gynecol 2003;21:437–40.

[60] Sherer DM, Miodovnik M, Bradley KS, et al. Intrapartum fetal head position II: comparison between transvaginal digital examination and transabdominal ultrasound assessment during the second stage of labor. Ultrasound Obstet Gynecol 2002;19:264–8.

[61] Henrich W, Dudenhausen J, Fuchs I, et al. Intrapartum translabial ultrasound (ITU): sonographic landmarks and correlation with successful vacuum extraction. Ultrasound Obstet Gynecol 2006;28:753–60.

[62] Zahalka N, Sadan O, Malinger G, et al. Comparison of transvaginal sonography with digital examination and transabdominal sonography for the determination of fetal head position in the second stage of labor. Am J Obstet Gynecol 2005;193:381–6.

[63] Ben-Haroush A, Melamed N, Kaplan B, et al. Predictors of failed operative vaginal delivery: a single-center experience. Am J Obstet Gynecol 2007;197:308, e301–5.

[64] Miksovsky P, Watson WJ. Obstetric vacuum extraction: state of the art in the new millennium. Obstet Gynecol Surv 2001;56:736–51.

[65] Chalmers JA, Chalmers I. The obstetric vacuum extractor is the instrument of first choice for operative vaginal delivery. Br J Obstet Gynaecol 1989;96:505–6.

[66] Whitlow BJ, Tamizian O, Ashworth J, et al. Validation of traction force indicator in ventouse devices. Int J Gynaecol Obstet 2005;90:35–8.

[67] Vacca A. Vacuum-assisted delivery: an analysis of traction force and maternal and neonatal outcomes. Aust N Z J Obstet Gynaecol 2006;46:124–7.

[68] Roshan DF, Petrikovsky B, Sichinava L, et al. Soft forceps. Int J Gynaecol Obstet 2005;88: 249–52.

[69] Leslie KK, Dipasquale-Lehnerz P, Smith M. Obstetric forceps training using visual feedback and the isometric strength testing unit. Obstet Gynecol 2005;105:377–82.

[70] Murphy DJ, Liebling RE, Verity L, et al. Early maternal and neonatal morbidity associated with operative delivery in second stage of labour: a cohort study. Lancet 2001;358:1203–7.

[71] Okunwobi-Smith Y, Cooke I, MacKenzie IZ. Decision to delivery intervals for assisted vaginal vertex delivery. BJOG 2000;107:467–71.

[72] Dupuis O, Moreau R, Silveira R, et al. A new obstetric forceps for the training of junior doctors: a comparison of the spatial dispersion of forceps blade trajectories between junior and senior obstetricians. Am J Obstet Gynecol 2006;194:1524–31.

[73] Cheong YC, Abdullahi H, Lashen H, et al. Can formal education and training improve the outcome of instrumental delivery? Eur J Obstet Gynecol Reprod Biol 2004;113:139–44.

ELSEVIER
SAUNDERS

CLINICS IN
PERINATOLOGY

Clin Perinatol 35 (2008) 85–99

Identifying Risk Factors
for Uterine Rupture

Jennifer G. Smith, MD, PhD*, Heather L. Mertz, MD,
David C. Merrill, MD, PhD

*Section on Maternal Fetal Medicine, Department of Obstetrics and Gynecology,
Wake Forest University, Medical Center Boulevard, Winston-Salem, NC 27157, USA*

Uterine rupture is perhaps one of the most feared intrapartum complications encountered by obstetricians. This catastrophic complication occurs most often in women attempting a vaginal birth after a prior cesarean delivery (VBAC). In women who undergo a trial of labor after one prior low transverse cesarean section, the incidence of uterine rupture is estimated to be less than 1%, whereas a trial of labor may be successful 60% to 80% of the time, depending on the indication for the initial cesarean section. Although the rate of uterine rupture is highest among women who are attempting a trial of labor, one must remember that there is an inherent risk of uterine rupture associated with a uterine scar. This risk is estimated as being between 0.0 and 0.16% [1–4]. The rate of cesarean delivery continues to rise, reaching an all-time high of 30.2% in 2005, a 46% increase since 1996 [5]. Thus, more women are entering subsequent pregnancies at increased risk for uterine rupture, whether or not they attempt a VBAC.

Concerns regarding the safety of VBAC have contributed to a decrease in the number of women attempting a trial of labor. The number of women attempting a vaginal delivery after cesarean has declined 67% since 1996, falling to only 9.2% in 2004 [6]. Although uterine rupture can result in major neonatal and maternal morbidity and mortality, obstetricians must remember that the overall risk of uterine rupture is very low and that an elective repeat cesarean section is not without risk. Each cesarean is a major abdominal surgery with inherent risks of bleeding, infection, and damage to surrounding structures. In addition to the operative risk, each uterine scar increases the risk of abnormal placentation in future pregnancies, thereby increasing the risk of major maternal morbidity including massive blood transfusion,

---

* Corresponding author.
E-mail address: jgsmith@wfubmc.edu (J.G. Smith).

0095-5108/08/$ - see front matter © 2008 Elsevier Inc. All rights reserved.
doi:10.1016/j.clp.2007.11.008

hysterectomy, and even death. In a prospective observational study of more than 39,000 women at term who had a history of a prior cesarean delivery, Spong and colleagues [1] reported that more maternal deaths occurred in women undergoing an elective cesarean than in those attempting a trial of labor. The ability to counsel patients effectively regarding their options for delivery after a prior cesarean section is an important responsibility of obstetricians. This article reviews the literature regarding uterine rupture to help obstetricians determine whether patients who have a history of prior cesarean section have an acceptable risk profile for attempting a trial of labor.

Rupture of the unscarred uterus

Although most uterine ruptures are associated with a trial of labor in a patient who has had a prior cesarean section, rupture of the nulliparous uterus is also possible. Spontaneous uterine rupture is an extremely rare event, estimated to occur in 1 of 8000 to 1 of 15,000 deliveries [7]. A recent review article by Walsh and colleagues [8] gives an excellent overview of the etiology of rupture of the primigravid uterus. Uterine rupture has been reported in women who have uterine anomalies secondary to a history of diethylstilbestrol exposure as well as bicornuate uteri. Maternal connective tissue disease, in particular Ehlers-Danlos syndrome, also has been associated with uterine rupture. Labor induction and augmentation with various agents also have been associated with rupture of the unscarred uterus. Another risk factor that has been associated with rupture of the unscarred uterus is abnormal placentation. The incidence of placenta accreta without a prior cesarean section or placenta previa has been estimated at 1 in 68,000 [8]. Although these events are rare, clinicians must remember that uterine rupture is a possibility in any laboring patient who exhibits abdominal pain, hypovolemia, and fetal compromise.

Uterine rupture in the primigravid patient: prior uterine surgery

In the most recent review of cases of uterine rupture, 31% of uterine ruptures occurred in women who had a history of prior uterine surgery, including myomectomy [8]. Classic teaching states that the risk of rupture is increased only if the uterine cavity is entered during myomectomy. Thus, women who have undergone removal of pedunculated or subserosal myomas are assumed to be at no increased risk of uterine rupture during subsequent pregnancies. Cases of uterine rupture, however, have been reported after laparoscopic myomectomy, the most common procedure used to remove pedunculated and subserosal myomas. In fact, 36% of the cases of uterine rupture that occurred following a prior uterine surgery occurred after a laparoscopic myomectomy [8]. A proposed explanation for this seemingly high rate of rupture following a laparoscopic procedure is that the suturing technique used in laparoscopic myomectomy is inferior to myomectomy site closure during an exploratory laparotomy. Other studies have reported that the risk of uterine rupture after laparoscopic myomectomy is no higher than 1%, but a large percentage of these patients underwent elective cesarean section, thus minimizing risk [9]. A recent study reports a success rate of 83% in women attempting a vaginal delivery after laparoscopic myomectomy [10]. All of these labors were managed as VBAC attempts, and there were no cases of uterine rupture. These data suggest that although uterine rupture is rare following laparoscopic myomectomy, it can occur, sometimes years after the procedure. To be most conservative, perhaps induction and augmentation of labor in women who have a history of laparoscopic myomectomy or laparotomy for pedunculated or subserosal myomas should be managed in a similar manner as VBAC attempts.

Uterine rupture associated with prior cesarean section: intrapartum predictors

Most uterine ruptures occur in women who have had a prior cesarean section. Therefore the remainder of this article focuses on these patients. The 2004 American College of Obstetricians and Gynecologists (ACOG) practice bulletin sets forth practice guidelines regarding candidates for an attempted VBAC [11]. Selection criteria include one previous low transverse cesarean delivery, a clinically adequate pelvis, no other uterine scars, no previous uterine rupture, a physician immediately available throughout active labor capable of monitoring labor and performing an emergency cesarean delivery, and the availability of anesthesia and personnel for emergency cesarean delivery.

Given the potential grave consequences for both mother and child in the event of an intrapartum uterine rupture, the obstetrician must be acutely aware of the clinical signs associated with uterine rupture. Clinical suspicion for uterine rupture is heightened by the presence of abdominal pain, vaginal bleeding, loss of fetal station, and/or nonreassuring fetal heart rate patterns. Unfortunately, by the time these clinical signs are present, major maternal and/or neonatal morbidity already may have occurred. Therefore, several investigators have attempted to describe intrapartum predictors of uterine rupture. Changes in the fetal heart rate pattern, especially fetal bradycardia and late decelerations, have been associated with uterine rupture, in some reports occurring in up to 87.5% of cases [12–15].

Early studies investigating fetal heart rate patterns in cases of uterine rupture were limited by a lack of controls. In a case-control study, however, Ridgeway and colleagues [16] investigated fetal heart rate patterns in cases of uterine rupture and were able to demonstrate that the only significant fetal heart rate pattern seen in cases of uterine rupture is bradycardia. Other clinical signs associated with uterine rupture in this study included abdominal pain, vaginal bleeding, loss of fetal station, and a palpable uterine defect. Most recently, Pryor and colleagues [17] at Wake Forest University reviewed 26 cases of confirmed full-thickness uterine rupture in a

case-controlled study design. The occurrence of mild and severe variable decelerations, late decelerations, fetal bradycardia, persistent abdominal pain,
vaginal bleeding, and uterine hyperstimulation at various time intervals before delivery were investigated. At less than 2 hours before delivery, mild
variable decelerations (odds ratio [OR], 15; 95% confidence interval [CI],
3.4–70), severe variable decelerations (OR, 64; 95% CI, 6–660), persistent
abdominal pain (OR, 45; 95% CI, 4.2–445), and uterine hyperstimulation
(OR, 5.9; 95% CI, 1.2–28.6) were more common in patients who experienced a uterine rupture. Persistent abdominal pain (defined as pain that
was continuously present and specifically noticed between contractions)
was more strongly correlated with uterine rupture than bradycardia or
late decelerations. Taken together, these studies suggest that in cases of uterine rupture, changes in fetal heart rate monitoring are probably the most reliable presenting clinical symptom, but persistent abdominal pain, especially
in the presence of severe variable decelerations, has a high predictive value
for uterine rupture. The authors suggest that mild and severe variable decelerations in the fetal heart rate tracing, persistent abdominal pain, and hyperstimulation are intrapartum factors that may signal the early phases or
initiation of uterine scar separation. These factors may be clinically useful
predictors of uterine rupture and may have the potential to aid in the prevention of uterine rupture in patients attempting VBAC. Such studies can
have a significant impact on the rate of uterine rupture in patients attempting VBAC, thus improving safety and potentially resulting in more patients
electing a trial of labor, with a subsequent reduction in the overall cesarean
section rate.

Uterine rupture associated with prior uterine incision: antepartum predictors

Given the catastrophic consequences that can be associated with an intrapartum uterine rupture, other investigators have attempted to predict an individual patient's risk of uterine rupture before labor based on various
antepartum variables. Important predictors that have been identified include
a prior spontaneous vaginal delivery, prior successful VBAC, maternal age,
maternal obesity, number of prior cesarean sections, the type of closure of
the prior uterine incision, gestational age at delivery, and the interpregnancy
interval.

First and foremost, evaluation of a woman considering a trial of labor
should document the type of prior uterine incision: low transverse, low vertical, classical, or unknown. The risk of uterine rupture differs significantly
depending on the location of the prior incision. The Maternal Fetal Medicine Units Network prospective observational study of 45,988 women
who had a singleton gestation estimates uterine rupture rates of 0.7% for
low transverse incisions and 2.0% for low vertical incisions [18]. A growing
number of patients are presenting a clinical challenge, in that they present

with an unknown scar. Clinicians then must infer which type of uterine incision is most likely, given the circumstances surrounding the delivery (eg, gestational age and indication for cesarean delivery). Landon and colleagues [18] reported a rupture rate of 0.5% for unknown scars, similar to that found for prior low transverse incisions. The risk of rupture with a T-shaped or classical incision is much higher, and ranges from 4% to 9% [11].

Perhaps another antepartum predictor that can be gleaned from the operative report is the type of uterine incision closure, specifically single versus double layer. Several studies have investigated this variable, with conflicting results. Initial studies suggested that the method of uterine incision closure did not influence VBAC success rates or uterine rupture rates [19,20]. In a retrospective review of 768 women who had a prior low transverse cesarean section, Durnwald and Mercer [21] reported an increase in uterine windows in the group with single-layer closure but failed to find an increase in the rate of uterine rupture. In an observational cohort study of 1980 women who had a prior low transverse cesarean section, however, Bujold and colleagues [22] demonstrated a fourfold increased risk of uterine rupture with single-layer uterine incision closure (OR, 3.95; 95% CI, 1.35–11.49). Most recently, Gyamfi and colleagues [23], in a retrospective chart review of more than 900 women attempting VBAC, reported that uterine rupture rates were eight times higher in women whose prior cesarean section incision had been closed with a single-layer closure than in those who had had a double-layer closure (8.6% versus 1.3%, respectively; $P = .015$). One drawback of this study is that it did not control for the type of induction and/or use of an augmentation agent in these trials of labor. The authors acknowledge that prostaglandins were used routinely during the period of this study, and their use may contribute to the overall high rupture rate reported. Randomized, controlled trials comparing the type of suture material used as well as the technique of closure are needed to answer this question definitively.

Intuitively, one would assume that if a woman who has a history of one cesarean section has an increased risk of uterine rupture, then two or more prior incisions would increase that risk further. This assumption may not be true. In a large multicenter prospective observational study, Landon and colleagues [24] demonstrated that the uterine rupture rate in women who had multiple (2–4) prior cesarean sections was no higher than that in women who had a single prior uterine incision (0.9% versus 0.7%; $P = .37$). Composite maternal morbidity (consisting of uterine rupture, endometritis, hysterectomy, transfusion, thromboembolic disease, and operative injury) was increased, however (OR, 1.35; 95% CI, 1.03–1.75). Additionally, there were no differences in perinatal outcomes. In a secondary analysis of a large, retrospective cohort study, Macones and colleagues [25] found that the risk of major maternal morbidity is increased in a trial of labor with a history of two prior cesarean sections. Current ACOG recommendations state that a trial of labor in a woman who has a history of two prior cesarean sections and no prior vaginal deliveries is contraindicated [11].

Several large studies have shown that women attempting a trial of labor who have a history of a prior successful vaginal delivery have a higher chance of successful VBAC and a decreased risk of uterine rupture. Landon and colleagues [26] demonstrated that a previous vaginal delivery was the most significant predictor of VBAC success (OR, 3.9; 95% CI, 3.6–4.3). Others have demonstrated a 60% to 80% reduction in the risk of uterine rupture in women who have had a previous successful vaginal delivery [27,28]. A large, retrospective cohort study recently reported that women who have a history of prior vaginal delivery and prior cesarean section have lower rates of major maternal morbidities with a trial of labor than women undergoing an elective repeat cesarean section [2]. Composite maternal morbidity, including uterine rupture, uterine artery laceration, and bladder and bowel injuries, however, was increased in women attempting a trial of labor without a history of successful vaginal delivery (relative risk, 2.71; 95% CI, 2.15–3.40) [2].

There are conflicting data regarding the effect of the interpregnancy interval on the risk of uterine rupture. A 12-year retrospective chart review of women who had one prior cesarean section and no prior vaginal delivery demonstrated a threefold increased risk of uterine rupture with an interdelivery interval of less than 18 months [29]. Bujold and colleagues [22] confirmed this finding and reported that an interdelivery interval of less than 24 months is associated with a two- to threefold increase in the risk of uterine rupture. On the other hand, Haung and colleagues [30] reported no difference in uterine rupture rates with interdelivery intervals less than or greater than 19 months. In the largest group of women studied to date, Landon and colleagues [24] have reported that an interdelivery interval of less than 2 years is associated with a higher rate of uterine rupture (OR, 2.05; 95% CI, 1.41–2.96). From the available data, it seems prudent to counsel patients interested in a trial of labor that a cesarean delivery within the previous 2 years may increase their risk of rupture above the generally quoted risk of less than 1%.

The gestational age at attempted VBAC also may contribute to the risk of uterine rupture and VBAC success rates. In a retrospective case review of more than 20,000 patients, Quinones and colleagues [31] described an increased VBAC success rate in preterm women and a trend toward lower uterine rupture rates (OR, 0.28; 95% CI, 0.07–1.17; $P = .08$). Durnwald and colleagues [32] compared women undergoing a preterm trial of labor versus a term trial of labor and found no difference in VBAC success rates but a significantly lower rate of uterine dehiscence (0.26% versus 0.67%; $P = .02$) and uterine rupture (0.34% versus 0.74%; $P = .03$) in preterm trials of labor. There were no cases of uterine rupture in women undergoing trial of labor at less than 32 weeks' gestation. It is possible that the thicker lower uterine segment present at earlier gestational ages is more resistant to rupture than the thin lower uterine segment found in term gestations.

Worldwide, more women are choosing to delay childbearing, and it is becoming clear that mothers of advanced maternal age are at increased risk for antepartum and intrapartum pregnancy-related complications [33]. Antepartum risks include diabetes, hypertensive disorders, and stillbirth [34]. Intrapartum risks include malpresentation and active-phase arrest disorders resulting in an increased risk of cesarean delivery. It also is recognized that older women are at increased risk of an adverse outcome during an attempted VBAC. In a 12-year retrospective chart review of women who had one prior cesarean delivery and no prior vaginal deliveries, Shipp and colleagues [35] were the first to report an increased risk of uterine rupture during a trial of labor for women over the age of 30 years (OR, 3.2; 95% CI, 1.2–8.4), even after controlling for confounders including induction of labor. In contrast, Bujold and colleagues [36] found a decreased rate of VBAC success in women older than 35 years but did not demonstrate a significant difference in the rate of uterine rupture. Recently, Kaczmarczyk [37], in a population-based cohort study of more than 300,000 Swedish women, reported that women older than 35 years had a twofold increased risk of uterine rupture compared with women aged 25 to 29 years. The physiologic mechanisms responsible for this finding are unclear but may suggest that older women do not heal as well as younger women.

Coincident with the increase in the number of women delaying childbearing is an increase in the use of assisted reproductive technology and subsequent increase in multifetal gestations. It is estimated that multiple gestations now account for 3.3% of all births in the United States [38]. Varner and colleagues [39] described maternal and neonatal outcomes in 412 women who had multiple gestations and a history of at least one prior cesarean delivery. They found no difference in the incidence of uterine rupture in women who underwent a twin trial of labor versus a singleton trial of labor (1.1% versus 0.7%; $P = .373$). Similarly, Ford and colleagues [40] found a similar rate of uterine rupture in women attempting a trial of labor with a twin versus a singleton pregnancy (0.9% versus 0.8%). The incidence of uterine rupture was significantly increased in women who failed a trial of labor, however (OR, 5.8; 95% CI, 1.3–25.8).

The incidence of obesity and morbid obesity is reaching epidemic proportions in the United States, with an estimated 66% of adults being affected. Obese women are at risk for many complications during pregnancy including increased risk of stillbirth [41], hypertensive disorders of pregnancy, and gestational diabetes. In addition to these risks, obese gravidas are at increased risk for cesarean section. Thus, many obese women will require counseling regarding the optimal mode of delivery after a prior cesarean section. A recent article by Hibbard and colleagues [42] investigated maternal morbidity stratified by body mass index category in women who had had one prior cesarean section undergoing a trial of labor. Morbidly obese women (ie, with a body mass index > 40 kg/m^2) were more likely to have a failed trial of labor. In addition, they have a fivefold increased risk of uterine rupture (2.1% versus 0.4%; 95% CI, 2.7–11.7). It is important to consider these data when counseling an obese patient who is interested in attempting a trial of labor.

A common finding associated with maternal obesity is fetal macrosomia. Although no studies to date have investigated the relationship of these two factors concurrently with success of an attempted VBAC or uterine rupture rates, several authors have investigated the relationship between fetal macrosomia and risk of uterine rupture. Zelop and colleagues [43] reviewed more than 2700 women who had a history of prior cesarean section and no prior vaginal delivery who attempted a trial of labor and whose infants had a birth weight of 4000 g or less versus women whose infants had a birth weight of more than 4000 g. Although women whose infants had a birth weight of less than 4000 g were more likely to have a failed trial of labor, the risk of uterine rupture was not significantly different between these groups (1.0% versus 1.6%; $P = .24$). Subgroup analysis of birth weights between 4000 g and 4250 g and more than 4250 g suggested an increased risk of rupture in women with larger babies, although this increase did not reach statistical significance (1% versus 2.4%; $P = .1$). This study, however, lacked sufficient power to detect a difference in rupture rates at birth weights higher than 4250 g because of the small sample size. Further study is necessary to provide practice guidelines for fetuses with an estimated fetal weight greater than 4250 g.

Other investigators have focused on the indication and the gestational age for the primary cesarean section to evaluate any association with risk of a subsequent trial of labor. Rochelson and colleagues [44] have suggested that a prior preterm cesarean delivery is associated with an increased risk of uterine rupture in a subsequent pregnancy. Varner and colleagues [45] report no significant difference in uterine rupture rates in women attempting a trial of labor whose prior cesarean section was secondary to multiple gestation.

One interesting technique currently under investigation is the use of ultrasound to measure the thickness of the lower uterine segment as an index of the risk for uterine rupture. One study found that a sonographic lower uterine segment thickness of 1.5 mm had a negative predictive value of 96.2% in predicting a paper-thin or dehisced lower uterine segment in women attempting a VBAC [46]. More research is necessary before this technique can be applied widely in clinical practice.

Providing appropriate counseling and informed consent to women who desire a trial of labor is an important responsibility. What can practitioners tell patients about their individual likelihood of uterine rupture? Macones and colleagues [47], in a secondary analysis of a large case-controlled study, identified 134 cases of uterine rupture and 670 controls. They compared clinical variables including prior vaginal delivery, two or more prior cesarean sections, birth weight, gestational age at delivery, and labor induction, among others. Using multivariable predictive models, they were unable to predict a uterine rupture based on antepartum variables. Therefore, although some antepartum factors seem statistically to increase or decrease an individual's risk for uterine rupture, this rare catastrophic event cannot be predicted accurately. Therefore, clinicians need to have a high index of suspicion when a patient who has a history of a prior cesarean section is laboring.

Uterine rupture associated with prior cesarean section: induction and augmentation of labor

Induction of labor is a common practice in the United States; it is estimated that nearly 22% of all deliveries are induced [6]. How does induction of labor affect the risk of uterine rupture in a patient who has a prior cesarean section? Several different agents are used routinely in the United States for induction and augmentation of labor: prostaglandin E1 analogues, prostaglandin E2 analogues, and pitocin.

Misoprostol, a prostaglandin E1 analogue, is a particularly attractive agent for the induction of labor because of its easy storage and its low cost. In patients who have a history of a prior cesarean section, however, its use has been associated with uterine hyperstimulation and increased rates of uterine rupture. A randomized trial was stopped because misoprostol was associated with an increased rupture rate when given to women who had a history of prior cesarean section [48]. Further studies have confirmed this finding. Lydon-Rochelle [49] reported that uterine rupture was almost 16 times more likely in women who had had one prior cesarean section who received prostaglandin E1 for induction of labor. In 2004, Landon and colleagues [18] reported results from a prospective, multicenter observational study of women undergoing a trial of labor versus repeat elective cesarean delivery. This study enrolled 45,988 women who had a history of cesarean delivery. Labor induction and augmentation were associated with a twofold increase in the risk of uterine rupture. The highest risk of rupture was in patients whose labor was induced with prostaglandins, with or without oxytocin (1.4%, versus 0.4% for spontaneous labor; $P < .001$). Macones and colleagues [27] conducted a multicenter, retrospective case-control study examining risk factors associated with uterine rupture in VBAC that showed that induction or augmentation of labor with oxytocin alone was not associated with an increased risk of rupture. If, however, a woman was exposed to a prostaglandin followed by oxytocin, the risk of uterine rupture was increased (OR, 4.54; 95% CI, 1.66–12.42; $P = .003$). Given these unacceptably high risks of uterine rupture, misoprostol should not be used for induction of labor in women who have a history of major uterine surgery, including cesarean section [50].

Unlike misoprostol, administration of oxytocin for labor induction and augmentation probably is safe. A meta-analysis of 11,417 trials of labor and 6147 elective repeat cesarean sections did not demonstrate an increased risk of uterine scar dehiscence or rupture in the labors in which oxytocin was used [51]. Goetzl and colleagues [52] compared oxytocin doses and duration of oxytocin use in women attempting a trial of labor. They found that neither the maximum dose of oxytocin nor the duration of oxytocin use was associated significantly with uterine rupture. Merrill and Zlatnik [53], in a randomized, double-blinded trial, were unable to demonstrate an increased rate of uterine rupture with a high-dose pitocin protocol (mean dose, 29.5 mU/min; maximum dose, 117 mU/min) used for either induction or augmentation of labor.

On the other hand, some studies have shown an increased risk of uterine rupture with oxytocin induction of labor after a prior cesarean section. This risk may be influenced by whether a woman has had a prior successful vaginal delivery. Zelop and colleagues [28] failed to demonstrate an increased rate of uterine rupture in women who received pitocin for labor augmentation. They did, however, find a 4.6-fold increased risk of uterine rupture with oxytocin induction of labor in women who had not had a prior vaginal delivery. Recently, Grobman and colleagues [54] studied 11,778 women who had one prior low transverse cesarean section and a singleton gestation who attempted a trial of labor; these investigators found that an increased rate of uterine rupture was seen only in women undergoing induction of labor who had no prior vaginal delivery (1.5% versus 0.8%; $P = .02$). An unfavorable cervix was associated with an increased risk of cesarean delivery but not with any other adverse outcomes. One shortcoming of this study is that it did not control for the method of induction or the maximum oxytocin doses used.

In contrast, Cahill and colleagues [55] recently reported their results of a secondary analysis of a retrospective multicenter cohort study that included more than 25,000 women who had a history of cesarean delivery to determine the association between intrapartum oxytocin doses and rates of uterine rupture. They demonstrated a dose–response relationship between maximum oxytocin dose and the incidence of uterine rupture. The highest risk of uterine rupture was with oxytocin doses greater than 20 mU/min (OR, 2.98; 95% CI, 1.51–5.90; $P = .002$). The present authors recently reported similar findings in their case-control study [17]. Patients who experienced a uterine rupture were exposed to an increased duration (8.7 versus 6.0 hours; $P < .001$) and maximum dose of oxytocin (11.6 versus 7.2 mU/min, $P < .001$). Thus, it seems that induction and augmentation of labor with oxytocin in women who have a history of prior cesarean section is probably safe, although close attention should be paid to the length of exposure and the maximum doses used.

Uterine rupture risk associated with a failed trial of labor

Women electing a trial of labor should be informed that their risk for maternal morbidity is increased if they do not have a successful VBAC. In a large, multicenter prospective study the rate of uterine rupture was 22 times higher in a failed trial of labor [18]. McMahon also reported a fivefold increase in major maternal complications in cases of failed trial of labor versus successful trial of labor [56]. Hibbard and colleagues [4] studied a total of

2450 women who had a history of prior cesarean section and compared outcomes of three groups: (1) women who had a successful VBAC (2) women who had a failed trial of labor, and (3) women who underwent elective cesarean section. They found that women who had a failed trial of labor had a rate of uterine rupture 8.9% higher than that of women who had a successful VBAC. They also exhibited a higher risk of chorioamnionitis, transfusion, and endometritis.

Uterine rupture associated with prior cesarean delivery: timing of elective repeat cesarean delivery

In an otherwise uncomplicated pregnancy, elective repeat cesarean delivery should be performed at 39 completed weeks of gestation to ensure fetal pulmonary maturity. Given the increased risk of uterine rupture associated with classical uterine incisions, however, the gestational age of delivery should be adjusted for these patients. The optimal time of delivery is still a matter of some debate. Most recently, Stotland and colleagues [57] published a decision analysis comparing four delivery strategies that included delivery at 39 weeks' gestation, delivery at 36 weeks' gestation without amniocentesis, amniocentesis at 36 weeks with delivery if fetal lung maturity was confirmed and antenatal steroid administration otherwise, and weekly amniocentesis until fetal lung maturity was confirmed with subsequent delivery. They concluded that delivery at 36 weeks without amniocentesis provided the lowest risk for uterine rupture with minimal risk of major complications. Further studies confirming this theoretical model are needed before clinical recommendations can be made. The present authors typically offer amniocentesis at 36 weeks with delivery if studies show fetal lungs are mature or expectant management until 37 weeks of gestation in cases of documented pulmonary immaturity at 36 weeks.

Uterine rupture and perinatal morbidity

Perinatal morbidity is another important consideration in counseling women who are candidates for a trial of labor. Landon and colleagues [18] reported that hypoxic-ischemic encephalopathy (0.46 cases per 1000 trials of labor) is more common among women who undergo a trial of labor than in those who elect a repeat cesarean section. Overall risk of adverse perinatal outcome in women attempting a trial of labor was estimated at 1 in 2000. Just as a failed trial of labor is associated with an increased risk of major maternal morbidity, it also is associated with an increase in composite major neonatal morbidities (sepsis, respiratory distress syndrome, pneumonia, acidosis, intraventricular hemorrhage, subgaleal bleeding, and trauma) (6.3% versus 2.8%; $P = .014$) [58]. Another recent publication investigating the risk of uterine rupture and adverse perinatal outcome from the Maternal Fetal Medicine Units Network reports that the overall risk of serious adverse perinatal outcome (defined as stillbirth, hypoxic ischemic encephalopathy, or neonatal death) was 0.27% regardless of mode of delivery [1]. They also reported that more maternal deaths occurred in women undergoing elective cesarean section without an indication than in women attempting a trial of labor.

Summary

Uterine rupture during a trial of labor remains a rare event, with an estimated occurrence of approximately 0.7% in women who have had one prior low transverse uterine incision. If a uterine rupture occurs, it can have catastrophic consequences for both mother and fetus. Clinicians need to assess each individual patient's risk of rupture during the informed consent process. Important variables to consider include prior uterine surgery, the indication for the prior cesarean section, type of prior uterine incision, type of uterine closure, maternal age, maternal obesity, gestational age of prior cesarean section, interpregnancy interval, prior successful vaginal delivery, prior successful VBAC, and estimated fetal weight. For women who have had a prior classical incision, delivery between 36 and 37 weeks with or without amniocentesis seems reasonable. It remains to be seen if antepartum assessment of the uterine scar by ultrasound will give clinicians an objective measure of a patient's risk of uterine rupture in a trial of labor.

When a woman decides to attempt a trial of labor after a prior cesarean section, the obstetrician must pay close attention to the potential intrapartum predictors of uterine rupture, including moderate and severe variable decelerations in the fetal heart rate, especially when seen in association with persistent abdominal pain. Data suggest that increased exposure to oxytocin may increase the risk of uterine rupture. Overall risk of maternal and perinatal morbidity is low with a trial of labor, although it is increased with a failed trial of labor. Perhaps over time more intrapartum factors will be found to be reliable predictors of uterine rupture. Alternatively, it may become possible to predict uterine rupture based on a patient's antepartum risk factors. Currently, there are no methods available to accurately predict uterine rupture. Therefore, potential candidates for a trial of labor should be selected based on antepartum criteria. This selection process should include appropriate counseling and informed consent. Although the overall incidence of uterine rupture during a trial of labor is low, vigilance and maintaining a high index of suspicion for uterine rupture are crucial when managing a patient with a history of a prior cesarean section.

References

[1] Spong CY, Landon MB, Gilbert S, et al. Risk of uterine rupture and adverse perinatal outcome at term after cesarean delivery. Obstet Gynecol 2007;110:801–7.

[2] Cahill AG, Stamilio DM, Obido AO, et al. Is vaginal birth after cesarean (VBAC) or elective repeat cesarean safer in women with a prior vaginal delivery? Am J Obstet Gynecol 2006;195: 1143–7.

[3] Mozurkewich EL, Hutton EK. Elective repeat cesarean delivery versus a trial of labor: a meta-analysis of the literature from 1989 to 1999. Am J Obstet Gynecol 2000;183(5):1187–97.

[4] Hibbard JU, Ismail MA, Wang Y, et al. Failed vaginal birth after a cesarean section: how risky is it? Am J Obstet Gynecol 2001;184:1365–73.

[5] Hamilton BE, Martin JA, Ventura SJ. Births: preliminary data for 2005. Natl Vital Stat Rep 2005;55:1–19.

[6] Martin JA, Hamilton BE, Menacker F, et al. Births: final data for 2004. Natl Vital Stat Rep 2006;55:1–101.

[7] Miller DA, Goodwin TM, Gherman RB, et al. Intrapartum rupture of the unscarred uterus [review]. Obstet Gynecol 1997;89:671–3.

[8] Walsh CA, Baxi LV. Rupture of the primigravid uterus: a review of the literature. Obstet Gynecol Surv 2007;62:327–34.

[9] Seracchioli R, Manuzzi L, Vianello F, et al. Obstetric and delivery outcome of pregnancies achieved after laparoscopic myomectomy. Fertil Steril 2006;86:159–65.

[10] Kumakiri J, Takeuchi H, Kitade M, et al. Pregnancy and delivery after laparoscopic myomectomy. J Minim Invasive Gynecol 2005;12(3):241–6.

[11] American College of Obstetricians and Gynecologists. Vaginal birth after previous cesarean delivery. ACOG Practice Bulletin 54. Washington, DC: ACOG; 2004.

[12] Leung AD, Leung EK, Paul RH. Uterine rupture after previous cesarean delivery: maternal and fetal consequences. Am J Obstet Gynecol 1993;169:945–50.

[13] Farmer RM, Kirschbaum T, Potter D, et al. Uterine rupture during trial of labor after previous cesarean section. Am J Obstet Gynecol 1991;165(4 Pt 1):996–1001.

[14] Ayres AW, Johnson TR, Hayashi R. Characteristics of fetal heart rate tracings prior to uterine rupture. Int J Gynaecol Obstet 2001;74:235–40.

[15] Yap OW, Kim ES, Laros RK Jr. Maternal and neonatal outcomes after uterine rupture in labor. Am J Obstet Gynecol 2001;184:1576–81.

[16] Ridgeway JJ, Weyrich DL, Benedetti TJ. Fetal heart rate changes associated with uterine rupture. Obstet Gynecol 2004;103:506–12.

[17] Pryor EC, Mertz HL, Beaver BW, et al. Intrapartum predictors of uterine rupture. Am J Perinatol 2007;24:317–21.

[18] Landon MB, Hauth JC, Leveno KJ, et al. Maternal and perinatal outcomes associated with a trial of labor after prior cesarean delivery. N Engl J Med 2004;351:2581–9.

[19] Chapman SJ, Owen J, Hauth JC. One- versus two-layer closure of a low transverse cesarean: the next pregnancy. Obstet Gynecol 1997;89:16–8.

[20] Hauth JC, Owen J, Davis RO. Transverse uterine incision closure: one versus two layers. Am J Obstet Gynecol 1992;167:1108–11.

[21] Durnwald C, Mercer B. Uterine rupture, perioperative and perinatal morbidity after single-layer and double-layer closure at cesarean delivery. Am J Obstet Gynecol 2003;189:925–9.

[22] Bujold E, Bujold C, Hamilton EF, et al. The impact of a single-layer or double-layer closure on uterine rupture. Am J Obstet Gynecol 2002;186:1326–30.

[23] Gyamfi C, Juhasz G, Gyamfi P, et al. Single-versus double layer uterine incision closure and uterine rupture. J Matern Fetal Neonatal Med 2006;19:639–43.

[24] Landon MB, Spong CY, Thom E, et al. Risk of uterine rupture with a trial of labor in women with multiple and single prior cesarean delivery. Obstet Gynecol 2006;108:12–20.

[25] Macones GA, Cahill A, Pare E, et al. Obstetric outcomes in women with two prior cesarean deliveries: is vaginal birth after cesarean delivery a viable option? Am J Obstet Gynecol 2005; 192:1223–8.

[26] Landon MB, Leindecker S, Spong CY, et al. The MFMU cesarean registry: factors affecting the success of trial of labor after previous cesarean delivery. Am J Obstet Gynecol 2005;193: 1016–23.

[27] Macones GA, Peipert J, Nelson DB, et al. Maternal complications with vaginal birth after cesarean delivery: a multicenter study. Am J Obstet Gynecol 2005;193:1656–62.

[28] Zelop CM, Shipp TD, Repke JT, et al. Effect of previous vaginal delivery on the risk of uterine rupture during a subsequent trial of labor. Am J Obstet Gynecol 2000;183:1184–6.

[29] Shipp TD, Zelop CM, Repke JT, et al. Interdelivery interval and risk of symptomatic uterine rupture. Obstet Gynecol 2001;97:175–7.

[30] Huang WH, Nakashima DK, Rumney PJ, et al. Interdelivery interval and the success of vaginal birth after cesarean delivery. Obstet Gynecol 2002;99:41–4.

[31] Quinones JN, Stamilio DM, Pare E, et al. The effect of prematurity on vaginal birth after cesarean delivery: success and maternal morbidity. Obstet Gynecol 2005;105:519–24.

[32] Durnwald CP, Rouse DJ, Leveno KJ, et al. The Maternal-Fetal Medicine Units cesarean registry: safety and efficacy of a trial of labor in preterm pregnancy after a prior cesarean delivery. Am J Obstet Gynecol 2006;195:1119–26.

[33] Montan S. Increased risk in the elderly parturient. Curr Opin Obstet Gynecol 2007;19:110–2.

[34] Reddy UM, Ko CW, Willinger M. Maternal age and the risk of stillbirth throughout pregnancy in the United States. Am J Obstet Gynecol 2007;195:764–70.

[35] Shipp TD, Zelop C, Repke JT, et al. The association of maternal age and symptomatic uterine rupture during a trial of labor after prior cesarean delivery. Obstet Gynecol 2002;99:585–8.

[36] Bujold E, Hammoud AO, Hendler I, et al. Trial of labor in patients with a previous cesarean section: does maternal age influence the outcome? Am J Obstet Gynecol 2004;190:1113–8.

[37] Kaczmarczyk M, Sparen P, Terry P, et al. Risk factors for uterine rupture and neonatal consequences of uterine rupture: a population-based study of successive pregnancies in Sweden. BJOG 2007;114:1208–14.

[38] Hoyert DL, Matthews TJ, Menacker F, et al. Annual summary of vital statistics: 2004. Pediatrics 2006;117:168–83.

[39] Varner MW, Leindecker S, Spong CY, et al. The Maternal Fetal Medicine Unit cesarean registry: trial of labor with a twin gestation. Am J Obstet Gynecol 2005;193:135–40.

[40] Ford AAD, Bateman BT, Simpson LL. Vaginal birth after cesarean delivery in twin gestations: a large, nationwide sample of deliveries. Am J Obstet Gynecol 2006;195:1138–42.

[41] Chu SY, Kim SY, Lau J, et al. Maternal obesity and risk of stillbirth: a metaanalysis. Am J Obstet Gynecol 2007;197:223–8.

[42] Hibbard JU, Gilbert S, Landon MB, et al. Trial of labor or repeat cesarean delivery in women with morbid obesity and previous cesarean delivery. Obstet Gynecol 2006;108:125–33.

[43] Zelop CM, Shipp TD, Repke JT, et al. Outcomes of trial of labor following previous cesarean delivery among women with fetuses weighing >4000g. Am J Obstet Gynecol 2001;185:903–5.

[44] Rochelson B, Pagano M, Conetta L, et al. Previous preterm cesarean delivery: identification of a new risk factor for uterine rupture in VBAC candidates. J Matern Fetal Neonatal Med 2005;18:339–42.

[45] Varner MW, Thom E, Spong CY, et al. Trial of labor after one previous cesarean delivery for multifetal gestation. Obstet Gynecol 2007;110:814–9.

[46] Cheung VY. Sonographic measurement of the lower uterine segment thickness in women with previous cesarean section. J Obstet Gynaecol Can 2005;27:674–81.

[47] Macones GA, Cahill AG, Stamilio DM, et al. Can uterine rupture in patients attempting vaginal birth after cesarean delivery be predicted? Am J Obstet Gynecol 2006;195:1148–52.

[48] Wing DA, Lovett K, Paul RH. Disruption of prior uterine incision following misoprostol for labor induction in women with previous cesarean delivery. Obstet Gynecol 1998;91:828–30.

[49] Lydon-Rochelle M, Holt VL, Easterling TR, et al. Risk of uterine rupture during labor among women with a prior cesarean delivery. N Engl J Med 2001;345:3–8.

[50] American College of Obstetricians and Gynecologists. Induction of labor for vaginal birth after cesarean delivery. ACOG Committee Opinion 342. Washington, DC: American College of Obstetricians and Gynecologists; 2006.

[51] Rosen MG, Dickinson JC, Westhoff CL. Vaginal birth after cesarean: a meta-analysis of morbidity and mortality. Obstet Gynecol 1991;77:465–70.

[52] Goetzl L, Shipp TD, Cohen A, et al. Oxytocin dose and the risk of uterine rupture in trial of labor after cesarean. Obstet Gynecol 2001;97:381–4.

[53] Merrill DC, Zlatnik FJ. Randomized, double-masked comparison of oxytocin dosage in induction and augmentation of labor. Obstet Gynecol 1999;455–63.

[54] Grobman WA, Gilbert S, Landon MB, et al. Outcomes of induction of labor after one prior cesarean. Obstet Gynecol 2007;109:262–9.

[55] Cahill AG, Stamilio DM, Odibo AO, et al. Does a maximum dose of oxytocin affect risk for uterine rupture in candidates for vaginal birth after cesarean delivery? Am J Obstet Gynecol 2007;197:495.e1–5.

[56] McMahon MJ, Luther ER, Bowes WA Jr, et al. Comparison of a trial of labor with an elective second cesarean section. N Engl J Med 1996;335:689–95.

[57] Stotland NE, LipschitzLS, Caughey AB. Delivery strategies for women with a previous classic cesarean delivery: a decision analysis. Am J Obstet Gynecol 2002;187:1203–8.

[58] El-Sayed YY, Watkins MM, Fix M, et al. Perinatal outcomes after successful and failed trials of labor after cesarean delivery. Am J Obstet Gynecol 2007;196:583.e1–5.

ELSEVIER
SAUNDERS

CLINICS IN
PERINATOLOGY

Clin Perinatol 35 (2008) 101–117

Medication Errors in Obstetrics

Toni A. Kfuri, MD, MPH, CMQ, FACOG[a],*,
Laura Morlock, PhD[a],
Rodney W. Hicks, PhD, RN[b],
Andrew D. Shore, PhD[c]

[a]*Department of Health Policy and Management, Johns Hopkins Bloomberg School of Public Health, 624 N. Broadway, Baltimore, MD 21205, USA*
[b]*Texas Tech University Health Sciences Center School of Nursing, Lubbock, TX 79430, USA*
[c]*Health Services Research and Development Center, The Johns Hopkins Bloomberg School of Public Health, 624 N. Broadway, Room 637, Baltimore, MD 21205, USA*

The provisional August 2007 National Vital Statistics report from the National Center for Health Statistics showed that in 2006 a total of 4,269,000 births were registered in the United States, slightly more than in 2005 [1]. After a downward trend in the 1990s, the total number of pregnancies in the United States has generally been increasing. The crude birth rate recently peaked at 16.7 per 1000 women and is now fluctuating between 13.9 and 14.4 per 1000 women [1]. Pregnancy risk factors are also on the rise. In 2004, 20% of obstetric patients had weight gains of more than 40 pounds [1], and pregnancy-associated hypertension and diabetes occurred among 4% of mothers (37.9% and 35.8% per 1000 births, respectively). The National Center for Health Statistics [1] also reports that the prevalence of diabetes rose by more than two thirds from 1990 to 2004 (from 21.3 to 35.8 per 1000 live births) and that the prevalence of chronic hypertension increased by almost one half since 1990 (6.5 in 1990 versus 9.6 in 2004). These increased risk factors together with the rise in maternal age [2] and chronic diseases point to a potential increase in medication prescriptions and use among the obstetric population, prompting concern regarding iatrogenic disease from medication errors in obstetrics.

* Corresponding author. P.O. Box 4303, Timonium, MD 21094.
E-mail address: akfuri@jhsph.edu (T.A. Kfuri).

0095-5108/08/$ - see front matter © 2008 Elsevier Inc. All rights reserved.
doi:10.1016/j.clp.2007.11.015 *perinatology.theclinics.com*

Prescribing and use of medications during pregnancy

Physicians do no harm

Obstetricians and perinatologists face a constant challenge in managing pregnant women who use medications because of the fear of teratogenicity and the potential for fetal harm as well as litigation. Drug use patterns during pregnancy are difficult to assess given that over 90% of pregnant patients take prescription medications and an equal number self-medicate with over-the-counter medications. Furthermore, 45% of pregnant women use herbal medications [3].

In 1979 the U.S. Food and Drug Administration (FDA) introduced a classification of fetal risks associated with the use of pharmaceuticals. Category D drugs are those "with positive evidence of human fetal risk, based on adverse reaction data." Category X drugs are those with "studies done on humans that have demonstrated fetal abnormalities and/or there is positive evidence of human fetal risk, based on adverse reaction data" [4]. A recent 2-year cross-sectional study of office visits by pregnant women [5] showed that there is considerable medication use of FDA class D and X medications. These medications account for 6.4% of prescriptions given at visits in private office-based practices and 2.9% of prescriptions in hospital settings. Class X drugs were most likely to include estrogens, medroxyprogesterone, warfarin, methotrexate, triazolam, simvastatin, and iodinated glycerol. Older pregnant women in the study were twice as likely to receive a class D or X medication when compared with younger patients. In a retrospective study, the medical records of delivered patients over a 4-year time span revealed that 5.8% of the patients had received an FDA class D or X medication early during pregnancy [6]. Furthermore, 1.1% of patients had received teratogenic medications during the 270 days before delivery. These drugs included carbamazepine, fluconazole, propylthiouracil, lithium, and tetracycline.

During the past 20 years, providers who care for pregnant women and the women themselves often have had inadequate information about the risks and benefits of a large number of prescribed teratogenic medications. Lo and Friedman [7] used standard clinical teratology resources to assess the risks of therapeutic treatment for 468 drugs approved by the FDA and concluded that between 1980 and 2000 the risk of teratogenicity was undetermined for 91.2% of the drugs. Despite limited data on prescription drugs, many physicians continue prescribing class X medications for pregnant women [8]. Some of these drugs clearly have no indications for use during pregnancy. In a recent 1-year study investigating the extent of self-reported use of prescription drugs during pregnancy, researchers found that prescription medication use was common among pregnant women. Four percent of the sampled cohort reported using FDA class D or X products, including dangerous medications such as tetracycline, doxycycline, isotretinoin, and cyclophosphamide. After adjusting for comorbid conditions, the study found that African American women were more likely than Caucasians to use a class D or X prescription drug during pregnancy. Women with less education were also more likely than college graduates to use such prescription medications [9].

There are definitely drug alternatives that are safer and carry lesser risks for the mother and fetus that providers could use. Examples include the replacement of tetracycline with penicillin and the replacement of sulfa medications with ampicillin. Providers should be well educated about potential teratogens. In addition, they must be extremely vigilant to weigh the advantages and risks associated with known teratogenic medications before allowing unnecessary exposure during pregnancy which could result in devastating fetal effects.

Isotretinoin, a potent human teratogen, is of particular concern because of its widespread popularity among young women and the dramatic increase in its use over the last decade. There are now three generic versions of this medication in the United States, further complicating the risk management of possible isotretinoin–exposed pregnancies. Four companies currently market this medication in the United States. They could jointly and voluntarily establish a consolidated mandatory registration and follow-up of all women who receive an isotretinoin prescription [10]. Such consolidated risk management has the potential of limiting the occurrence of exposed pregnancies and avoiding devastating fetal effects and possible subsequent litigation.

A recent study using a mother-baby record linkage based on data from the General Practice Research Database from the United Kingdom identified a large cohort of ($> 80,000$) pregnant women and concluded that 1 in every 164 women received an FDA class X prescription in early pregnancy [11]. These results should alert physicians to review all prescriptions early in pregnancy and to be aware and cautious regarding the possibility of prescribing a class X medication.

How to effectively decrease the dispensing of class D and X medications was the focus of a recent randomized trial in which usual care patterns were compared with a pharmacist's intervention. A computerized tool was used by pharmacists to alert physicians when a prescription was associated with an FDA class D or X product [12]. The study found that patients in the intervention group were dispensed 2.9% of class D or X products, whereas the usual care group received 5.5% of these products ($P < .001$). Prescribing contraindicated medication to pregnant patients is a serious but preventable error that can be easily controlled in early prenatal care visits, when a thorough history taking can avert a potentially serious problem not only for the patient but also for her progeny.

Patients do no harm

Known teratogens can be traced with respect to their associated fetal effects through pharmacoepidemiologic research. For over-the-counter medication use in pregnancy, such a known association may not be sufficient to guide behavior because of the absence of prescriptions or the means to follow patients over time. The FDA has mandated that drug labels clearly describe the drug's potential injury to the unborn as well as its potential ill effect on the mother. Despite such warnings, many antepartum patients opt to take popular over-the-counter medications. Such medication use during pregnancy is extremely common [13] and most often includes analgesics, decongestants, and antihistamines. For example, in one study, 15% of patients took ibuprofen, with one third of the medication consumed in the third trimester [3]. Empiric evidence of whether such exposures are safe is lacking. Studies are needed to examine the possible associations between over-the-counter medications and birth defects to develop the evidence necessary to inform pregnant women and their providers about potential risks.

The American College of Obstetricians and Gynecologists (ACOG) April 2006 Committee Opinion on the "Safe Use of Medication" stresses the point that "clinicians should assist the patient in understanding the medical condition for which a medication has been prescribed" and suggests that one engage the patient in her own care [14]. This committee opinion also emphasizes that medication ordering errors are the leading cause of medical errors and that physicians should be familiar with medications before prescribing them to their obstetric patients. Safe practices will help avoid medication use errors by maintaining up-to-date references on current medications, understanding the appropriate indications, considering alternatives, and increasing awareness of special situations that may affect the efficacy of prescribed medications or the interactions of specific agents with other medications that are used concomitantly by the patient.

Depression and pregnancy

A growing number of women of reproductive age use psychotropic medications, with evidence suggesting that pregnant women over 35 years of age are twice as likely to use antidepressants as those under 35 years of age [15]. The estimated prevalence of depression during pregnancy is 10% to 16% [16]. A large cohort study of Dutch pregnant patients (N = 20,007) found that, during the first trimester, 2% of all pregnant women were taking antidepressants, and 1.8% were also taking anxiolytics during the second and third trimesters. Paroxetine and fluoxetine were the most frequently used antidepressants during pregnancy [16]. A more recent, larger, 4-year cohort study from the Tennessee Obstetric Medicaid program revealed an even higher exposure to antidepressants. The proportion of pregnancies with antidepressant use increased from 5.7% in 1999 to 13.4% in 2003 [8].

Psychotropic medications have many potential adverse side effects and deserve special attention, especially among pregnant women. There is much uncertainty and debate concerning the safety of antidepressant use in pregnancy. Maternal concerns surround preterm labor and postnatal withdrawal symptoms as well as the increased fetal risks of cardiovascular malformations and persistent pulmonary hypertension [16]. It is imperative that maternal health providers be well versed in the pharmacology of psychotropic drugs and remain vigilant given that a considerable number of newborns are exposed to such agents and may need special care in the immediate neonatal period. Although psychotropic drugs are necessary in some cases, in many others nonpharmacologic treatments offer valid alternatives for the pregnant woman. The noxious effects of antidepressants and anxiolytics should urge providers of obstetric care to look for possible alternatives. These options might include enhancing the efficacy of alternative treatments through early detection, monitoring for mood disorders beginning in the earliest stages of pregnancy, and the concerted efforts of multidisciplinary teams.

It is imperative to examine drug-prescribing patterns for obstetric patients and to examine carefully those medications prescribed and used in addition to prenatal vitamins and iron and folic acid supplements. The over-the-counter use of analgesics, antihistamines, and antacids by pregnant women in response to physiologic changes affecting their bodies, together with the daily long-term use of medications for chronic illnesses and more recently the increased use of psychotropic drugs, makes the obstetric patient an increasing challenge. Exposure to such a "polypharmacy" places the pregnant patient at high risk for medication errors.

Scope of the problem during labor and delivery

The medication use process in the labor and delivery area deserves attention and vigilance because of the continuous emergent and sometimes unexpected nature of the laboring process. During labor and delivery, pain medication may include narcotics, conduction anesthesia, or local blocks. Labor induction and augmentation will always necessitate some exposure to drugs. A patient in labor may also need intravenous fluids and, possibly, the use of general anesthesia. The ACOG issued a Committee Opinion on preventing medication errors in the urgent surgical environment where orders are given verbally, making them vulnerable to misinterpretation or misapplication [17]. Critical information must be available and constantly updated to all members of the care team. A contemporaneous documentation is also necessary for maintaining patient safety.

One recent study identified 164 medication errors in an obstetric hospital [18], the majority involving oral and parenteral antibiotics and analgesics. Another cohort study of 425 obstetric patients [19] identified a 2% risk for an adverse drug event, most commonly associated with "system problems" such as failure of medication delivery or order implementation. This study concluded that quality problems are common and should be targets for improvement [19]. Table 1 lists a series of case reports and other studies [20–27] on

Table 1
Series of case reports on medication errors in obstetrics

Study	Drug	Error	Type of error	Adverse effects
Pocock and Chen 2006 [20]	Antibiotic prophylaxis for infective endocarditis	Not AHA/ACOG regimens	Wrong medication/wrong dose/wrong timing	Intrapartum infection Chorioamnionitis
Glover et al 2004 [21]	Codeine for analgesia	Add: paroxetine	Drug-drug interaction	Lower analgesic efficiency
Glover et al [21]	Central nervous system depressant	Kava	Drug-drug interaction	Severe depression
Glover et al [21]	Oral contraceptives	St. John's wort	Drug-drug interaction	Bleeding
Reedy et al 1992 [22]	Prostaglandin E_1	Prostaglandin F_{2alpha}	Wrong medication	Disseminated intravascular coagulation, ventricular tachycardia, hypotension
Joy et al 2005 [23]	Nevirapine for HIV and pregnancy	Started in third trimester	Incorrect timing	Hepatitis/renal failure/rash/eosinophilia
Fujii and Numazaki 2002 [24]	Propofol for emesis in cesarean section	Suboptimum dose, 0.5 mg/kg/h	Incorrect dose	Nausea/vomiting/retching/no sedation
Simpson 2006 [25]	$MgSO_4$ for preterm labor	16 g bolus of $MgSO_4$	Overdose $4\times$	Maternal death
Goodman et al 2006 [26]	$MgSO_4$ for preeclampsia	8.7 g through the epidural space	Incorrect route	Malaise/disorientation
Goodman et al 2006 [26]	$MgSO_4$	9.6 g through the epidural space	Incorrect route/wrong medication	Arrest of labor/fetal tachycardia/cesarean section
Bilal et al 2002 [27]	Antimicrobials for nosocomial infection	Drug resistant pathogens	Wrong medication/wrong dose	Multiple-drug resistant pathogens/UTI MRSA endemic nursery

Abbreviation: UTI MRSA, urinary tract infection with methicillin-resistant *Staphylococcus aureus.*
Courtesy of Toni A. Kfuri, MD, MPH, CMQ, Timonium, MD.

medication errors involving obstetric patients, some with severe if not fatal consequences. These case reports document various types of errors, including the wrong dose, wrong timing, or wrong medication. Some adverse effects included liver or kidney damage, bleeding, and maternal death.

Medication errors can be costly. Economic data on medication errors and adverse drug reactions have been generated through examining medical malpractice information using Pennsylvania Health Insurance Company's closed claims data [28]. Excluding the costs of litigation, an adverse drug reaction may cost up to $2500 in additional hospital resources, and a preventable medication error may cost almost $4500 [28]. Data from the National Practitioner Data Bank [29] indicate that $184,986 was the mean medical malpractice payment associated with medication-related malpractice claims in the United States in 2002. Information from this data bank also reveals that 10,408 payments were made due to medication-related malpractice in the United States during 2002. Diagnostic, therapeutic, and communication issues were the most common factors identified in a retrospective "cause and effect" analysis of closed claims in obstetrics and gynecology [30].

An analysis of medication errors in obstetrics using data from the MEDMARX program

For more than 15 years, the United States Pharmacopeia (USP) has operated several nationally recognized, voluntary, medication error reporting programs. MEDMARX, an Internet accessible, anonymous, medication error reporting program, began in 1998 and is currently licensed through subscriptions to hospitals and related health systems for use in quality improvement activities aimed at improving safe medication use. This program contains more than 1.3 million medication error records collected during 1998 to 2005 from more than 870 hospitals. The USP uses patterns identified from this reporting system in the standards-setting process to address issues with medication nomenclature, packaging, storage, and labeling.

A survey by Savage and colleagues [31] regarding the utility of MEDMARX was developed and mailed to 550 hospitals and health care systems that used the medication error reporting program. Most participating facilities (94%) generated reports from the medication error database, and 75% used this information to identify many opportunities for improving their medication use system. It was concluded that the implementation of this voluntary, on-line reporting system led to an increase in the number of reported medication errors and to improvements in the medication use process.

Methods

The authors examined a 36-month (January 1, 2003 through December 31, 2005) sample of MEDMARX medication error reports that identified at least one medication product associated with inpatient obstetric patients in the labor and delivery area, the obstetric recovery room, or the maternity ward. For each report, we examined the severity of the error using the National Coordinating Council for Medication Error Reporting and Prevention's (NCC MERP's) Index for Categorizing a Medication Error [32]. Other medication error data fields examined included the phase of the medication use process in which the error originated, the level of staff identified as having made the initial error, the type of error, and the product associated with the error. The main objective of the analysis was to compare the medication error profiles for the three obstetric inpatient locations. Because medication error reports are "clustered" by reporting facility, differences across the inpatient locations were tested for statistical significance using the Rao-Scott modified chi-square test which takes into consideration the clustered nature of the data [33]. Given the anonymous nature of MEDMARX data, this study received exempt status from our institutional review committee.

Results

During the study period, MEDMARX received 4583 obstetric medication error reports, which represented about 4.8% of all reports submitted over the same time period. Errors occurred in each of the reporting locations (Table 2), with 48% taking place in the labor and delivery area, about 5% in the recovery room, and 47% in the maternity ward. The percentages of errors reported from the labor and delivery area were comparable with that in a previous report based on MEDMARX data [34], although there was some increase in the number and percentage of error reports from maternity wards and fewer from recovery areas. What is more significant is the total number of errors reported—3775 obstetric errors within the earlier 4-year period [34] in comparison with 4583 obstetric medication errors within the more recent 3-year time frame.

Table 2
Number of medication errors reported to MEDMARX during two reporting periods by error location

| Reporting period | Error location | | | |
	Labor/delivery, number (%)	Maternity ward, number (%)	Obstetric recovery room, number (%)	Total, number (%)
August 1998–December 2002[a]	1844 (48.9)	1560 (41.3)	371 (9.8)	3775 (100)
January 2003–December 2005	2218 (48.4)	2143 (46.8)	222 (4.8)	4583 (100)

[a] *Data from* Beyea SC, Kobokovich LJ, Becker SC, et al. Medication errors in the LDRP. AWHONN Lifelines 2004;8:130–40.

Error severity

The majority of reports to voluntary reporting systems such as MED-MARX involve errors that result in no patient harm (so-called "near misses"), with the objective of identifying vulnerabilities in systems of care that need to be remedied to prevent future patient harm. The great majority of obstetric medication errors reported to the system during this time period did not result in patient harm; however, 3.2% (146 of 4583) were identified as harmful (Table 3). Harmful medication errors included 122 that involved temporary harm and required a patient care intervention, 18 that were associated with temporary harm that required initial or prolonged hospitalization, 3 that involved permanent patient harm, and an additional 3 that required intervention necessary to sustain life. Significantly ($P < .001$) more harmful medication errors of all categories were reported from labor and delivery areas than from maternity wards or obstetric recovery rooms.

Origin of medication errors

For each of the three clinical areas, some errors originated in each of the phases of the medication use process (Table 4), although the great majority ($> 70\%$) in all three clinical areas occurred while administering medications to patients. Across all three locations, approximately 5% of medication errors originated during the prescribing phase, 13% during transcribing, 8% during dispensing, and almost 1% during patient monitoring. An analysis

Table 3
Harmful and nonharmful medication errors by error location

Degree of harm experienced by patient	Error location			
	Labor/delivery, number (%)	Maternity ward, number (%)	Obstetric recovery room, number (%)	Total, number (%)
No harm	2125 (95.8)	2094 (97.7)	218 (98.2)	4437 (96.8)
Harm[a]	93 (4.2)	49 (2.3)	4 (1.8)	146 (3.2)[b]
Category E	76	43	3	122
Category F	13	4	1	18
Category G	2	1	0	3
Category H	2	1	0	3
Total (row %)	2218 (48.4)	2143 (46.8)	222 (4.8)	4583 (100)

[a] Based on the National Coordinating Council for Medication Error Reporting and Prevention Index (A through I); ratings of E through I are considered indicative of patient harm. Category E = error may have contributed to or resulted in temporary harm to the patient and required intervention. Category F = error may have contributed to or resulted in temporary harm to the patient and required initial or prolonged hospitalization. Category G = error may have contributed to or resulted in permanent patient harm. Category H = error required intervention necessary to sustain life.

[b] Differences among error locations between harmful and no harm events are significant at the $P < .001$ level based on a Rao-Scott modified chi-square test.

Data from Medication errors reported to the MEDMARX database from January 1, 2003, through December 31, 2005.

Table 4
Phase in the medication use process where errors originated by error location

Phase in the medication use process where the error originated[a]	Labor and delivery, number (%)	Maternity ward, number (%)	Obstetric recovery room, number (%)	Total number of errors, number (%)
Prescribing	135 (6.1)	91 (4.2)	7 (3.2)	233 (5.1)
Transcribing	223 (10.1)	324 (15.1)	39 (17.6)	586 (12.8)
Dispensing	184 (8.3)	191 (8.9)	16 (7.2)	391 (8.5)
Administering	1651 (74.5)	1524 (71.1)	158 (71.2)	3333 (72.8)
Monitoring	23 (1.0)	13 (0.6)	2 (0.9)	38 (0.8)
Total (row %)	2216 (48.4)	2143 (46.8)	222 (4.8)	4581 (100.0)

[a] Differences among error locations are significant at the $P < .01$ level based on a Rao-Scott modified chi-square test.

Data from Medication errors reported to the MEDMARX database from January 1, 2003, through December 31, 2005.

of all medication errors resulting in patient harm also indicated that the great majority (72%) were associated with errors during the medication administration phase (data not shown). In comparing the three clinical settings, the proportion of errors originating during prescribing was highest in labor and delivery, whereas the proportion of transcribing errors was highest in obstetric recovery rooms ($P < .01$).

Staff identified as associated with the initial error

Hospital staff members in direct contact with the patient are also involved with the medication use process. These personnel encompass physicians, residents, and nursing staff as well as pharmacists and their technicians. The MEDMARX data indicate that most types of hospital personnel were responsible for one or more medication errors during this time period (Table 5). Physicians, pharmacists, and nurses (both licensed practical and registered nurses) formed the majority of responsible personnel. Registered nurses were associated with the greatest number of errors (78.2%), a pattern that is internally consistent with the finding that most medication errors originate during the medication administration process. Although registered nurses are associated with the majority of medication errors in all three clinical settings, they are involved in proportionately fewer errors reported from obstetric recovery rooms than from the other two locations ($P < .001$).

Types of medication errors

The most common types of errors reported to MEDMARX from the three clinical settings combined (Table 6) included omission errors (32% of all errors), followed by errors involving improper doses (17%) or wrong timing (17%) and unauthorized drugs (16%). Less frequent were errors involving extra doses (5%), incorrect preparations (3%), wrong administration techniques (3%), wrong patients (2%), administration by the wrong route

Table 5
Level of staff associated with the initial medication error

Level of staff associated with the initial error[a]	Error location			
	Labor and delivery, number (%)	Maternity ward, number (%)	Obstetrics recovery room, number (%)	Total, number (%)
Registered nurse	1788 (80.6)	1659 (77.5)	135 (60.8)	3582 (78.2)
Physician	121 (5.5)	85 (4.0)	11 (5.0)	217 (4.7)
Pharmacist	90 (4.1)	68 (3.2)	10 (4.5)	168 (3.7)
Licensed practical nurse/vocational nurse	54 (2.4)	94 (4.4)	6 (2.7)	154 (3.4)
Nursing personnel, nonspecific	44 (2.0)	82 (3.8)	11 (5.0)	137 (3.0)
Unit secretary/ clerk	21 (0.9)	32 (1.5)	9 (4.1)	62 (1.4)
Post-baccalaureate nurse	26 (1.2)	23 (1.1)	5 (2.3)	54 (1.2)
Pharmacy technician	20 (0.9)	26 (1.2)	1 (0.5)	47 (1.0)
Pharmacy personnel, nonspecific	8 (0.4)	19 (0.9)	4 (1.8)	31 (0.7)
Other personnel	46 (2.1)	53 (2.5)	30 (13.6)	129 (2.8)
Total (row %)	2218 (48.4)	2143 (46.8)	222 (4.8)	4581 (100.0)

[a] Differences among error locations are significant at the $P < .001$ level based on a Rao-Scott modified chi-square test.

Data from Medication errors reported to the MEDMARX database from January 1, 2003, through December 31, 2005.

(2%), or wrong dosage forms (1%). By location, the highest omission rate (46%) was associated with errors reported from obstetric recovery rooms ($P < .001$). The labor and delivery area had the highest percentage (20%) of improper dose/quantity errors ($P < .001$). An earlier analysis of types of medication errors reported to the MEDMARX system [33] also found a predominance of omission errors, with the percentages of these errors in labor and delivery settings and maternity wards similar to the findings in our study of a later time period; however, the earlier analysis found a lower percentage (33%) of omission errors reported from obstetric recovery rooms than that reported (46%) during the time period of our study.

An analysis of types of errors resulting in patient harm suggests that the highest proportions of these errors are most likely to result from omission errors (27%), improper doses or quantities (27%), and unauthorized or wrong medications (22%).

Pharmaceutical products involved in errors

The ten most commonly reported pharmaceutical products associated with obstetric medication errors during the study period are displayed in

Table 6
Selected types of medication errors by location

Type of error	Labor and delivery, number (%)	Maternity ward, number (%)	Obstetric recovery room, number (%)	Total, number (%)	P value[a]
Omission error	655 (29.5)	728 (34.0)	103 (46.4)	1486 (32.4)	P < .001
Wrong time	373 (16.8)	390 (18.2)	24 (10.8)	787 (17.2)	NS
Improper dose/ quantity	438 (19.7)	319 (14.9)	28 (12.6)	785 (17.1)	P < .0001
Unauthorized/ wrong drug	376 (17.0)	332 (15.5)	38 (17.1)	746 (16.3)	NS
Extra dose	93 (4.2)	141 (6.6)	14 (6.3)	248 (5.4)	P < .05
Drug prepared incorrectly	70 (3.2)	75 (3.5)	7 (3.2)	152 (3.3)	NS
Wrong administration technique	88 (4.0)	57 (2.7)	3 (1.4)	148 (3.2)	P < .01
Wrong patient	42 (1.9)	50 (2.3)	5 (2.3)	97 (2.1)	NS
Wrong route	35 (1.6)	41 (1.9)	4 (1.8)	80 (1.7)	NS
Wrong dosage form	14 (0.6)	18 (0.8)	1 (0.5)	33 (0.7)	NS

[a] Tests of statistical significance are based on Rao-Scott modified chi-square tests. NS indicates not significant at P < .05.

Data from Medication errors reported to the MEDMARX database from January 1, 2003, through December 31, 2005.

Table 7. Antibiotics, including ampicillin, cefazolin, and gentamicin, formed the largest therapeutic class (26% of all products associated with errors), followed by opioid analgesics including meperidine, oxycodone, and acetaminophen (18%), and non-steroidal anti-inflammatory drugs and tocolytics, including magnesium sulfate.

The most commonly reported obstetric drugs resulting in harmful medication errors were also identified (Fig. 1). The most common obstetric

Table 7
Top ten medications associated with obstetric medication errors

Generic name	Count
Ampicillin	381
Oxytocin	250
Ibuprofen	243
Cefazolin	236
Oxycodone and acetaminophen	183
Ketorolac	155
Magnesium sulfate	146
Terbutaline	116
Gentamicin	111
Meperidine	98

Data from Medication errors reported to the MEDMARX database from January 1, 2003, through December 31, 2005.

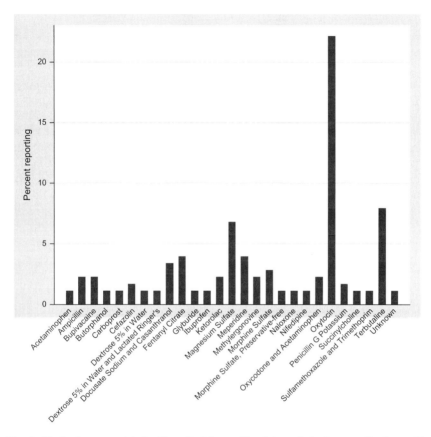

Fig. 1. Medications associated with patient harm. The data exclude those medications with only one occurrence. (*Data from* Medication errors reported to the MEDMARX database from January 1, 2003, through December 31, 2005.)

medication was oxytocin (22% of all medications associated with patient harm), a medication used across the three clinical areas of obstetrics. Primarily used to induce or augment labor, its effects are dose related and require continuous monitoring, sometimes with invasive modalities such as an intrauterine pressure device and fetal electrode. Terbutaline and magnesium sulfate were the other two medications most commonly involved in harmful outcomes to the patient. All products associated with two or more harmful errors are displayed in Fig. 1 to alert providers of obstetric care to the potential for harm when using these medications.

Discussion

The findings highlighted in this article suggest that obstetricians and perinatologists face a number of challenges for safe medication use during pregnancy. Furthermore, evidence of in-hospital medication errors from obstetric services has been provided by national medication error data voluntarily submitted from many hospitals. Secondary analysis of data from large reporting systems provides an economically efficient means of studying the iatrogenic impact of medication errors experienced by obstetric patients. The data provide fresh insight into the nature of medication errors in obstetrics, especially regarding the medication use process, the most common types of errors reported, the most commonly reported products overall, as well as those that resulted in patient harm. Providers and staff working within health care organizations should be well aware that a substantial number of patients experience medication errors that can result in serious injuries.

The percentages of errors reported from the labor and delivery area are comparable with that in a previous report using MEDMARX data [34] except for an increase in the number and percentage of error reports from maternity wards and fewer reports from recovery areas. Although the number of errors increased from the previous study, the results could be attributed to more facilities participating, a more enhanced willingness to report errors, or better error detection methods. No firm conclusion can be drawn to infer that patients are less safe; rather, the openness to report such events could be responsible and should be applauded.

The medication use process is complex and follows a sequence of identifiable steps. The prescriber selects the product based on a patient assessment. Nursing personnel often transcribe the order. The pharmacist reviews the order and releases the product for clinical use. Finally, the patient receives the medication. More than 70% of obstetric medication errors reported originated in the "administering node" of the medication use process. Although this high percentage may indicate better reporting of errors in this phase of the medication use process, there are also fewer opportunities in the administration phase to detect and correct errors before they reach the patient. Medication administration must be an important focal area for interdisciplinary quality improvement activities.

Providers and other staff members involved in obstetric care should seek all opportunities and avenues for improvement in medication errors management. The seven recommendations promulgated by the Institute of Medicine (IOM) report, "Preventing Medication Errors," are likely to be helpful in this regard [35]. The purpose of this study, sponsored by the Centers for Medicare and Medicaid services, was to develop action agendas for reducing medication errors based on incidence, costs, and available evidence of prevention strategies. The IOM committee estimated that "on average, a hospital patient is subject to at least one medication error per day, with considerable variation in error rates" [35]. The committee also identified "enormous gaps in the knowledge base with regard to medication errors" and suggested that a key approach for reducing medication errors is "establishing and maintaining a strong provider-patient partnership." Although

Table 8
Reported implemented actions consistent with the IOM recommendations and results achieved in medication safety

Study	Action implemented	IOM recommendation	Results improvement
Costello et al 2007 [36]	Pharmacy-led medication safety team	#3: Active monitoring	Increased reporting Decrease in error
Savage et al 2005 [31]	On-line reporting	#3: Effective use of technology	Increased reporting Improved process
Kuperman et al 2007 [37]	Computer physician order entry/clinical decision support Medication related	#3: Active monitoring	Dosing guidance Drug-drug interaction
Grotting 2002 [38]	Barcode-enabled point-of-care	#3: Technology use	Increased reporting errors Causation insight
Poon et al 2006 [39]	Pharmacy barcode	#3: Technology use	Less adverse drug events by 74%
Skibinski et al 2007 [40]	Pharmacy computer Point-of-care products	#5:Automated dispensing system Process time	Identify failure modes Standard processes Increased accuracy
Donyai et al 2007 [41]	E-prescribing	#7: Unable E-script	Reduced prescribing errors (3% to <1.9%)
Franklin et al 2007 [42]	E-prescribing barcode	#7: Unable E-script #3: Technology use	Script errors: 3.8% to 2% Adverse drug events: 7% to 4.3%

advocating for the adoption of a safety culture and the further use of health information technology, the IOM report places emphasis on seven recommendations [35] to reduce errors aimed at consumers and providers, the federal government, and other stakeholders. Early adopters of the IOM prevention strategies have had fair to good results in reducing medication errors as summarized in Table 8. Whether it is a "pharmacist-led medication team" [36], an on-line reporting and active monitoring system, the use of clinical decision supports, or pharmacy "barcoding" [39,40] or "e-prescribing," these institutions are implementing technologies that it is hoped will lead to the next level of medication safety.

References

[1] Hamilton BE, Martin JA, Ventura SJ. Births: preliminary data for 2005. Natl Vital Stat Rep 2006;55:1–18.
[2] Nabukera S, Wingate MS, Alexander GR, et al. First-time births among women 30 years and older in the United States: patterns and risk of adverse outcomes. J Reprod Med 2006;51: 676–82.
[3] Glover DD, Amonkar M, Rybeck BF, et al. Prescription, over-the-counter, and herbal medicine use in a rural, obstetric population. Am J Obstet Gynecol 2003;188:1039–45.

[4] Food and Drug Administration, Health and Human Services. Requirements on content and format of labeling for human prescription drug and biological products. Final rule. Fed Regist 2006;71:3921–97.

[5] Lee E, Maneno MK, Smith L, et al. National patterns of medication use during pregnancy. Pharmacoepidemiol Drug Saf 2006;15:537–45.

[6] Andrade SE, Raebel MA, Morse AN, et al. Use of prescription medications with a potential for fetal harm among pregnant women. Pharmacoepidemiol Drug Saf 2006;15:546–54.

[7] Lo WY, Friedman JM. Teratogenicity of recently introduced medications in human pregnancy. Obstet Gynecol 2002;100:465–73.

[8] Cooper WO, Hickson GB, Ray WA. Prescriptions for contraindicated category X drugs in pregnancy among women enrolled in TennCare. Paediatr Perinat Epidemiol 2004;18:106–11.

[9] Riley EH, Fuentes-Afflick E, Jackson RA, et al. Correlates of prescription drug use during pregnancy. J Womens Health (Larchmt) 2005;14:401–9.

[10] Honein MA, Lindstrom JA, Kweder SL. Can we ensure the safe use of known human teratogens? The iPLEDGE test case. Drug Saf 2007;30:5–15.

[11] Hardy JR, Leaderer BP, Holford TR, et al. Safety of medications prescribed before and during early pregnancy in a cohort of 81,975 mothers from the UK general practice research database. Pharmacoepidemiol Drug Saf 2006;15:555–64.

[12] Raebel MA, Carroll NM, Kelleher JA, et al. Randomized trial to improve prescribing safety during pregnancy. J Am Med Inform Assoc 2007;14:440–50.

[13] Werler MM, Mitchell AA, Hernandez-Diaz S, et al. Use of over-the-counter medications during pregnancy. Am J Obstet Gynecol 2005;193:771–7.

[14] American College of Obstetricians and Gynecologists. ACOG Committee Opinion: safe use of medication. Number 331, April 2006. Obstet Gynecol 2006;107:969–72.

[15] Ververs T, Kaasenbrood H, Visser G, et al. Prevalence and patterns of antidepressant drug use during pregnancy. Eur J Clin Pharmacol 2006;62:863–70.

[16] Kallen B, Otterblad Olausson P. Antidepressant drugs during pregnancy and infant congenital heart defect. Reprod Toxicol 2006;21:221–2.

[17] American College of Obstetricians and Gynecologists. ACOG Committee Opinion Number 328: patient safety in the surgical environment. Obstet Gynecol 2006;107:429–33.

[18] Little JA, Velazquez MB, Rayburn WF. Reported medication errors in obstetric inpatients in 1 hospital. J Reprod Med 2003;48:818–20.

[19] Forster AJ, Fung I, Caughey S, et al. Adverse events detected by clinical surveillance on an obstetric service. Obstet Gynecol 2006;108:1073–83.

[20] Pocock SB, Chen KT. Inappropriate use of antibiotic prophylaxis to prevent infective endocarditis in obstetric patients. Obstet Gynecol 2006;108:280–5.

[21] Glover DD, Rybeck BF, Tracy TS. Medication use in a rural gynecologic population: prescription, over-the-counter, and herbal medicines. Am J Obstet Gynecol 2004;190:351–7.

[22] Reedy MB, McMillion JS, Engvall WR, et al. Inadvertent administration of prostaglandin E1 instead of prostaglandin F2 alpha in a patient with uterine atony and hemorrhage. Obstet Gynecol 1992;79:890–4.

[23] Joy S, Poi M, Hughes L, et al. Third-trimester maternal toxicity with nevirapine use in pregnancy. Obstet Gynecol 2005;106:1032–8.

[24] Fujii Y, Numazaki M. Dose-range effects of propofol for reducing emetic symptoms during cesarean delivery. Obstet Gynecol 2002;99:75–9.

[25] Simpson KR. Minimizing risk of magnesium sulfate overdose in obstetrics. MCN Am J Matern Child Nurs 2006;31:340.

[26] Goodman EJ, Haas AJ, Kantor GS. Inadvertent administration of magnesium sulfate through the epidural catheter: report and analysis of a drug error. Int J Obstet Anesth 2006;15:63–7.

[27] Bilal NE, Gedebou M, Al-Ghamdi S. Endemic nosocomial infections and misuse of antibiotics in a maternity hospital in Saudi Arabia. APMIS 2002;110:140–7.

[28] Benjamin DM, Pendrak RF. Medication errors: an analysis comparing PHICO's closed claims data and PHICO's event reporting trending system (PERTS). J Clin Pharmacol 2003;43:754–9.

[29] National Practitioner Data Bank for Adverse Information on Physicians and Other Health Care Practitioners. Medical malpractice payments reporting requirements–HRSA: notice of proposed rulemaking. Fed Regist 1998;63:71255–7.

[30] White AA, Pichert JW, Bledsoe SH, et al. Cause and effect analysis of closed claims in obstetrics and gynecology. Obstet Gynecol 2005;105:1031–8.

[31] Savage SW, Schneider PJ, Pedersen CA. Utility of an online medication-error-reporting system. Am J Health Syst Pharm 2005;62:2265–70.

[32] National Coordinating Council for Medication Error Reporting and Prevention (NCC MERP). National Coordinating Council for Medication Error Reporting and Prevention (NCC MERP), about medication errors (1996). Available at: www.nccmerp.org. Accessed August 1, 2004.

[33] Rao JNK, Scott AJ. On simple adjustments to chi-square tests with survey data. The Annals of Statistics 1987;15:385–97.

[34] Beyea SC, Kobokovich LJ, Becker SC, et al. Medication errors in the LDRP. AWHONN Lifelines 2004;8:130–40.

[35] Institute of Medicine. Preventing medication errors: quality chasm series. Washington, DC: National Academy Press; 2006.

[36] Costello JL, Torowicz DL, Yeh TS. Effects of a pharmacist-led pediatrics medication safety team on medication-error reporting. Am J Health Syst Pharm 2007;64:1422–6.

[37] Kuperman GJ, Bobb A, Payne TH, et al. Medication-related clinical decision support in computerized provider order entry systems: a review. J Am Med Inform Assoc 2007;14: 29–40.

[38] Grotting JB. Reducing medication errors at the point of care. Trustee 2002;55:21.

[39] Poon EG, Cina JL, Churchill W, et al. Medication dispensing errors and potential adverse drug events before and after implementing bar code technology in the pharmacy. Ann Intern Med 2006;145:426–34.

[40] Skibinski KA, White BA, Lin LI, et al. Effects of technological interventions on the safety of a medication-use system. Am J Health Syst Pharm 2007;64:90–6.

[41] Donyai P, O'Grady K, Jacklin A, et al. The effects of electronic prescribing on the quality of prescribing. Br J Clin Pharmacol 2007;41(4):1–7.

[42] Franklin BD, O'Grady K, Donyai P, et al. The impact of a closed-loop electronic prescribing and administration system on prescribing errors, administration errors and staff time: a before-and-after study. Qual Saf Health Care 2007;16:279–84.

ELSEVIER
SAUNDERS

CLINICS IN
PERINATOLOGY

Clin Perinatol 35 (2008) 119–139

Computer-Related Medication Errors in Neonatal Intensive Care Units

John Chuo, MD, MS[a],*,
Rodney W. Hicks, PhD, RN[b]

[a]*Robert Wood Johnson Medical School, University of Medicine and Dentistry of New Jersey,
One Robert Wood Johnson Place, New Brunswick, NJ 08903, USA*
[b]*Texas Tech University Health Sciences Center, Lubbock, TX, USA*

The Institute of Medicine reports "To Err is Human" and "Crossing the Quality Chasm: A New Health System for the 21st Century" invigorated a national effort to improve the reporting of medication errors. The purpose of voluntary reporting is to identify patterns of system failures so that measures that will mitigate the risks and hazards patients encounter in the health care system can be recommended [1,2]. The Patient Safety and Quality Improvement Act of 2005 called for the creation of Patient Safety Organizations to facilitate data collection, analysis, and dissemination, all of which depend on technology, to improve the health care process [3]. During the last 8 years, the application of technology to medication usage processes has increased, but its effect on iatrogenic medication errors are mixed [4–8]. Such integration of technology into processes that affect patient safety is especially apparent in the neonatal ICU (NICU), where health care delivery depends heavily on the use of computers [9]. This article discusses what is known about technology usage in the NICU and its impact on medication errors. Among solutions put forth to improve patient safety during the past decade, computerized prescriber order entry (CPOE) has attracted influential support from the federal government, the Institute of Medicine, and numerous patient safety advocates; it has also been the focus of controversies. This article lso analyzes computer-related NICU medication errors and CPOE errors reported to the MEDMARX database (U.S. Pharmacopeia Convention, Inc., Rockville, Maryland, USP). Finally, it describes key areas

This article was supported in part by U.S. Pharmacopeia, Rockville, MD.
* Corresponding author.
E-mail address: chuojo@umdnj.edu (J. Chuo).

for evaluating technology in the NICU medication use process (MUP) and reviews the implications of technology use for health policy in terms of dollar cost versus patient safety benefits.

Medication errors

Medication errors account for as many as 7000 iatrogenic deaths in the United States each year [1]. From the US Food and Drug Administration (FDA) database, known as "MedWatch," investigators analyzed 7111 pediatric adverse medication error reports received over 5 years between November 1997 and December 2002 [10] and showed an increased vulnerability of younger children, especially those less than 1 year old, to medication errors. In this patient population, 30% of medication errors can lead to disability lasting longer than 6 months, and 15% lead to death [11]. Adverse drug events are reported to occur three times more often in children than in adults, and as many as 17% of these errors can originate in the NICU [12,13]. According to a report by Kaushal and Bates [12], the NICU has the highest number of preventable iatrogenic medication errors, with three of five pediatric adverse drug events occurring in neonates. A 12-month study in a NICU identified the incidence of medication errors as 1.6 to 26.5 per 1000 NICU days [14]. In a European study examining the NICU medication error records for 1 year, researchers concluded that as many as 24% of events were either moderate or severe [15].

Technology and the neonatal ICU medication use process

Although the epidemiology of neonatal medication errors seems to be limited when compared with other populations, this population seems to be at greater risk of medication errors than older children [16]. Neonatal practitioners often face unique challenges in the MUP, for which technology is well suited to assist in decision-making. The MUP is a systems approach that describes the general flow of how medications are ordered, dispensed, and administered (Fig. 1). Without doubt, information technology plays an important role in the prevention of NICU medication errors throughout the MUP. Recently, researchers in New Zealand explored imperfections in the MUP through a series of expert panel failure mode and effects analyses. The panel identified 72 failures attributable to 193 causes; the vulnerabilities existed throughout the MUP.

Prescribing

At the point of prescribing, technology uses include CPOE systems with clinical decision support systems. Early estimates of medication errors suggested that nearly half of the errors originated with prescribers [17]. CPOE systems (1) avoid errors in handwriting, (2) ensure accurate calculations, (3)

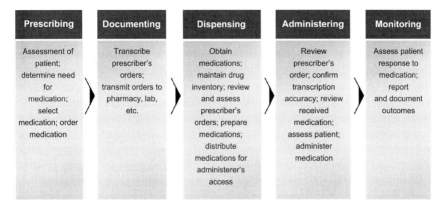

Fig. 1. The medication use process. (*Courtesy of* US Pharmacopeia, Inc., Rockville, MD; with permission.)

eliminate incomplete orders, (4) provide the prescriber with standardized dosage, (5) detect duplicate therapies, and (6) assist with route selections. Systems that have clinical decision support systems provide extra support by providing allergy alerts, signaling drug–drug interactions, assessing laboratory values, and alerting providers when doses exceed normal pre-established dose limits [17]. CPOE systems also can remove the need for manual transcription of orders (the second phase of the MUP) and thus reduce the opportunity for errors to be introduced during transcription. A prospective cohort study by Shulman and colleagues [18] comparing errors from written and CPOE orders showed a reduction in error with CPOE. Armed with this information, in 2002, the Leapfrog Group called on hospitals to adopt CPOE systems as the standard of prescribing care. In the most recent 2007 survey (n = 1285), only 10% of the hospitals met the standard [19].

One study reported the benefits of CPOE in the NICU setting. The researchers compared various MUP outcomes of two medications before and after implementation of a commercial CPOE system. There were significant reductions in the turnaround times after implementation of the CPOE system for caffeine. Accuracy of gentamicin dosing also increased with the CPOE system. The authors concluded that even with the complexities of NICU, the use of CPOE systems can improve the MUP.

Proponents of technology usage, including support at the federal level, have advocated the use of CPOE systems to reduce medication errors [20] but admit that errors may increase if implementation is flawed or when major systemic changes are made without adequate preparation [7,21]. To assess the true effects of CPOE on medication errors, researchers favor studies that compare paper and CPOE ordering methods directly [22]. Attempts to standardize practice by embedding clinical guidelines into CPOE systems have had disappointing results; those incorporating patient-specific information seem more promising [23,24].

Transcribing

Nursing personnel begin the transcription phase of the MUP when the orders are copied manually from the original order onto another source, such as the Kardex or hand-written medication administration record. At the end of the transcription phase, copies of the original order are sent to the pharmacy (either hand carried or sent through the pneumatic tube system) or are scanned for pharmacy processing (eg, by faxing or copying).

In a recent sample of 510 hospitals, researchers found that nearly one quarter still used handwritten medication administration records, and in smaller hospitals (<50 beds) the percentage increased to more than 40%. Since 1999 there has been a gradual decline in the percentage of handwritten medication administration records and a shift toward computer-generated medication administration records [25].

Dispensing

The dispensing phase begins with a pharmacist's review of the order and continues until the product is ready for patient use. Technology used in the dispensing phase includes pharmacy information systems, automated dispensing devices, robotic fills, and other equipment. Pharmacy information systems often communicate with the hospital's information system for admission, discharge, and transfer notices and for financial purposes (eg, billing). Pharmacy information systems also can create a printed medication administration record, either on demand or through batch processing (eg, nightly).

Automated dispensing devices are another form of technology used during the dispensing phase of the MUP. Automated dispensing cabinets are storage devices that electronically dispense medications and offer simultaneous tracking of the doses retrieved. The use of automated dispensing devices increased steadily between 1999 and 2005, and many now link directly to the pharmacy computer system to improve safety by controlling access to medications authorized on the patient profile [25]. Recently, several NICU patients died after receiving the wrong dose of heparin. The adult formulation of heparin (rather than heparin-lock solution) had been placed erroneously within the NICU's automatic dispensing device. As a result of the mis-stocking error, a nurse withdrew and administered up to a 1000-fold excessive dose to six patients, several of whom subsequently died [26].

A recent report showed that pharmacists monitor medication therapy in more than 90% of all hospitals. Eighty-seven percent of hospitals routinely monitor serum drug levels and provide pharmacists with access to laboratory data to track patient profiles. More than 70% of hospitals have medication reconciliation programs [27].

Administering

The administering phase of the MUP begins as the person preparing to administer the medication compares the original order with the medication administration record and obtains the medication. In the NICU, the most common technological devices used in the administering phase of the MUP are the infusions devices, which include syringe pumps and infusion pumps. Infusion devices are a source of iatrogenic error in the NICU population. For example, intralipid infusion errors were the subject of a recent study in which researchers explored 266 case reports from 55 different institutions [28]. More than 90% of the errors resulted from inaccurate programming of an infusion device (eg, selecting the wrong volume to be infused or the wrong rate of the infusion or failing to turn the pump on). An additional threat is the use of multiple infusion devices, in which parameters for one product are swapped with another.

"Smart pumps" are the newest generation of infusion pumps. These devices integrate clinical guidelines with a point-of-care computer [25]. Smart pump use varies by hospital size, but there is a general trend toward adoption of these devices. Threats to the effectiveness of smart pumps involve user interactions and inaccurate drug libraries.

Another technology available for preventing medication errors is bar-code medication administration. This technology involves placing a unique identifier (bar code) on a drug package. The bar code is machine readable by an optical scanner. The patient also has a unique bar code on the identification bracelet. Before drug administration, the user scans both the drug package and the patient to verify the administration against the medication profile. This ability is particularly important in the administration phase of the MUP, where there are the fewest opportunities for preventing a medication error before it reaches the patient [29].

Bar-code medication administration is not error proof for a number of reasons. In a recent study, researchers reported a number of areas in which technology failed to prevent a medication error. For example, the medication packages could be labeled with the incorrect bar code when medications are repackaged within a facility. Some packages did not contain barcode labels. Another failure occurred when optical scanners could not read locally produced bar codes [29]. Although this study did not report errors by the NICU setting, it is logical to assume that the same failures could occur within the NICU.

Medication error reporting

USP is a practitioner-based organization that sets legally enforceable standards addressing the strength, purity, labeling, packaging, and storage of therapeutic products. USP has more than 30 years of experience in operating various voluntary reporting programs for purposes of integrating findings into the standards-setting process to fulfill its public health mission. The two medication error reporting programs are the USP- Institute for Safe Medication Practices (ISMP) Medication Errors Reporting (MER)

Program and MEDMARX. The USP-ISMP MER Program began in 1991 and currently accepts reports of medication errors from any clinician or member of the public from any site. Since its inception, the program has amassed more than 12,000 reports, many coming from community pharmacies, home health agencies, hospitals, and patients. USP reviews and codes each report before entering the information into a database. USP shares copies of the reports with manufacturers and the FDA.

Based on the experiences of the MER program, consultation with the National Coordinating Council for Medication Error Report and Prevention (NCC MERP), and interactions with other national thought leaders, USP designed and deployed MEDMARX in August 1998 as an anonymous, voluntary medication error reporting program for hospitals and related health systems. MEDMARX refers to participating hospitals and related health systems as "facilities," and each facility has a unique facility identification number. Reporters are facility employees who submit medication error data to MEDMARX. Because of the significant size of the database, which now contains more than 1.3 million medication error records, participating facilities (now numbering more than 770) can collect, analyze, compare, and disseminate their medication error data, including the practical solutions taken in response to the error, to other subscribing facilities. Facilities can use the collective learning of all participating facilities as part of ongoing quality improvement efforts aimed at improving safe medication use.

MEDMARX collects medication error data in a standardized format through a series of required and optional fields. Part of the standardized format includes the NCC MERP definition of a medication error. According to NCC MERP, "A medication error is any preventable event that may cause or lead to inappropriate medication use or patient harm while the medication is in the control of the health care professional, patient, or consumer. Such events may be related to professional practice, health care products, procedures, and systems, including prescribing; order communication; product labeling, packaging, and nomenclature; compounding; dispensing; distribution; administration; education; monitoring; and use" [30].

Methods

Given the anonymous nature of the data, the authors received an exempt status from an institutional review committee. USP staff used Crystal Reports, version 9 (Crystal Decisions, Inc., San Jose, California) via open database connectivity drivers to query the MEDMARX program. These drivers allowed the Crystal Reports application to access the data stored within the various data tables (regardless of the underlying database management system). Selected medication error variables were included in this study. The primary criteria were that MEDMARX received the medication error record between the dates of January 1, 2001 and December 31, 2005,

NICU was the location of error, and the error involved either computer entry or CPOE. Other variables include the error severity, as measured by the NCC MERP Index for Categorizing Medication Errors. This scale has a reported kappa value of $k = 0.62$ [9]. Each record also was analyzed for the type of error, phase of the MUP, patient outcome, product involved in the error, staff type identified as having made the original error, and actions taken. Demographics of the participating facilities included bed size, type, and owner. The researchers then exported each of the Crystal Reports to worksheet format for importation to Statistica version 7.1, (Stat-Soft, Tulsa, Oklahoma).

Results

The MEDMARX program contained 343 NICU medication errors associated with either computer entry (n = 298) or CPOE (n = 45). These records came from 48 institutions, most of which were either community hospitals or academic medical centers.

Error category (severity)

As indicated by the NCC MERP Index for Categorizing Medication Errors (Table 1), about one third of computer entry errors reached patients (categories C–E; 34%); some required interventions to preclude harm, and others resulted in harm (categories D and E; 7%). In contrast, more than 75% of CPOE errors were recognized before reaching the patient (category A or B errors).

Medication use process

NICU medication errors occurred throughout the MUP, although there were differences between computer entry and CPOE errors (Table 2). As a percentage, computer entry errors (9%) originating during the prescribing phase

Table 1
Comparison between computer entry errors and computerized physician order entry errors in the neonatal ICU

Category	Computer entry error		Computerized physician order entry	
	n	%	n	%
A	13	4.4	3	6.7
B	184	61.7	31	68.9
C	80	26.8	8	17.8
D	16	5.4	2	4.4
E	5	1.7	1	2.2
F	0	0	0	0
G	0	0	0	0
H	0	0	0	0
I	0	0	0	0
Total	298	100	45	100

Table 2
Medication use process [a]

	Computer error		Computerized physician order entry	
Phase of process	n	%	n	%
Procurement	1	<1	0	0
Prescribing	27	9.5	32	76.2
Transcribing/documenting	176	61.8	5	11.9
Dispensing	46	16.1	1	2.4
Administering	33	11.6	4	9.5
Monitoring	2	<1	0	0

[a] Node is not applicable to category A cases.

were reported less often than those associated with CPOE (71%). Conversely, a greater percentage of errors originated during transcribing/documenting for computer errors (59%) than during CPOE (11%). In the dispensing phase there also were more computer entry errors (15%) than CPOE errors (2%).

Error type

There were differences between computer entry errors and CPOE in the patterns of errors reported (Table 3) Computer entry errors had a great percentage of improper dose/quantity, wrong time, and extra dose errors than did CPOE errors. The frequency of two types of errors (prescribing error and wrong dosage form) differed greatly between CPOE and computer entry.

Contributing factors

The contributing factors that seem to play a greater role in CPOE errors include distractions (4.7%–56%), staff inexperience (5.1%–52%),

Table 3
Error type

	Computer error		Computerized physician order entry	
Error type	n	%	n	%
Improper dose/quantity	108	36.2	12	26.7
Wrong time	64	21.5	2	4.4
Omission error	39	13.1	5	11.1
Extra dose	19	6.4	0	0
Unauthorized/wrong drug	19	6.4	4	8.9
Prescribing error	17	5.7	28	62.2
Wrong dosage form	16	5.4	10	22.2
Wrong route	13	4.4	1	2.2
Drug prepared incorrectly	10	3.6	1	2.2
Wrong patient	10	3.6	1	2.2
Mislabeling	3	1	0	0
Wrong administration technique	3	1	0	0
Expired product	1	<1	0	0

insufficient staffing ($< 1\%–12\%$), and workload ($3.3\%–8\%$). Furthermore, 4% of errors seem also to be related to patient transfer and cross-coverage issues (Table 4).

Action to patients

Most computer-related medication errors resulted in no significant action to patients (Table 5) For errors not related to CPOE usage that led to actions, the top three involved the laboratory test performed, drug therapy initiated/changed, and observation initiated/increased. CPOE errors were associated more frequently with vital signs monitoring ($4.2\%–8.3\%$) and delay in diagnosis and treatment ($5.6\%–8.3\%$) and were associated less often with laboratory test performed ($16.9\%–8.3\%$) and drug therapy change ($22.5\%–16.7\%$).

Actions toward staff

Without CPOE usage, most response to errors involved informing the member of the staff who made the error or was involved in the error. With CPOE usage, response involving education and training increased ($6.5\%–\%21.4\%$). Patients' physicians were informed more often as well (Table 6).

Discussion

This study examined NICU medication errors involving either computer entry or CPOE, two important technologies that aim to reduce the burden of iatrogenic errors. Data were reported voluntarily by 48 facilities to a national medication error reporting program.

Table 4
Factor contributing to medication error

Contributing factor	Computer error		Computerized physician order entry	
	n	%	n	%
Computer system/network	9	4.2	1	4
Distractions	10	4.7	14	56
Imprinting, identification failure	1	<1	0	0
No 24-hour pharmacy	1	<1	0	0
None	174	80	2	8
Similar patient names	3	1.4	0	0
Shift change	6	2.8	2	8
Inexperienced staff	11	5.1	13	52
Insufficient staffing	2	<1	3	12
Workload increase	7	3.3	2	8
Agency/temporary staff	7	3.3	0	0
Patient transfer	0	0	1	4
Cross coverage	0	0	1	4

Table 5
Action to patient

Action	Computer error		Computerized physician order entry	
	n	%	n	%
Delay in diagnosis/treatment	4	5.6	1	8.3
Drug therapy initiated/changed	16	22.5	2	16.7
Laboratory test performed	12	16.9	1	8.3
None	41	57.7	5	41.7
Observation initiated/increased	7	9.9	1	8.3
Vital signs monitoring initiated/increased	3	4.2	1	8.3
Diagnostic tests done	0	0	1	8.3

Error category

The apparent reduction in the percentage of errors that reached the patient (categories C–E) versus the percentage of errors that did not reach the patient (category A or B) may result from the clinical support alerts embedded in CPOE systems that verify weight-based dosing, verify prescription orders against acceptable dose ranges, and assess for patient allergies. These alerts inform clinicians of potential errors at the point of action so that errors can be avoided.

Error node, type, and factors

There were fewer transcribing errors with CPOE systems than computer entry systems because physicians prescribe the medication orders directly in CPOE. Even so, most CPOE errors occur in the prescribing phase of the MUP. Fewer of these prescribing errors involved wrong dosing and time (perhaps because of the formulary clinical support features embedded in CPOE); more errors involved the wrong dosage form (eg, liquid versus tablets). Because CPOE implementation involves a steep learning curve and

Table 6
Action toward staff

Action	Computer error		Computerized physician order entry	
	n	%	n	%
Communication process enhanced	10	4.3	0	0
Computer software modified/obtained	3	1.3	1	7.1
Education/training provided	15	6.5	3	21.4
Informed patient's physician	18	7.8	6	42.9
Informed patient/caregiver of error	1	<1	0	0
Informed staff who made the initial error	201	87	9	64.3
Informed staff involved in error	45	19.5	4	28.6
None	12	5.2	1	7.1

increased workload for staff, it is not surprising that the chief factors contributing to CPOE errors are inadequate staffing, lack of experience, and workload burden. The authors' review of the literature shows that even in the best CPOE implementations there may be a delay of more than 6 months before the return on investment can begin to be seen [31–34]. These findings support the notion that implementation of CPOE systems requires much attention to the prescribing activities, such as training prescribers on the proper use of the software. Although automated error-check systems may prevent errors from reaching patients, prescribing errors still occur at an undesirable level.

Action toward staff and patient

CPOE errors seem to result in fewer patient interventions, a finding that is consistent with the finding that more CPOE errors are caught before they can reach and harm patients. Of interest, CPOE errors have slightly increased delay in diagnosis and treatment and vital sign monitoring. Reasons for these trends are unclear. It is interesting that CPOE errors are reported to the patient's physician more readily than computer entry errors, probably because most prescribing errors are made by the physicians themselves.

The finding that action toward staff after CPOE errors involved more staff education and less "individual reprimanding" (as with computer entry errors) probably reflects the current shifts in quality improvement strategies. During the last 10 years, the focus of health care quality improvement has been redirected toward group education with emphasis on correcting systemic problems associated with the errors and taking corrective focus off the individual [35–40]. This strategy seems to be working: enlisting staff as proponents of a hospital's patient safety programs helps facilitate buy-in from their colleagues [41].

Evaluation of technology

Embedding technology into key areas of health care delivery requires significant expertise in managing workflow processes, information technology, cultural change, and staff workspace [42]. The implementation process imposes a tremendous political and financial burden. Here the authors summarize a strategy for evaluating emerging technology for the MUP in the NICU in terms of five categories: context, unit attributes, personnel, performance, and cost.

Context

Context involves determining the needs and workflow of the unit. Planning committees often create use-cases to model each node of the MUP to define the functional requirements of each phase. How realistic the models are and how effectively the technology can deliver the required functions determines the usability of the technology and the opportunities for error that may arise. Many earlier medication management computer systems have been modeled after adult MUPs and are not likely to work without being adjusted to the unique context of the NICU environment. The authors' finding that error rates in both computer entry and CPOE are highest in the prepharmacy nodes (prescribing and transcribing) supports the notion that, in the NICU, the prescribing phase has complex needs and workflows, and failure to address these needs perfectly introduces more opportunities for error. NICU prescription orders rely heavily on patient weight and on gestational and chronologic age. These dosing rules are incorporated in very few of the clinical decision support modules embedded in today's pharmacy and CPOE systems. The technological barrier stems from the need to access the critical information from non-CPOE systems such as daily nurse flow sheets (assuming that they are electronic). Some systems allow the prescriber to enter the information, but such entry complicates and adds precious time to the usage process. Medication alerts concerning therapeutic and harmful drug levels in the neonatal population are different from those in adults. Certain antibiotics that are used routinely in adults, such as ceftriaxone, are contraindicated in hyperbilirubinemic infants, but obtaining a warning against this usage requires an interface with the hospital's laboratory system [43]. Another example is the reported association of ranitidine with neonatal late-onset sepsis [44]. Other important contextual NICU issues to consider when evaluating CPOE technology are (1) the high volume of orders per day and per patient; (2) emergency code situations in which physicians need medications immediately but cannot physically enter the medication orders into the CPOE system; and (3) the fact that most daily NICU orders are placed in the morning and are expected to be executed early in the day, so that well-constructed order sets that can be performed quickly by physicians, pharmacy, and nursing as well as a flexible but safe signature mechanism are highly desirable. Technological adaptation to the unit's context often requires willingness by the administration and staff to change policies and processes, either permanently or temporarily [45]. Defining this "adaptation gap" between human and technology and creating a strategy with contributions from both sides is essential.

The authors' data show that although current CPOE technology can reduce computer entry errors at the transcribing and dispensing nodes, there still is difficulty in preventing prescribing errors. One reason for the rate of high prescribing errors in CPOE could be that physicians must struggle with details of ordering medications that formerly were managed by pharmacists (eg, distinguishing between medications with similar names or using proprietary names versus generic names). A system that guards against such errors would be valuable.

As early adopters of computer systems for medication management, pharmacy suites have either automated and/or standardized dispensing procedures to take advantage of emerging technology. Therefore, the MUP dispensing phase seems to produce fewer opportunities for error than the prescription phase. Entry errors committed in the dispensing phase were mistaken entries of incorrect patient information or medication order components. The frequency of these errors decreased with the use of CPOE systems that reduced the need for manual entry.

Medication administration in the NICU has unique features because of the special needs of the neonatal population. For example, lipids typically run as a separate infusion drip in neonates (in adults, lipids can be mixed with the parenteral nutrition). This practice has led to serious errors when the lipid infusion rate has been confused with the parenteral rate [28]. Very sick infants often require multiple intravenous medications that run concurrently at similar rates, introducing potential infusion rate errors. Neonates are more vulnerable to the adverse effects of certain medications (eg, fentanyl should be given over a longer period to avoid rigid chest syndrome). Because of the high workload of nurses, who have little time to perform complex calculations to check dosing, technology aimed at medication reconciliation and "smart" infusion pumps that are preprogrammed with standard concentrations, dose range limits, and weight-based dose calculators have been most useful [46,47]. Smart pumps can check dose inputs automatically, either by (1) using logic algorithms that check for data consistency (ie, that the desired total volume is always greater than rate entered), (2) wireless synchronization with a computerized order entry system, or (3) weight-based checking. The potential for such features to prevent errors is tempered by the complexity of programming such pumps. Hence, their impact on serious medication error rates remains unclear [48,49].

Unit attributes

Unit attributes including statistics and culture, such as workload, staffing, the availability of information technology resources, and architectural layout, affect how much and quickly technology will be accepted and used. Invariably, a successful implementation window depends partly on the extent and availability of resources such as extra staffing, technical support, and readiness for unanticipated events [36].

In units where CPOE is not used, written physician orders are transcribed by unit clerks and are verified by nurses. The checking mechanism between the clerk and nurse is prone to error when workload increases and staffing is insufficient, possibly explaining the authors' finding that transcription errors dominated computer entry errors. CPOE technology helps reduce this type of error, but its effects on patient outcome remain debatable [6,7,50–56]. Unit characteristics such as average census, average patient acuity, the medical team construct, and computer availability are important considerations when customizing technology such as CPOE to the prescription phase of the MUP. When census and acuity are high, ordering medications must take minimal time without sacrificing accuracy. The use of order sets within CPOE systems has made drug ordering easier and safer [57–59]. Prebuilt order sets in the CPOE system for common scenarios such as admission, discharge, and procedures, as well as NICU-specific order entry systems, have been helpful [60,61]. At Somerset Medical Center, a NICU "convenience order set" in the CPOE that contains 85% to 90% of all possible orders that might be placed on a daily basis in the NICU has saved the team precious time by removing the need to search for the orders in the CPOE databank.

The physical layout of the unit (eg, proximity of the infant beds to each other and degree of noise) can contribute to the distractions that may interrupt the medical team during rounds. The authors' data support other reports that distraction is a frequent reason for medication errors, especially at the prescription and administration phases [62]. Collins and colleagues [63] report associations between CPOE errors and interruptions during clinical communication; such interruptions occur in as many as 35% of clinical communications [64]. Dispensing errors are reported to correlate with distraction and workload [65,66]. Poor location of computer equipment can increase workflow disruption [67]. Questions to consider are whether prescribers will have to wait for an available computer, whether computers will be available at the bedside, and whether mobile wireless computing is available. Nevertheless, interruptions in a busy NICU often are unavoidable and frequently convey important information. Therefore the user's expected short attention span should be factored into the training and usage strategy for a technology. Training sessions should be terse, showing only relevant neonatal content and needs. A frequent complaint is that the CPOE system times out too quickly and forces the user to repeat the login process. The entire system should be intuitive to the NICU user. Integration of the CPOE system with other technological aspects of the unit, such as the patient medical record, laboratory systems, and radiology systems, is a critical part of the decision support component of the CPOE [36]. Finally, critical determinants of success are the institutional leadership's involvement and commitment, the funding and resources dedicated to the implementation process, and the ability to rally staff in support of the patient safety mission of the institution [36,68–74].

Personnel

Medication errors occur when technology is deployed within the MUP without a clear understanding of the technology's target audiences (ie, "used by whom" and "for whom"). Koppel and colleagues' [21] report outlines the possible CPOE-related errors. For instance, CPOEs are used by health care workers to prescribe medications for pharmacists to dispense. Hence, the CPOE system should allow physicians to prescribe medications quickly in a format that is readable by the pharmacist. Pharmacists use automated dispensing systems to deliver medications for nurses to administer. The medication label should correspond to the correct patient and should be simple for nurses to read and verify. Invariably, audience analyses must reflect the context and unit culture.

The training strategy and how the system will be used depend on (1) the intended user's role (house staff, attending, nurse, resident, locum tenens, or pharmacist) and (2) his/her encounter frequency. Training methods include classroom lectures, focus groups, computer-based training, one-on-one training, just-in-time training, and reference documents. Residents are reported to be best trained by classroom and computer-based methods, whereas attending physicians are trained better by focus groups and one-on-one sessions [75]. House staff and hospitalists seem to embrace CPOE more readily than community physicians and locum tenens, perhaps because community physicians use the system less frequently and resist having to learn multiple systems if they attend different hospitals. House staff performs and is more familiar with the daily operations of the unit and may master the learning curve quickly enough to appreciate the potential benefits of the technology. The training strategy depends on how much the user will use the system. It would be impractical for residents rotating through the NICU unit for a month at a time to have a week-long training period or to train them long before they start the rotation. Even more difficult is the training of locum tenens; currently, there is no good solution to this problem other than perhaps using a strategy that includes online, just-in-time training. On the other hand, it may be prudent to have a more detailed training course for nurse practitioners who will be attending the unit consistently so that they can learn to maximize the benefits of the system. Of note, Petersen [76] associated house-staff discontinuity of care with an increase risk of preventable adverse events. The authors' own data showed a 4% CPOE error rate relating to patient transfer of care, but the reason for this error is unclear.

Studies using distributed resource modeling to study the cognitive demands of CPOE on users suggest that prescription errors can result from malconfigurations and lack of intuitive design in the ordering program [77,78]. Minimizing the unnecessary cognitive burden of the nonclinical aspects of CPOE can help reduce errors. For instance, admission order sets with order items arranged in a mnemonic sequence familiar to most clinicians would avoid the user's having to reorient to the order set's layout. Convenience order sets should arrange the most common orders first to minimize scrolling. Medications that sound and look alike should have some distinguishing feature when they are displayed together on the screen. Medication error alerts should be triggered judiciously; excessive alarms can desensitize recipients, slow workflow to a crawl, cause more errors, and kill a CPOE implementation [79].

Computerized medication management systems are deeply rooted in the MUP dispensing phase. During the last decade, pharmacists have taken an increasingly important role in monitoring and reporting medication error and have been responsible for most of the category A and B error detections [27].

Performance

The performance history of a particular technology offers valuable information, and it is tempting to believe that results at an outside site can be repeated at the home site. Without a thorough comparative analysis of context, facility characteristics, and staffing between the home site and the outside site (the source of the results), false expectations can lead to disappointing outcomes. In short, important differences exist between the MUPs of academic and community hospitals, between adult and children's hospitals, and between inpatient and outpatient settings [80–82]. Lessons certainly can be learned, however, from studying how the implementation process of a CPOE system affected its ability to help prevent iatrogenic medication errors at the outside site.

Han and colleagues [7] draw special attention to this point in an important 2005 report associating CPOE implementation with increased mortality rate. The report sparked important debate that emphasized the importance of preimplementation workflow analysis and of human-centered designs [8].

Health policy perspective: money spent on technology versus patient safety

Expenses involving new technology are one of the five top drivers of increasing health care cost [83]. The cost of implementing a CPOE system depends on the location and on the pre-existing computer system. Ohsfeldt and colleagues [84] report the initial cost of implementing CPOE ranges from $1.3 million to $4.4 million. Poon and colleagues' [85] estimates range from $2 to $5 million for small hospitals and from $10 to $30 million for larger hospitals. These numbers translate to a substantial portion of the hospital's operating budget (19%–30%). The annual maintenance the system is estimated to cost an additional 3.4% to 14% of the hospital's budget, and more for rural hospitals [84]. Although CPOE may increase the efficiency of patient care [86], its ability to decrease cost per admission remains unclear. Studies that attempt to quantify the impact of CPOE on hospital operating costs have shown equivocal cost savings [84] and have even suggested that costs and errors may increase during the early implementation phases [87]. Although a large volume of supporting literature shows that a successfully implemented CPOE system can reduce iatrogenic medication errors at all phases of the MUP, only about 2% of all hospitals in the United States have adopted CPOE fully [4,19,33,88]. A simulation study by Ohsfeldt and colleagues [84] estimated that in rural hospitals CPOE implementation would increase operating cost substantially, without a substantial cost savings from improved efficiency and patient safety. For larger hospitals, the results are more optimistic, and savings in patient care cost and revenue enhancement seem to offset CPOE costs. Even larger hospitals consider the risks seriously, because of the implementation difficulties and the sizable cost involved. Of note, the analyses (value stream mapping and cost scrutinies) typically are hospital centric and do not account for the cost of medication errors outside the hospital. Such cost may become apparent only when analyses involve larger hospital networks or insurance provider network. Hence, insurance providers and those who "see the benefits" have begun to provide incentives for implementation of CPOEs (eg, pay for performance), encouraging adoption by smaller hospitals that otherwise see the technology as a cost burden [89,90].

Limitations of this study

The study presented in this manuscript has numerous limitations. First, all data came from voluntarily reported medication errors. Voluntary reporting generally is considered to result in fewer errors being reported and thus may not be truly representative of all NICU errors. Second, this study did attempt to correlate the errors with institutional characteristics, meaning that the possibility of nesting remains present. The absence of denominator data hindered the analysis. Therefore, no statistical comparisons are offered. Additionally, the data have not been reviewed or recoded. A more comprehensive comparison with non–computer-related medication errors in the MUP would be valuable.

Summary

Iatrogenic medication errors in the NICU are common in pediatrics and impose a formidable health risk to neonates. Among all participants in the MUP, pharmacists have been among the earliest adopters of technology for error prevention. As dispensing technology became more effective in preventing errors, prescription and transcription errors became even more prominent. Addressing such prepharmacy errors has been the intention of CPOE advocates. Although CPOE seems to have reduced transcription errors (eg, wrong-quantity and -time prescription errors) that reach patients, it has limitations. Its implementation requires the dedication of a tremendous amount of institutional resources and organizational leadership. Even with sufficient resources and support, many hospitals have demonstrated that, even with the best intentions, a flawed implementation can fail quickly. The reasons for failure have been the subject of much discourse concerning organizational culture, human-centered function design, cost-effective analysis, use case modeling, and human cognition and learning. Borrowing from such notable work and their own data analysis, the authors propose a strategy that evaluates technology intended to prevent iatrogenic mediation errors in the NICU covering five areas of concern: context, unit attributes, personnel, performance, and cost.

References

[1] Kohn LT, Corrigan JM, Donaldson MS. To err is human: building a safer health system. Washington, DC: National Academy Press; 2000.
[2] Institute of Medicine Committee on Quality of Health Care in America. Crossing the quality chasm: a new health system for the 21st century. Washington, DC: National Academy Press; 2001.

[3] Agency for Healthcare Research and Quality. The Patient Safety and Quality Improvement Act of 2005. 2005; Available at: http://www.ahrq.gov/qual.psoact.htm. Accessed October 2007.

[4] King WJ, Paice N, Rangrej J, et al. The effect of computerized physician order entry on medication errors and adverse drug events in pediatric inpatients. Pediatrics 2003;112(3):506–9.

[5] Kaushal R, Bates DW. Information technology and medication safety: what is the benefit? Qual Saf Health Care 2002;11(3):261–5.

[6] Del Beccaro MA, Jeffries HE, Eisenberg MA, et al. Computerized provider order entry implementation: no association with increased mortality rates in an intensive care unit. Pediatrics 2006;118(1):290–5.

[7] Han YY, Carcillo JA, Venkataraman ST, et al. Unexpected increased mortality after implementation of a commercially sold computerized physician order entry system. Pediatrics 2005;116(6):1506–12.

[8] Sittig DF, Ash JS, Zhang J, et al. Lessons from "unexpected increased mortality after implementation of a commercially sold computerized physician order entry system". Pediatrics 2006;118(2):797–801.

[9] Forrey RA, Pedersen CA, Schneider PJ. Interrater agreement with a standard scheme for classifying medication errors. Am J Health Syst Pharm 2007;64(2):175–81.

[10] Moore TJ, Weiss S, Kaplan ST, et al. Reported adverse drug events in infants and children under 2 years of age. Pediatrics 2000;11(5):E53–9.

[11] Fernandez CV, Gillis-Ring J. Strategies for the prevention of medical error in pediatrics. J Pediatr 2003;143(2):155–62.

[12] Kaushal R, Bates DW, Landrigan C, et al. Medication errors and adverse drug events in pediatric inpatients. JAMA 2001;285(16):2114–20.

[13] Ross LM, Wallace J, Paton JY. Medication errors in a paediatric teaching hospital in the UK: five years operational experience. Arch Dis Child 2000;83(6):492–7.

[14] Simpson JH, Lynch R, Grant J, et al. Reducing medication errors in the neonatal intensive care unit. Arch Dis Child 2004;89(6):F480–2.

[15] Frey B, Buettiker V, Hug M, et al. Does critical incident reporting contribute to medication error prevention? Eur J Pediatr 2002;161(11):594–9.

[16] Kunac DL, Reith DM. Identification of priorities for medication safety in neonatal intensive care. Drug Saf 2005;28(3):251–61.

[17] Shojania KG, Duncan BW, MacDonald KM, et al. Making health care safer. A critical analysis of patient safety practices. Evidence report/technology assessment number 43. Rockville (MD): Agency for Healthcare Research and Quality; 2001.

[18] Shulman R, Singer M, Goldstone J, et al. Medication errors: a prospective cohort study of hand-written and computerised physician order entry in the intensive care unit. Crit Care 2005;9(5):R516–21.

[19] Computer physician order entry, factsheet 2007. Available at: www.leapfroggroup.org/media/file/leapfrog-computer_physician_order_Entry_fact_sheet.pdf. Accessed October 2007.

[20] Kaushal R, Shojania KG, Bates DW. Effects of computerized physician order entry and clinical decision support systems on medication safety: a systematic review. Arch Intern Med 2003;163(12):1409–16.

[21] Koppel R, Metlay JUP, Cohen A, et al. Role of computerized physician order entry systems in facilitating medication errors. JAMA 2005;293(10):1197–203.

[22] Spooner SA. Literature review. Cocitnews. Elk Grove Village (IL): The Council on Clinical Information Technology; 2006. p. 19.

[23] Asaro PV, Sheldahl AL, Char DM. Physician perspective on computerized order-sets with embedded guideline information in a commercial emergency department information system. AMIA Annu Symp Proc 2005;6–10.

[24] Asaro PV, Sheldahl AL, Char DM. Embedded guideline information without patient specificity in a commercial emergency department computerized order-entry system. Acad Emerg Med 2006;13(4):452–8.

[25] Pedersen CA, Schneider PJ, Scheckelhoff DJ. ASHP national survey of pharmacy practice in hospital settings: dispensing and administration—2005. Am J Health Syst Pharm 2006;63(4): 327–45.

[26] Vecchione A. Heparin overdoses bring changes. Available at: http://www.drugtopics.com/drugtopics/issue/issueDetail.jsp?id = 10588. Accessed March 2007.

[27] Pedersen CA, Schneider PJ, Scheckelhoff DJ. ASHP national survey of pharmacy practice in hospital settings: monitoring and patient education—2006. Am J Health Syst Pharm 2007; 64(5):507–20.

[28] Chuo J, Lambert G, Hicks RW. Intralipid medication errors in the neonatal intensive care unit. Jt Comm J Qual Patient Saf 2007;33(2):104–11.

[29] Cochran GL, Jones KJ, Brockman J, et al. Errors prevented by and associated with bar-code medication administration systems. Jt Comm J Qual Patient Saf 2007;33(5):293–301, 245.

[30] National Coordinating Council for Medication Error Reporting and Prevention. Available at: www.nccmerp.org. Accessed January 16, 2007.

[31] Kaushal R, Jha AK, Franz C, et al. Return on investment for a computerized physician order entry system. J Am Med Inform Assoc 2006;13(3):261–6.

[32] Agrawal A. Return on investment analysis for a computer-based patient record in the outpatient clinic setting. J Assoc Acad Minor Phys 2002;13(3):61–5.

[33] Mekhjian HS, Kumar RR, Kuehr L, et al. Immediate benefits realized following implementation of physician order entry at an academic medical center. J Am Med Inform Assoc 2002; 9(5):529–39.

[34] Taylor R, Manzo J, Sinnett M. Quantifying value for physician order-entry systems: a balance of cost and quality. Healthc Financ Manage 2002;56(7):44–8.

[35] Silow-Carroll S, Alteras T, Meyer JA. Hospital quality improvement: strategies and lessons from U.S. Hospitals 2007. Available at: http://www.commonwealthfund.org/publications/publications_show.htm?doc_id=471265#areaCitation. Accessed October 2007.

[36] Ash JS, Stavri PZ, Kuperman GJ. A consensus statement on considerations for a successful CPOE implementation. J Am Med Inform Assoc 2003;10(3):229–34.

[37] Leape LL. Foreword: preventing medical accidents: is "systems analysis" the answer? Am J Law Med 2001;27(2–3):145–8.

[38] Leape LL. A systems analysis approach to medical error. J Eval Clin Pract 1997;3(3): 213–22.

[39] Leape LL, Bates DW, Cullen DJ, et al. Systems analysis of adverse drug events. ADE Prevention Study Group. JAMA 1995;274(1):35–43.

[40] Horns KM, Loper DL. Medication errors: analysis not blame. J Obstet Gynecol Neonatal Nurs 2002;31(3):347–54.

[41] Kemelgor B, Mears P. HR's role in the CQI process. Journal for Quality and Participation 1995;18(6):66–71.

[42] Lehmann CU, Kim GR. Computerized provider order entry and patient safety. Pediatr Clin North Am 2006;53(6):1169–84.

[43] Waknine Y. FDA safety changes: Advicor, Rocephin, Tindamax. Available at: www.Medscape.com. Accessed October 2007.

[44] Bianconi S, Gudavalli M, Sutija VG, et al. Ranitidine and late-onset sepsis in the neonatal intensive care unit. J Perinat Med 2007;35(2):147–50.

[45] Upperman JS, Staley P, Friend K, et al. The introduction of computerized physician order entry and change management in a tertiary pediatric hospital. Pediatrics 2005;116(5): E634–42.

[46] Brannon TS. Ad hoc versus standardized admixtures for continuous infusion drugs in neonatal intensive care: cognitive task analysis of safety at the bedside. AMIA Annu Symp Proc 2006;862.

[47] Larsen GY, Parker HB, Cash J, et al. Standard drug concentrations and smart-pump technology reduce continuous-medication-infusion errors in pediatric patients. Pediatrics 2005; 116(1):E21–5.

[48] Bratton SL. Medication errors reduced with smart-pump infusion. American Academy of Pediatrics Grand Rounds 2005;14(6):68A–9A.

[49] Rothschild JM, Keohane CA, Cook EF, et al. A controlled trial of smart infusion pumps to improve medication safety in critically ill patients. Crit Care Med 2005;33(3):533–40.

[50] Ammenwerth E, Talmon J, Ash JS, et al. Impact of CPOE on mortality rates—contradictory findings, important messages. Methods Inf Med 2006;45(6):586–93.

[51] Jacobs BR, Brilli RJ, Hart KW. Perceived increase in mortality after process and policy changes implemented with computerized physician order entry. Pediatrics 2006;117(4): 1451–2, author reply 1455–6.

[52] Keene A, Ashton L, Shure D, et al. Mortality before and after initiation of a computerized physician order entry system in a critically ill pediatric population. Pediatr Crit Care Med 2007;8(3):268–71.

[53] Longhurst C, Sharek P, Hahn J, et al. Perceived increase in mortality after process and policy changes implemented with computerized physician order entry. Pediatrics 2006;117(4): 1450–1, author reply 1455–6.

[54] O'Reilly M, Talsma AN, VanRiper S, et al. An anesthesia information system designed to provide physician-specific feedback improves timely administration of prophylactic antibiotics. Anesth Analg 2006;103(4):908–12.

[55] Rosenbloom ST, Harrell FE, Lehmann CU, et al. Perceived increase in mortality after process and policy changes implemented with computerized physician order entry. Pediatrics 2006;117(4):1452–5, author reply 1455–6.

[56] Wu RC, Laporte A, Ungar WJ. Cost-effectiveness of an electronic medication ordering and administration system in reducing adverse drug events. J Eval Clin Pract 2007;13(3):440–8.

[57] Bobb AM, Payne TH, Gross PA. Viewpoint: controversies surrounding use of order sets for clinical decision support in computerized provider order entry. J Am Med Inform Assoc 2007;14(1):41–7.

[58] Kuperman GJ, Bobb A, Payne TH, et al. Medication-related clinical decision support in computerized provider order entry systems: a review. J Am Med Inform Assoc 2007;14(1): 29–40.

[59] Payne TH, Hoey PJ, Nichol P, et al. Preparation and use of preconstructed orders, order sets, and order menus in a computerized provider order entry system. J Am Med Inform Assoc 2003;10(4):322–9.

[60] Waitman LR, Pearson D, Hargrove FR, et al. Enhancing computerized provider order entry (CPOE) for neonatal intensive care. AMIA Annu Symp Proc 2003;1078.

[61] Campbell MA. Development of a clinical pathway for near-term and convalescing premature infants in a level II nursery. Adv Neonatal Care 2006;6(3):150–64.

[62] Gladstone J. Drug administration errors: a study into the factors underlying the occurrence and reporting of drug errors in a district general hospital. J Adv Nurs 1995;22(4):628–37.

[63] Collins S, Currie L, Bakken S, et al. Interruptions during the use of a CPOE system for MICU rounds. AMIA Annu Symp Proc 2006;895.

[64] Alvarez G, Coiera E. Interruptive communication patterns in the intensive care unit ward round. Int J Med Inform 2005;74(10):791–6.

[65] Carnahan BJ, Maghsoodloo S, Flynn EA, et al. Geometric probability distribution for modeling of error risk during prescription dispensing. Am J Health Syst Pharm 2006;63(11): 1056–61.

[66] Creating effective reporting systems. Available from: http://anesthesiology.med. miami.edu/Library/MPSC%20docs/MPSC%20docs/Code%2015-FinalReport.pdfhttp:// anesthesiology.med.miami.edu/Library/MPSC%20docs/MPSC%20docs/Section%2036-1. pdf. Accessed October 2007.

[67] Cheng CH, Goldstein MK, Geller E, et al. The effects of CPOE on ICU workflow: an observational study. AMIA Annu Symp Proc 2003;150–4.

[68] Cohen AB, Hanft RS, Encinosa WE, et al. Technology in American health care: policy directions for effective evaluation and management. University of Michigan Press; 2004.

[69] Reineck C. Models of change. J Nurs Adm 2007;37(9):388–91.
[70] Clarke JR, Lerner JC, Marella W. The role for leaders of health care organizations in patient safety. Am J Med Qual 2007;22(5):311–8.
[71] Jeffs L, Law M, Baker GR. Creating reporting and learning cultures in health-care organizations. Can Nurse 2007;103(3):16–7, 27–8.
[72] Winokur SC, Beauregard KJ. Patient safety: mindful, meaningful, and fulfilling. Front Health Serv Manage 2005;22(1):17–32.
[73] Nicklin W, Mass H, Affonso DD, et al. Patient safety culture and leadership within Canada's academic health science centres: towards the development of a collaborative position paper. Can J Nurs Leadersh 2004;17(1):22–34.
[74] Nicklin W, McVeety JE. Canadian nurses' perceptions of patient safety in hospitals. Can J Nurs Leadersh 2002;15(3):11–21.
[75] Brisset PR, Gilman CS, Morgan MT, et al. Who are your CPOE users and how do you train them? Lessons learned at Cedars-Sinai Health System. MedInfo 2004. IOS Press. Copyrighted, International Medical Informatics Association.
[76] Petersen LA, Brennan TA, O'Neil AC, et al. Does housestaff discontinuity of care increase the risk for preventable adverse events? Ann Intern Med 1994;121(11):866–72.
[77] Horsky J, Kaufman DR, Patel VL. The cognitive complexity of a provider order entry interface. AMIA Annu Symp Proc 2003;294–8.
[78] Horsky J, Kaufman DR, Oppenheim MI, et al. A framework for analyzing the cognitive complexity of computer-assisted clinical ordering. J Biomed Inform 2003;36(1–2):4–22.
[79] Connolly C. Cedars-Sinai doctors cling to pen and paper. Washington Post. March 2005:A1.
[80] Computerized physician order entry: costs, benefits, and challenges. A case study approach 2003. Available at: www.leapfroggroup.org/media/file/leapfrog-CPOE_Costs_Benefits_Challenges.pdf. Accessed October 2007.
[81] Abboud PA, Ancheta R, Mckibben M, et al. Impact of workflow-integrated corollary orders on aminoglycoside monitoring in children. Health Informatics J 2006;12(3):187–98.
[82] Ash JS, Sittig DF, Seshadri V, et al. Adding insight: a qualitative cross-site study of physician order entry. Int J Med Inform 2005;74(7–8):623–8.
[83] Goetghebeur MM, Forest S, Hay JW. Understanding the underlying drivers of inpatient cost growth: a literature review. Am J Manag Care 2003;9:SP3–12.
[84] Ohsfeldt RL, Ward MM, Schneider JE, et al. Implementation of hospital computerized physician order entry systems in a rural state: feasibility and financial impact. J Am Med Inform Assoc 2005;12(1):20–7.
[85] Poon EG, Blumenthal D, Jaggi T, et al. Overcoming the barriers to the implementing computerized physician order entry systems in US hospitals: perspectives from senior management. Health Aff 2004;23(4):184–90.
[86] Cordero L, Kuehn L, Kumar RR, et al. Impact of computerized physician order entry on clinical practice in a newborn intensive care unit. J Perinatol 2004;24(2):88–93.
[87] Berger RG, Kichak JP. Computerized physician order entry: helpful or harmful? J Am Med Inform Assoc 2004;11(2):100–3.
[88] Bates DW, Teich JM, Lee J, et al. The impact of computerized physician order entry on medication error prevention. J Am Med Inform Assoc 1999;6(4):313–21.
[89] Classen DC, Avery AJ, Bates DW. Evaluation and certification of computerized provider order entry systems. J Am Med Inform Assoc 2007;14(1):48–55.
[90] Traynor K. Anthem quality program rewards Virginia Hospitals 2005; Available at: http://www.ashp.org/s_ashp/article_news.asp?CID=167&DID=2024&id=10317. Accessed October 2007.

ELSEVIER
SAUNDERS

Clin Perinatol 35 (2008) 141–161

Medication Errors in Neonates

Theodora A. Stavroudis, MD[a,*],
Marlene R. Miller, MD, MSc[b,c,d],
Christoph U. Lehmann, MD[a,e,f]

[a]Eudowood Neonatal Pulmonary Division, Department of Pediatrics,
Johns Hopkins University School of Medicine, Baltimore, MD, USA
[b]Department of Pediatrics, Johns Hopkins University
School of Medicine, Baltimore, MD, USA
[c]Department of Health Policy and Management, Johns Hopkins University
Bloomberg School of Public Health, Baltimore, MD, USA
[d]National Association of Children's Hospitals and Related Institutions,
401 Wythe Street, Alexandria, VA 22314, USA
[e]Department of Dermatology, Johns Hopkins University
School of Medicine, 600 North Wolfe Street, Baltimore, MD 21287, USA
[f]Division of Health Sciences Informatics, Johns Hopkins University
School of Medicine, 2024 E MONUMNT 1-201, Baltimore, MD 21287, USA

The phrase "primum non nocere," Latin for "first do no harm," is a professional ideal of medicine that emerged three to four centuries BC in the Hippocratic Oath, one of the oldest documents in medicine whose principles are still held sacred by health care providers worldwide. Despite the pledge to hold steadfast to this principle of nonmaleficence, the now well-known 1999 report *To Err is Human* by the Institute of Medicine noted that harm from medical error continues to plague medicine in the twenty-first century [1]. Since the release of this report, reduction and prevention of medical errors has become a national priority. Leaders in the field of patient safety, such as the Joint Commission on Accreditation of Healthcare Organizations (JCAHO), the Leapfrog Group, and the Institute for Healthcare Improvement (IHI), have risen to the challenge of defining and outlining the problems and solutions surrounding medical errors [2–4]. This article focuses on a small subset of medical errors: the medication errors that affect the care of the neonate.

* Corresponding author. Division of Neonatology, Johns Hopkins Hospital, 600 North Wolfe Street/Nelson 2-133, Baltimore, MD 21287.
  E-mail address: tstavro1@jhmi.edu (T.A. Stavroudis).

0095-5108/08/$ - see front matter © 2008 Elsevier Inc. All rights reserved.
doi:10.1016/j.clp.2007.11.010

Defining medication errors

A variety of definitions for medication errors exist in the literature, and recent efforts have been made to adopt uniform descriptions and classification systems [5–7]. The National Coordinating Council for Medication Error Reporting and Prevention defines a medication error as "any preventable event that may cause or lead to inappropriate medication use or patient harm while the medication is in the control of the health care professional, patient, or consumer. Such events may be related to professional practice, health care products, procedures, and systems, including prescribing; order communication; product labeling, packaging, and nomenclature; compounding; dispensing; distribution; administration; education; monitoring; and use" [8]. This is to be differentiated from an adverse drug event, which is an injury that results from medication use that may include expected adverse drug reactions or side effects [9,10].

To help describe medication errors, the National Coordinating Council for Medication Error Reporting and Prevention developed a nationally recognized taxonomy for medication error reports in 1998 with the following categories: medication classification, error setting, personnel involved in the incident, type of error, cause of error, contributing factors, and patient outcome. Error categories reflecting degree of harm are listed in Table 1 [8].

Neonates: a vulnerable population

The neonatal intensive care unit (NICU) is a clinical environment burdened with challenges that frequently may lead to adverse outcomes and medical errors. The severity and critical nature of illness, intricacy of treatment, immaturity of the newborn physiology, difficulty of multidisciplinary care, complexity of communication, and the changing technology that continues to shape and advance neonatal care make neonates a unique and vulnerable patient population.

Neonates are at further risk for harm from medication errors because of rapidly changing body size parameters (over the course of a hospitalization an infant may double or triple their birth weight); off-label drug usage; inability to communicate with providers; and changing developmental systems affecting drug absorption, distribution, metabolism, and excretion [11–16]. For instance, patients in the NICU are at increased risk for 10- to 100-fold dosing errors because of the necessary calculations involved in the ordering of medications and dilution of stock drugs [17]. In addition, as many as 80% of drugs used in the NICU are prescribed off-label [12,18–22]. With 4.1 million babies born in the United States each year and an admission rate of 5.6% to NICUs (range between 2% and 6.6%), the impact of medication errors among neonates can be substantial [23–25].

Table 1
National Coordinating Council for Medication Error Reporting and Prevention error category classification for medication errors

Degree of harm	Error category	Definition
No error, no harm	A	Circumstances or events that have the capacity to cause error
Error, no harm	B	An error occurred, but the error did not reach the patient
	C	An error occurred that reached the patient, but did not cause patient harm
	D	An error occurred that reached the patient and required monitoring to confirm that it resulted in no harm to the patient or required intervention to preclude harm
Error, harm	E	An error occurred that may have contributed to or resulted in temporary harm to the patient and required intervention
	F	An error occurred that may have contributed to or resulted in temporary harm to the patient and required initial or prolonged hospitalization
	G	An error occurred that my have contributed to or resulted in permanent patient harm
	H	An error occurred that required an intervention necessary to sustain life
Error, death	I	An error occurred that may have contributed to or resulted in the patient's death

The incidence of medication errors among neonates

Given the complexity of care, frequency of patient hand-offs, and environments with sensory overload (eg, visual and auditory alarms, telephones, pagers, and so forth), the occurrence of medication errors in NICUs is not unexpected. Although various means have been used to determine the extent of medication errors in medicine including chart reviews, occurrence reports, "trigger" event methodologies, and patient-family surveys, published estimates of medication errors in neonates are few. Regardless of the methods used to discover and describe medication errors, all reveal that medication errors are common, substantial, and preventable within the NICU. Furthermore, they demonstrate the need to use standardized definitions and a universal taxonomy to classify and characterize medication errors.

Retrospective or concurrent chart review

This method of adverse event (AE) and adverse drug event detection was used by Brennan and colleagues [26] in the Harvard Medical Practice Study in 1991, and later by other well-recognized studies demonstrating the pervasiveness of medication errors throughout medicine [27]. Limitations of chart review methods include bias of error types with skewing toward detection of prescribing errors as opposed to dispensing and administering errors, lack of completeness of the medical records, difficulty of ascertaining data from medical records because of legibility and conflicting entries, time and personnel demands of conducting the review, and lack of consistency in applying the standardized definitions to the discovered medication error.

While applying the chart review method in their study of pediatric medication errors, Kaushal and colleagues [27] found that errors were frequent in the NICU (91 per 100 admissions), and moreover, were more likely to be associated with harm. Errors with the potential to cause harm were eight times more likely to occur in the NICU compared with adults in the hospital setting. In addition, when compared with neonates in other wards of the hospital, potential adverse drug event rates (not to be confused with error rates) were more common among NICU patients, 46 per 100 admissions compared with 9 per 100 admissions.

Occurrence reports

To delineate and understand further the factors involved in medication errors, the safety community has established and analyzed reports made to centralized reporting systems [1,28–36]. These reporting systems were modeled after the successful error reporting systems used in aviation, where incidents or "near misses" are reported to NASA's Aviation Safety Reporting System and accidents that result in death, serious injury, or substantial damage to aircraft are reported to the National Transportation Safety Board and the Federal Aviation Administration. Although relatively inexpensive to establish and sustain, one limitation of error reporting systems is potential bias in event recollection and error type submission. Furthermore, reporting systems can be time intensive and perceived to be punitive by staff. Nevertheless, this methodology can provide insight into medication errors.

The Vermont Oxford Network (VON) is comprised of 54 hospitals. In a study of 1230 medical errors submitted to the VON's NICQ.org anonymous, Internet-based, voluntary reporting system, Suresh and colleagues [33] found that medication errors comprised 47% of medical error reports affecting the care of the newborn. Ninety-five percent of medical error reports named the NICU as the location for the error, with the remaining 5% of errors taking place in such locations as the delivery room, mother's room, step-down unit, operating room, and during neonatal transports. The study reported that 31% of reported medication errors occurred in the administering of the medicine; 25% in dispensing; 16% in ordering; 12% in transcribing; and 1.4% in monitoring. Furthermore, the study showed that protocol deviations, inattention, communication problems, distraction, and poor teamwork were significant contributing factors in reported medication errors. Although actual harm to the patient was reported in 27% of reports, fortunately only few medication errors resulted in serious harm to the patient (1.9%) and death (0.2%).

Other studies also have used incident reporting systems to determine the occurrence of medication errors [34–36]. However, lack of consistency in application of error classification schemes and varying methods of error reporting make it difficult to compare these studies. Nevertheless, they emphasize the added vulnerability of NICU patients and show that medication errors are common in this area of the hospital. For instance, Ross and colleagues [34] determined that NICU medication errors accounted for 17% of all pediatric medication error reports made over 5 years in a teaching hospital in the United Kingdom. Simpson and colleagues [35] found a rate of 24.1 errors per 1000 neonatal activity days in their study of NICU medication errors. And finally, Kanter and colleagues [36] determined that there were 1.2 reported medical errors, including medication errors, per 100 discharges for premature neonates at community hospitals in over 20 states in the United States.

Trigger-based methods

Recently, use of the "trigger" methodology has been shown to be a more sensitive method to identify an AE than other strategies, and triggers have been heralded as one of the most promising methods to use in error detection [37–39]. Triggers are defined as "occurrences, prompts, or flags found on review of the medical record that 'trigger' further investigation to determine the presence or absence of an adverse event" [38]. Trigger tools do not detect all medication errors, but they are a good screening tool (high sensitivity, low specificity). For example, an algorithm may look for the use of a D10W bolus in a patient on insulin. If this combination is found, the chart may be flagged as a potential medication error involving insulin.

Sharek and colleagues [40] applied this methodology to the NICU with the following trigger list: nosocomial infection; antibiotic use; accidental extubations; hypotension; respiratory arrest; death; catheter infiltration or skin burn; naloxone use; anticoagulant (enoxaparin, warfarin, or heparin drip) administration; rising serum creatinine; necrotizing enterocolitis; seizures; phenobarbital; electrolyte abnormality; abnormal cranial imaging; hyperglycemia; and unplanned return to surgery. They found 0.74 AEs per patient, and demonstrated that patients less than 28 weeks gestation and less than 1500 g at birth had higher AE rates than other NICU patients. Fifty-six of all AE were considered preventable, and 22.7% of the AEs resulted in either permanent harm, necessity to provide interventions to sustain life, or death (Harm Categories G–I). The authors also pointed out that only 8% of AEs were identified in hospital-based occurrence reports, again highlighting the strength of the trigger-based approach over reporting tools in identifying patients at risk for harm. Although Sharek's trigger list encompassed events not related to medication errors per se (eg, respiratory arrest, unplanned extubations, nosocomial infections), the trigger list did include medications, some of which are included in the Institute for Safe Medication Practices (ISMP) List of High Alert-Medications [41,42].

Patient and family error reporting

Nationally, there have been many initiatives and endorsements by groups, such as the American Academy of Pediatrics and JCAHO, to encourage patient and family participation in error reporting and disclosure [43,44]. Parent-led ventures, such as the Josie King Safety Program at Johns Hopkins Medical Institutions, also have demonstrated the value of this approach to patient safety [45,46]. Patient and family member perceptions of inpatient quality of care have been examined in a variety of pediatric settings [47–51] and have drawn attention to the need for improvement in communication [49], standardization of nursing protocols and procedures [49], discharge planning [47], parental teaching of medication administration and side effects [47], and pain management [47]. More importantly, patient and family participation has initiated and precipitated a change in safety culture [45,46].

Among neonates, studies have shown that participation in the care of their infant in the NICU is desired by parents and is a source of empowerment, parental bonding, and communication enhancement among all caregivers [50,51]. In the VON study, medical error reports were queried to discern family member involvement. Twenty-four of the 1256 reports involved a parent or family member in the event. This study revealed that not only could family members be contributors to medication errors in the NICU setting, but also be key players in the discovery and investigation of these errors and prevention of harm to their infants [33]. Additional work is needed further to delineate parental and family member perspectives on errors and their role in error prevention in the NICU. At least one such effort is currently underway (Pamela Donohue, PA, ScD, personal communication, 2007).

Types of errors and strategies for improvement

Wrong drug dose

Dosing errors are among the most common pediatric medication errors, accounting for approximately 28% of AEs, and constituting up to 34% of potential adverse drug events [27]. Rapidly changing body parameters, such as weight, may predispose pediatric patients to dosing errors. In addition, the need to dose medications by the patient's weight or body surface area requires health care providers to perform calculations, which may further increase the potential for dosing errors [52].

Several studies bring attention to dosing errors in pediatrics [53–55]. In one study, pharmacists reviewed all orders and all reported medication errors. Thirty-seven percent of errors occurred in patients less than 1 month of age, and 49.7% of errors occurred in the NICU [53]. Most of these errors reflected dosing errors with 55.1% of errant orders being overdosed and 26.9% underdosed [53].

The vulnerability of NICU patients to dosing errors also has been described by Simpson and colleagues [35], who reported that 49% of

NICU medication errors were caused by inaccurate prescribing, such as incorrect dose (37 errors); wrong dosing units (five errors); and incomplete prescriptions (14 cases). Two cases of drug overdose in their study included a 10-fold dose miscalculation, with one involving an opiate overdose for which naloxone had to be administered [35]. In their review of pediatric intensive care unit (PICU) and NICU critical incidents, Frey and colleagues [54] determined that 60% of medication error reports involved incorrect drug dosing [54]. In addition, they revealed that 13% of drug incidents were caused by decimal point errors, highlighting the need for accurate drug calculations in pediatric patients. This concept was delineated further by Carroll and colleagues [55], who found that 27.7% of NICU progress notes by resident physicians contained incorrect documentation of medications (incorrect medications, missing medications, missing doses, and incorrect doses), and 13.3% had discrepancies in patient weight. As anticipated, documentation errors were more likely to be found in the records of patients with longer lengths of stay in the NICU.

Dosing errors also were found in a study by Raju and colleagues [15], who reviewed medication errors that reached patients in the NICU and pediatric PICU. Wrong dosing errors were found in 13.7% of reports, and omission errors were found in 12.4% of reports [15]. Ross and colleagues [34] also found similar rates of dosing errors on their review of reports made to a pediatric hospital over 5 years in the United Kingdom: 14.8% incorrect dose administered, 13.8% extra dose given, and 12.3% dose omitted.

A variety of measures to prevent dosing errors have been explored including computerized prescription writing tools, updated formularies for handheld devices, and dose-range checks in computerized provider order entry (CPOE) systems [56–70]. In addition, computer-assisted total parenteral nutrition programs, Web-based pediatric arrest medication and continuous infusion calculators, and computerized antibiotic management programs have been introduced to assist health care providers with calculations and dosing administration [71–77]. Independent redundant checks at different stages of medication-order processing, such as ordering, dispensing, and administering, also have been instituted to prevent harm from human error [78]. By using various system changes, dosing medication errors may be reduced in the health care setting.

Wrong strength or concentration, dosage form

Although pediatric patients are at risk for errors resulting from incorrect medication-dosage forms, studies have found that these types of errors have not generated a great portion of medication error reports. In their study of medication errors in the NICU and pediatric ICU, Raju and colleagues [15] found that 8.3% of errors resulted because of wrong preparation of medications. Ross and colleagues [34] found that administration of the incorrect strength of a drug was found in only 0.5% of medication errors, and an incorrect intravenous concentration was administered in 10.3% of cases.

Neonates in hospitals are served by the same pharmacy that dispenses medications to older children and adults. Selecting the wrong dosage form is a systems error caused by the required stocking of varying dosage forms. Unlike adults, where weights range by a factor of 5 (40–200 kg), children have much larger weight ranges (0.5–200 kg) with a factor of 400. This necessitates a larger number of concentrations to be stocked, increasing the likelihood of an error. Different concentrations may be manufactured in very similar appearing packages leading to additional systemic errors. A recent high profile example of wrong concentration leading to infant deaths was the 1000-fold heparin overdose of six NICU patients in Indianapolis [79].

Assortments of methods have been proposed and used to combat medication errors secondary to using the wrong preparation of medicines. To avoid misinterpreting drug names and doses, "tall man" lettering can be used by manufacturers on packaging and labeling, pharmacy on shelf labels, and information technology systems on computer software [80,81]. Tall man lettering highlights dissimilar letters in two names that may otherwise look or sound alike and has been recently applied to medication usage (eg, DOBUTamine versus DOPamine). This strategy also can be used to decipher various concentration forms of a medication (eg, twenty-FIVE mg/100 mL versus FIFTY mg/100 mL).

Other methods of preventing errors that arise from using the wrong preparation of medications include CPOE, bar coding, dispensing robots, and automated alerts [55,65–67,69,70,82–91]. In addition, standardized drug concentrations and smart-pump technology have been used in intensive care settings to minimize errors that result from incorrect calculations and ad hoc preparations [92–97]. Although studies have shown that these methods have reduced the risk associated with drug ordering, preparation, and administration, new risks for errors can be introduced by using these technologies.

Monitoring errors: drug-drug interactions, documented allergy, and clinical

Few studies have brought attention to monitoring errors in pediatrics, likely reflecting the difficulty in discovering the occurrence of these errors. Suresh and colleagues [33] reported that 0.2% of medical error reports in the NICU were the consequence of a failure to act on results of monitoring or testing. Although this was not exclusive to medication error reports, the finding does highlight that monitoring errors are not reported frequently. This may be a sign of the limitations of voluntary, error-reporting systems in that reports may be biased by the health care providers that are making the error reports, and that are unaware that a delay in follow-up of test results is considered a medical error that can result in harm.

Errors in drug-drug interactions and drug allergies also have been explored. In their retrospective chart review of pediatric patient errors, Kaushal and colleagues [27] found that 1.3% of pediatric medication errors involved a known allergy to the medication for the patient. Folli and colleagues [53] also report that 1.9% of error reports found on review of orders by pharmacists were caused by drug-drug interactions and 0.4% of patients had a documented drug allergy to the medication ordered. Although reported medication errors that have been attributed to drug allergies and drug interactions are few, the potential for harm to a patient from these types of errors can be significant, and mechanisms reinforcing the avoidance of these errors should be incorporated in safety efforts.

Medication errors also may result as a consequence of not properly monitoring the administration of medications. Vincer and colleagues [98,99] found that 32 of 313 incidents in the NICU were caused by improper monitoring of an intravenous infusion. Labeling errors have been implicated in error reports, comprising 9.9% of incident reports in a pediatric hospital in the United Kingdom [34].

CPOE, tall man labeling, and automated alerts can help prevent medication errors caused by drug-drug interactions, allergies, and breakdowns in clinical monitoring [55,65–67,69,70,80,81,88–91]. Other approaches can include implementing clinical decision support systems that remind physicians to order the appropriate laboratory tests and alert physicians of abnormal laboratory values [98]. Future studies are needed to characterize and measure the occurrence of monitoring errors, so that more strategies can be devised to prevent harm from these types of errors.

Wrong patient

Patient misidentification can occur among neonates given the high rate of multiple births and the practice of using "BB" (baby boy) or "BG" (baby girl) instead of a first name, resulting in similarities in patient names. It has been estimated that 50% of patients on any given day are at risk of such an error, and that this may be a consequence of similarities in standard identifiers [100]. Although Kaushal and colleagues [27] found that only 0.16% of pediatric medication errors involved the wrong patient, Simpson and colleagues [35] found that one quarter of serious medication errors in the NICU involved patient misidentification. In addition, Suresh and colleagues [33] reported that 11% of NICU errors involved misidentification. In the United Kingdom, 3.9% of errors involved the wrong patient [34]. Patient misidentification plays an important role in medication errors in the NICU and is an aspect of care that should be addressed by NICU safety initiatives.

Provider order entry has been used to help decrease errors caused by patient misidentification. Provider order entry systems may increase the problem of misidentification, however, especially if they have poorly designed interfaces. At the Johns Hopkins Hospital, an increase in error reports for orders on the wrong patient was noted with provider order entry. In settings where providers use mobile computers and move between patients, such as in the ICUs, providers may forget to change the patient context in the provider order entry system and enter orders on the incorrect patient as they move from bed to bed. At Johns Hopkins, the increase in wrong patient errors required a redesign of the provider order entry interface and an additional confirmation of the patient identification at time of order submission (Christoph Lehmann, MD, personal communication, 2007). The phenomenon of wrong patient errors has been described as one of the unintended consequences of provider order entry [101].

The application of automatic identification technologies, such as bar coding, automated dispensing machines, and radiofrequency identification (RFID), also has been investigated in a variety of medical settings to help prevent medical and medication errors caused by misidentification [82–86,102–108]. Bar code technology has been used by the pharmacy to identify and track medications and by nursing to identify and document patient medication administration. Bar codes allow rapid processing of information to ensure compliance with the "five rights" of the medication process (right patient, right drug, right time, right dose, right route) [85]. Use of barcode technology has been reported to decrease administration errors by 80% [102].

With RFID systems, objects can be tagged with RFID chips storing unique identification codes, and tracked passively by wireless devices in a local network. The information and location of patients or objects (eg, medications, pumps, endotracheal tubes) can be known automatically at any time [103–107]. Among neonates, this technology has been applied mostly in labor and delivery units, where neonates have RFID cord clamps placed on their umbilical cords to help prevent abductions [109]. Although patient confidentiality concerns have been raised with the use of this technology, RFID systems have wide-reaching applications in the health care industry, particularly in streamlining medication reconciliation and analyzing operational inefficiencies and workflow.

Wrong route of administration, technique, rate, duration, or time

Patients in the NICU also may be at risk for medication errors caused by improper administration of drugs, and administrative errors may be underreported based on the method used to detect medication errors, such as the retrospective or concurrent chart review methods [110,111]. Nevertheless, administrative errors have been found to be frequent in intensive care settings, and this has also been found to be true in the NICU. In their retrospective chart review, Kaushal and colleagues [27] found that medications were given at the incorrect frequency in 9.4% of cases and by the wrong route in 18% of cases. Fifty-five percent of drugs given by the wrong route were intravenous drugs, followed by oral drugs in 21% of cases, and inhaled drugs in 7.5% according to error reports. Folli and colleagues [53] also found errors in wrong route of administration (1.9%) and drug intravenous incompatibility (2.7%) in their evaluation of errors in two children's hospitals. Ross and colleagues [34] report that 15.8% of medication errors were caused by incorrect intravenous infusion rates, and 4.4% of errors were caused by wrong route of administration.

Timing of medication administration also has been implicated in administrative errors. Simpson and colleagues [35] found that 19 of 75 NICU medication errors were categorized as incorrect dosing intervals, most commonly for gentamicin. In 30 other cases, medication errors were a result of administrative errors; in eight cases, the medication was given either by wrong route or too quickly; and in six cases, the medication was delayed from being given [35]. Similar results were found by Raju and colleagues [15], whose report indicated that most errors that reached the patient were caused by the wrong timing of medication administration (21.6%) and incorrect rate of drug administration (13.7%). They also found that the wrong technique was implicated in 13% of error reports, and the wrong route involved in 4.1% of errors. Errors in timing of medication administration also were found by Vincer and colleagues [98], who reported that 52 of 313 medication error incidents were a result of failing to give a medication on schedule in the NICU.

Because medication errors caused by incorrect route, timing, rate, duration, and technique have been found to be frequent in the NICU, they have been targets for intervention to improve health care delivery. Technologies, such as bar codes, automated alerts, RFIDs, and safety pumps, have been investigated as potential solutions [82–86,88–90,101–107,110]. Further research is needed to delineate the human factors involved in administration errors and their potential solutions.

Wrong drug

Wrong drug administration has been implicated in NICU medication errors. Kaushal and colleagues [27] found that 8.4% of medical errors reported the use of the wrong medication. Folli and colleagues [53] found 5.6% of medication error reports citing the use of the wrong drug, and Raju and colleagues [15] found that 13.3% of reports implicated the administration of an unauthorized drug to a patient. Frey and colleagues [54] report that 11 out of 62 reports were caused by wrong medication use, and Ross and colleagues [34] found that 12.3% of pediatric medication errors in the United Kingdom involved the wrong drug.

Efforts have been taken to aid in the correct identification of medications used in the ICU. Tall man labeling system has been used to assist in the reduction of these types of errors [80,81]. In March 2001, the Office of Generic Drugs embarked on a project aimed at encouraging manufacturers to revise the appearance of 16 similar medication name pairs in hopes of reducing errors resulting from name confusion [112].

Drugs involved in medication errors

Drugs involved in medication errors have been described in the pediatric literature. Although this problem is not exclusive to the NICU, a good portion of these medications involve antibiotics and parenteral nutrition (used in neonates). Frequent use of a medication results in more frequent errors. One definition of risk is: Risk = frequency of occurrence × harm. Attention must be paid to medications that are used commonly and medications that have narrow therapeutic windows. Efforts have been made to distinguish medications that are more harmful if used incorrectly. For example, Folli and colleagues [53] reported that digoxin, antibiotics, parenteral nutrition, and fluids and electrolytes accounted for 18 of 27 "potentially lethal" medication errors and for 47 of the 147 "serious" medication errors in pediatrics. A summary of drugs involved in pediatric medication error reports is shown in Table 2. A list of medications involved in harmful medication error reports at the Johns Hopkins Hospital NICU is shown in Box 1.

Table 2
Medications involved in pediatric and neonatal ICU medication errors

Medication	Simpson et al, [35] % Parenteral medications involved in pediatric medication errors	Kaushal et al, [27] % Pediatric error reports/% adverse drug events	Ross et al, [34] % Medications involved in pediatric medication errors
Antibiotics, anti-infectives		20/28	44
Gentamicin	33		
Benzyl penicillin	16		
Vancomycin	14		
Tazocin	3		
Analgesics and sedatives[a]		16/17	
Morphine	10		4.60
Electrolytes and fluids, parenteral nutrition[a]		25/15	16.50
Bronchodilators		7.1/15	
Aminophiline	5		
Insulin[a]	6		3.70
Immunizations	5		
Inotropes[a]			5.50
Anticancer drugs[a]			10.10
Steroids			4.60
Other		27/31	11
Missing		3.7/0	

[a] Denotes Institute for Safe Medication Practices high-alert medication.

Box 1. List of medications involved in high-risk errors (D–I) at the Johns Hopkins Hospital NICU (July 2004–September 2007 in descending order by frequency)

- Narcotics
- Electrolytes and total parenteral nutrition
- Vasopressive agents
- Antibiotics other than gentamicin
- Intralipids
- Gentamicin
- Caffeine
- Albuterol
- Heparin
- Furosemide
- Phenobarbital

High-alert medications are drugs that have an increased risk of causing patient harm when used in error [41,42]. In 1995, a list of high-alert medications was created by the ISMP after reviewing data on serious medication errors in 161 health care organizations. Since that time, the list has undergone multiple revisions based on harmful errors reported in the literature and input from safety experts [42]. This list of medications also has become part of the IHI's Save Five Million Lives campaign [113]. To date, the ISMP list of high-alert medications has not been evaluated in the neonatal population; however, one such study is underway (Theodora Stavroudis, MD, personal communication, 2007).

Total parenteral nutrition

A unique issue in the NICU is the administration of total parenteral nutrition. As many as 25% of medication errors have been attributed to fluid and electrolyte solutions [27]. Moreover, these errors may result in death [114]. Computerized total parenteral nutrition programs have been implemented to reduce these medication errors, and have shown reductions in calculation errors (100%); osmolality outside the allowed range (88%–91%); and knowledge deficit (84%–100%) [71].

Patients in the NICU are also at risk for harm from intralipid errors. Chuo and colleagues [115] found 266 out of 7329 NICU medication error reports involved intralipids. Reports were submitted to the Medmarx database by 55 hospitals between January 1, 2000, and December 31, 2005. Most errors took place during the administering phase of medication processing (93.2%); involved improper dosing (69.3%); and took place in the evening hours (27.4%). Most errors (96.3%) did not result in harm to the patient.

This study highlights the role of human factors in the administration of continuous medication infusions. Continuous infusions are a part of NICU care that warrants further study.

Safety culture

A strong institutional safety culture has been associated with improved quality of care [116]. Creating and sustaining a culture of safety requires commitment and participation of all stakeholders including leadership, health care team members, and patients. Furthermore, it requires an understanding of the systemic aspects of health care delivery (Fig. 1) [117]. Although the topic of safety culture is vast and outside the scope of this article, a few of the safety initiatives as they pertain to the NICU are highlighted.

The VON is a well-known leader in NICU patient safety, and toward this aim has created the Evidence-Based Quality Improvement Collaborative for Neonatology and the Neonatal Intensive Care Quality Improvement Collaborative Year 2007 (NIC/Q2007), where 47 institutions in North America work together on safety initiatives [118,119]. "Four Key Habits" have been identified by this group for clinical improvement: (1) change, (2) evidence-based practice, (3) collaborative learning, and (4) systems thinking. This group has supported the testing and implementation of potentially better practices in the care of the newborn and disseminates this information to their members by resource kits and a series of Internet-based collaboratives [118].

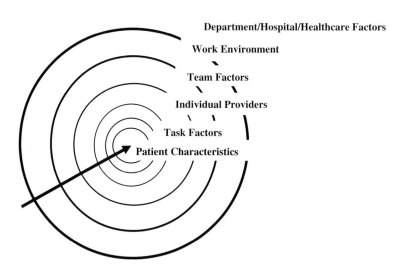

Fig. 1. The hierarchy of systems that influence patient care. (*Adapted from* Randolph AG, Pronovost P. Reorganizing the delivery of intensive care could improve efficiency and save lives. J Eval Clin Pract 2002;8:1–8; with permission.)

On a local level, patient safety rounds have been used to promote a team approach in identifying, prioritizing, and implementing safety initiatives [116–123]. At the Johns Hopkins Hospital, monthly NICU Safety Rounds take place at the bedside with the chief of pediatrics, director of information of technology, pediatric safety leadership, pediatric pharmacists, NICU nurses, and NICU physicians. This multidisciplinary approach has led to many changes within the Children's Center that enhance patient safety. Thirty-five percent of the completed problems were classified as Care Coordination/Records, 27% as Equipment Safety Situation/Preventative Maintenance, 21.4% as Equipment/Supplies/Devices, 3.8% as Error Related to Procedure/Treatment/Test, and 3.8% as Medication Error [120]. At Johns Hopkins, the NICU safety team meets monthly to discuss patient safety issues, such as medication errors, unplanned extubations, and

---

Box 2. Modified List of JCAHO's 2008 patient safety goals pertaining to medication errors

- Improve the accuracy of patient identification (use at least two patient identifiers)
- Improve the effectiveness of communication among caregivers
  Read back the verbal orders or test results
  Standardize a list of abbreviations and symbols that are not to be used
  Improve the timeliness of reporting and receipt of critical test results and values
- Improve the safety of using medications
  Identify and review look-alike and sound-alike drugs
  Label all medications on and off the sterile field
  Reduce errors associated with the use of anticoagulation therapy
- Accurately and completely reconcile medications across the continuum of care
  Compare the patient's current medications with those ordered for the patient
  Communicate the patient's medications to the next provider of service when a patient is referred or transferred to another setting, and review the complete list of medications to the patient on discharge
- Encourage patients' active involvement in their own care as a patient safety strategy
  Define and communicate the means for patients and their families to report concerns about safety and encourage them to do so

implementation of various technologies in the NICU (Christoph Lehmann, MD, personal communication, 2007).

On a national level, leaders in the field of patient safety have initiated movements to promote safety and prevent harm from medication errors. The IHI's Save Five Million Lives campaign highlights the prevention of medication errors from high-alert medications [113]. In addition, JCAHO's 2008 Patient Safety Goals encompass objectives that apply to medication error prevention [78]. A list of these objectives is provided in Box 2.

Summary

Medication errors are common in the NICU, and most errors can be prevented. A variety of measures and methods exist to help reduce the potential for harm to patients from medication errors and include such technologies as CPOE, bar codes, safety pumps, tall man labeling, Internet-based calculators, and RFID. More work is needed to delineate further the factors involved in NICU medication errors, so that targets for intervention can be established, validated, and maintained in a timely, efficient, and resource-effective way.

Acknowledgments

The authors thank Panagiotis K. Ordoulidis for his assistance in the preparation of this article.

References

[1] Institute of Medicine. To err is human: building a safer health system. Washington, D.C.: National Academy Press; 1999.
[2] The Leapfrog Group. Available at: http://www.leapfroggroup.org. Accessed September 29, 2007.
[3] The Joint Commission on Accreditation of Healthcare Organizations. Available at: http://www.jointcommission.org/. Accessed September 18, 2007.
[4] The Institute for Healthcare Improvement. Available at: http://www.ihi.org/IHI/. Accessed September 18, 2007.
[5] Wilson DG, McArtney RG, Newcombe RG, et al. Medication errors in paediatric practice: insights from a continuous quality improvement approach. Eur J Pediatr 1998;157(9): 769–74.
[6] Cimino MA, Kirschbaum MS, Brodsky L, et al. Child health accountability I. Assessing medication prescribing errors in pediatric intensive care units. Pediatr Crit Care Med 2004;5(2):124–32.
[7] Rothschild JM, Landrigan CP, Cronin JW, et al. The Critical Care Safety Study: the incidence and nature of adverse events and serious medical errors in intensive care. Crit Care Med 2005;33(8):1694–700.

[8] National Coordinating Council for Medication Error Reporting and Prevention Taxonomy of Medication Errors, Copyright 1998. Available at: http://www.nccmerp.org/pdf/taxo2001-07-31.pdf. Accessed September 18, 2007.

[9] Agency for Healthcare Research and Quality Patient Safety Network Glossary. Available at: http://www.psnet.ahrq.gov/glossary.aspx. Accessed September 29, 2007.

[10] Walsh KE, Kaushal R, Chessare JB. How to avoid paediatric medication errors: a user's guide to the literature. Arch Dis Child 2005;90(7):698–702.

[11] Kozer E, Scolnik D, Keays T, et al. Large errors in the dosing of medications for children. N Engl J Med 2002;346:1175–6.

[12] Conroy S, Choonara I, Impicciatore P, et al. Unlicensed and off-label drug use in pediatric wards in different European countries. BMJ 2000;320:79–82.

[13] Levine SR, Cohne MR, Blanchard NR, et al. Guidelines for preventing medication errors in pediatrics. J Pediatr Pharmacol Ther 2001;6:426–42.

[14] Frey B, Buettiker V, Hug MI, et al. Does critical incident reporting contribute to medication error prevention? Eur J Pediatr 2002;161(11):594–9.

[15] Raju TN, Kecskes S, Thornton JP, et al. Medication errors in neonatal and paediatric intensive care units. Lancet 1989;2(8659):374–6.

[16] Gray JE, Goldmann DA. Medication errors in the neonatal intensive care unit: special patients, unique issues. Arch Dis Child Fetal Neonatal Ed 2004;89:472–3.

[17] Chappell K, Newman C. Potential tenfold drug overdoses on a neonatal unit. Arch Dis Child Fetal Neonatal Ed 2004;89:483–4.

[18] Cuzzolin L, Atzei A, Fanos V. Off-label and unlicensed prescribing for newborns and children in different settings: a review of the literature and a consideration about drug safety. Expert Opin Drug Saf 2006;5(5):703–18.

[19] Avenel S, Bomkratz A, Dassieu G, et al. The incidence of prescriptions without marketing product license in a neonatal intensive care unit. Arch Pediatr 2000;7(2):143–7.

[20] Barr J, Brenner-Zada G, Heiman E, et al. Unlicensed and off-label medication use in a neonatal intensive care unit: a prospective study. Am J Perinatol 2002;19:67–72.

[21] Pandolfini C, Bonati M. A literature review on off-label drug use in children. Eur J Pediatr 2005;164(9):552–8.

[22] Shaw SS, Hall M, Goodman DM, et al. Off-label drug use in hospitalized children. Arch Pediatr Adolesc Med 2007;161(3):282–90.

[23] The U.S. Department of Health and Human Services Centers for Disease Control and Prevention. Available at: http://www.cdc.gov/nchs/pressroom/06facts/births05.htm. Accessed September 18, 2007.

[24] Stankaitis JA, Brill HR, Walker DM. Reduction in neonatal intensive care unit admission rates in a Medicaid managed care program. Am J Manag Care 2005;11(3):166–72.

[25] Reece EA, Lequizamon G, Silva J, et al. Intensive interventional maternity care reduces infant morbidity and hospital costs. J Matern Fetal Neonatal Med 2002;11(3):204–10.

[26] Brennan TA, Leape LL, Laird NM, et al. Incidence of adverse events and negligence in hospitalized patients: results of the Harvard Medical Practice Study I. N Engl J Med 1991;324:370–6.

[27] Kaushal R, Bates DW, Landrigan C, et al. Medication errors and adverse drug events in pediatric inpatients. JAMA 2001;285:2114–20.

[28] Institute of Medicine. Crossing the quality chiasm: a new health system for the 21st century. Washington, DC: National Academy Press; 2001.

[29] Kivlahan C, Sangster W, Nelson K, et al. Developing a comprehensive electronic adverse event reporting system in an academic health center. Jt Comm J Qual Improv 2002;28:583–94.

[30] Joint Commission on Accreditation of Healthcare Organizations. Our commitment to patient safety: sentinel event policy. Available at: www.jointcommission.org/PatientsSafety/facts_patient_safety.htm. Accessed May 14, 2007.

[31] US Pharmacopeia: Medmarx. Available at: www.medmarx.com//index.jsp. Accessed May 14, 2007.

[32] Wu AW, Pronovost P, Morlock L. ICU incident reporting systems. J Crit Care 2002;17:86–94.

[33] Suresh G, Horbar J, Plsek P, et al. voluntary anonymous reporting of medical errors for neonatal intensive care. Pediatrics 2004;113:1609–18.

[34] Ross LM, Wallace J, Paton JY. Medication errors in a paediatric teaching hospital in the UK: five years operational experience. Arch Dis Child 2000;83:492–7.

[35] Simpson JH, Lynch R, Grant J, et al. Reducing medication errors in the neonatal intensive care unit. Arch Dis Child Fetal Neonatal Ed 2004;89:F480–2.

[36] Kanter DE, Turenne W, Slonim AD. Hospital-reported medical errors in premature neonates. Pediatr Crit Care Med 2004;5(2):119–23.

[37] Resar RK, Rozich JD, Simmonds T, et al. A trigger tool to identify adverse events in the intensive care unit. Jt Comm J Qual Saf 2006;32(10):585–90.

[38] Rozich JD, Haraden CR, Resar RK. Adverse drug event trigger tool: a practical methodology for measuring medication related harm. Qual Saf Health Care 2003;12:194–200.

[39] Resar RK, Rozich JD, Classen DC. Methodology and rationale for the measurement of harm with trigger tools. Qual Saf Health Care 2003;12:39–45.

[40] Sharek PJ, Horbar JD, Mason W, et al. Adverse events in the neonatal intensive care unit: development, testing, and findings of an NICU-focused trigger tool to identify harm in North American NICUs. Pediatrics 2006;118:1332–40.

[41] Cohen MR, Kilo CM. High-alert medications: safeguarding against errors. In: Cohen MR, editor. Medication errors 5.1–5.40. Washington, D.C.: American Pharmaceutical Association; 1999.

[42] The Institute for Safe Medication Practice List of High Alert-Medications. Available at: www.ismp.org. Accessed September 19, 2007.

[43] Stucky ER. American Academy of Pediatrics: Committee on Drugs and Committee on Hospital Care. Prevention of medication errors in the pediatric inpatient setting. Pediatrics 2003;112:431–6.

[44] Joint Commission on Accreditation of Healthcare Organizations. Speak up initiatives. Available at: http://www.jointcommission.org/PatientSafety/SpeakUp. Accessed September 20, 2007.

[45] Kennedy P, Pronovost P. Shepherding change: how the market, healthcare providers, and public policy can deliver quality care for the 21st century. Crit Care Med 2006;34(3):S1–6.

[46] King S. Our story. Pediatr Radiol 2006;36:284–6.

[47] Homer CJ, Marino B, Cleary PD, et al. Quality of care at a children's hospital: the parent's perspective. Arch Pediatr Adolesc Med 1999;153(11):1123–9.

[48] Co JP, Ferris TG, Marino BL, et al. Are hospital characteristics associated with parental views of pediatric inpatient care quality? Pediatrics 2003;111(2):308–14.

[49] Sobo EJ, Billman G, Lim L, et al. A rapid interview protocol supporting patient-centered quality improvement: hearing the parent's voice in a pediatric cancer unit. Jt Comm J Qual Improv 2002;28(9):498–509.

[50] Hurst I. Vigilant watching over: mothers' actions to safeguard their premature babies in the newborn intensive care nursery. J Perinat Neonatal Nurs 2001;15(3):39–57.

[51] Wigert H, Johansson R, Berg M, et al. Mothers' experiences of having their newborn child in a neonatal intensive care unit. Scand J Caring Sci 2006;20:35–41.

[52] Rowe C, Koren T, Koren G. Errors by paediatric residents in calculating drug doses. Arch Dis Child 1998;79(1):56–8.

[53] Folli HL, Poole RL, Benitz WE, et al. Medication error prevention by clinical pharmacists in two children's hospitals. Pediatrics 1987;79:718–22.

[54] Frey B, Kehrer B, Losa M, et al. Comprehensive critical incident monitoring in a neonatal-pediatric intensive care unit: experience with the system approach. Intensive Care Med 2000;26:69–74.

[55] Carroll AE, Tarczy-Hornoch P, O'Reilly E, et al. Resident documentation discrepancies in a neonatal intensive care unit. Pediatrics 2003;111:976–80.

[56] Kushniruk A, Triola M, Stein B, et al. The relationship of usability to medical error: an evaluation of errors associated with usability problems in the use of a handheld application for prescribing medications. Medinfo 2004;11:1073–6.

[57] Kushniruk AW, Triola MM, Borycki EM, et al. Technology induced error and usability: the relationship between usability problems and prescription errors when using a handheld application. Int J Med Inf 2005;74:519–26.

[58] Clauson KA, Seamon MJ, Clausen AS, et al. Evaluation of drug information databases for personal digital assistants. Am J Health Syst Pharm 2004;61(10):1015–24.

[59] Lehmann CU, Kim GR. Computerized provider order entry and patient safety. Pediatr Clin North Am 2006;53:1169–84.

[60] Stengel D, Bauwens K, Walter M, et al. Comparison of handheld computer-assisted and conventional paper chart documentation of medical records: a randomized, controlled trial. J Bone Joint Surg Am 2004;86-A(3):553–60.

[61] Roukema K, Los RK, Bleeker SE, et al. Paper versus computer: feasibility of an electronic medical record in general pediatrics. Pediatrics 2006;117(1):15–21.

[62] Kirk RC, Li-Meng Goh D, Packia J, et al. Computer calculated dose in paediatric prescribing. Drug Saf 2005;28(9):817–24.

[63] Walton R, Dovey S, Harvey E, et al. Computer support for determining drug dose: systematic review and meta-analysis. BMJ 1999;318(7189):984–90.

[64] Giannone G. Computer-supported weight-based drug infusion concentrations in the neonatal intensive care unit. Comput Inform Nurs 2005;23(2):100–5.

[65] Ali NA, Mekhjian HS, Kuehn PL, et al. Specificity of computerized physician order entry has a significant effect on the efficiency of workflow for critically ill patients. Crit Care Med 2005;33(1):110–4.

[66] Koppel R. Role of computerized physician order entry systems in facilitating medication errors. JAMA 2005;293:1197–203.

[67] Cordero L, Kuehn L, Kumar RR, et al. Impact of computerized physician order entry on clinical practice in a newborn intensive care unit. J Perinatol 2004;24(2):88–93.

[68] McAlearney AS, Chisolm D, Veneris S, et al. Utilization of evidence-based computerized order sets in pediatrics. Int J Med Inf 2005;75(7):501–12.

[69] Waitman LR, Pearson D, Hargrove FR, et al. Enhancing computerized provider order entry for neonatal intensive care. AMIA Annu Symp Proc 2003;1078.

[70] Kaushal R, Jha AK, Franz C, et al. Return on investment for a computerized physician order entry system. J Am Med Inform Assoc 2006;13(3):261–6.

[71] Lehmann CU, Conner KG, Cox JM. Preventing provider errors: online total parenteral nutrition calculator. Pediatrics 2004;113(4):748–53.

[72] Brown CL, Garrison NA, Hutchison AA. Error reduction when prescribing neonatal parenteral nutrition. Am J Perinatol 2007;24(7):417–27.

[73] Costakos DT. Of lobsters, electronic medical records, and neonatal total parenteral nutrition. Pediatrics 2006;117(2):e328–32.

[74] Blackledge CG Jr, Veltri MA, Matlin C, et al. Patient safety in emergency situations: a web-based pediatric arrest medication calculator. J Healthc Qual 2006;28(2):27–31.

[75] Lehmann CU, Kim GR, Gujral R, et al. Decreasing errors in pediatric continuous intravenous infusions. Pediatr Crit Care Med 2006;7(3):225–30.

[76] Johns Hopkins University Division of Infectious Diseases. Johns Hopkins point-of-care information technology (POC-IT) antibiotic guide. Available at: http://www.hopkins-abxguide.org. Accessed September 27, 2007.

[77] Evans RS, Pestotnik SL, Classen DC, et al. A computer-assisted management program for antibiotics and other antiinfective agents. N Engl J Med 1998;338(4):232–8.

[78] The Joint Commission. 2008 National Patient Safety Goals Hospital Program. Available at: http://www.jointcommission.org/PatientSafety/NationalPatientSafetyGoals/08_hap_npsgs.htm. Accessed September 29, 2007.

[79] Hospital procedures questioned after death of two babies. Available at: http://abcnews.go. com/WNT/Health/story?id=2465287&page=1. Accessed September 27, 2007.

[80] Filik R, Purdy K, Gale A, et al. Labeling of medicines and patient safety: evaluating methods of reducing drug name confusion. Hum Factors 2006;48(1):39–47.

[81] Bates DW, Gawande AA. Improving safety with information technology. N Engl J Med 2003;348(25):2526–34.

[82] Cummings J, Bush P, Smith D, et al. UHC bar-coding task force. Am J Health Syst Pharm 2005;62(24):2626–9.

[83] Perrin RA, Simpson N. RFID and bar codes: critical importance in enhancing safe patient care. J Healthc Inf Manag 2004;18(4):33–9.

[84] Wright AA, Katz IT. Bar coding for patient safety. N Engl J Med 2005;353(4):329–31.

[85] Paoletti RD, Suess TM, Lesko MG, et al. Using bar-code technology and medication observation methodology for safer medication administration. Am J Health Syst Pharm 2007; 64(5):536–43.

[86] Poon EG, Cina JL, Churchill WW, et al. Effect of bar-code technology on the incidence of medication dispensing errors and potential adverse drug events in a hospital pharmacy. AMIA Annu Symp Proc 2005;1085.

[87] Perini VJ, Vermeulen LC Jr. Comparison of automated medication-management systems. Am J Hosp Pharm 1994;51(15):1883–91.

[88] Glassman PA, Simon B, Belperio P, et al. Improving recognition of drug interactions: benefits and barriers to using automated drug alerts. Med Care 2002;40(12):1161–71.

[89] Rind DM, Safran C, Phillips RS, et al. Effect of computer-based alerts on the treatment and outcomes of hospitalized patients. Arch Intern Med 1994;154(13):1511–7.

[90] Raschke RA, Gollihare B, Wunderlich TA, et al. A computer alert system to prevent injury from adverse drug events: development and evaluation in a community teaching hospital. JAMA 1998;280(15):1317–20.

[91] Glassman PA, Belperio P, Simon B, et al. Exposure to automated drug alerts over time: effects on clinicians' knowledge and perceptions. Med Care 2006;44(3):250–6.

[92] Larsen GY, Parker HB, Cash J, et al. Standard drug concentrations and smart-pump technology reduce continuous-medication-infusion errors in pediatric patients. Pediatrics 2005;116(1):e21–5.

[93] Bullock J, Jordan D, Gawlinski A, et al. Standardizing IV infusion mediation concentrations to reduce variability in medication errors. Crit Care Nurs Clin North Am 2006; 18(4):515–21.

[94] Roman N. Innovative solutions: standardized concentrations facilitate the use of continuous infusions for pediatric intensive care unit nurses at a community hospital. Dimens Crit Care Nurs 2005;24(6):275–8.

[95] Brannon TS. Ad hoc versus standardized admixtures for continuous infusion drugs in neonatal intensive care: cognitive task analysis of safety at the bedside. AMIA Annu Symp Proc 2006:862.

[96] JCAHO's compliance expectations for standardized concentrations. Rule of Six in pediatrics does not meet requirements. Jt Comm Perspect 2004;24(5):11.

[97] Apkon M, Leonard J, Probst L, et al. Design of a safer approach to intravenous drug infusions: failure mode effects analysis. Qual Saf Health Care 2004;13(4):265–71.

[98] Vincer MJ, Murray JM, Yuill A, et al. Drug errors and incidents in a neonatal intensive care unit: quality assurance activity. Am J Dis Child 1989;143:737–40.

[99] Mekhjian H, Saltz J, Rogers P, et al. Impact of CPOE order sets on lab orders. AMIA Annu Symp Proc 2003:931.

[100] Gray JE, Suresh G, Ursprung R, et al. Patient misidentification in the neonatal intensive care unit: quantification of risk. Pediatrics 2006;117:e43–7.

[101] Ash JS, Gorman PN, Lavelle M, et al. A cross-site qualitative study of physician order entry. J Am Med Inform Assoc 2003;10(2):188–200.

[102] Kaushal R, Bates DW. Information technology and medication safety: what is the benefit? Qual Saf Health Care 2002;11(3):261–5.

[103] Testa M, Pollard J. Safe pill-dispensing. Stud Health Technol Inform 2007;127:139–46.

[104] Cavalleri M, Morstabilini R, Reni G. A wearable device for a fully automated in-hospital staff and patient identification. Conf Proc IEEE Eng Med Biol Soc 2004;5:3278–81.

[105] Shindo A, Matsuda A, Tani S, et al. Construction of a safety management system for drug use by using an RFID tag. Stud Health Technol Inform 2006;122:770.

[106] Reicher J, Reicher D, Reicher M. Use of radio frequency identification (RFID) tags in bedside monitoring of endotracheal tube position. J Clin Monit Comput 2007;21(3):155–8.

[107] Wicks AM, Visich JK, Li S. Radio frequency identification applications in hospital environments. Hosp Top 2006;84(3):3–8.

[108] Crane J, Crane FG. Preventing medication errors in hospitals through a systems approach and technological innovation: a prescription for 2010. Hosp Top 2006;84(4):3–8.

[109] Nahirny C. Trends in infant abductions. J Healthc Prot Manage 2005;21(2):95–9.

[110] Miller MR, Clark JS, Lehmann CU. Computer based medication error reporting: insights and implications. Qual Saf Health Care 2006;15(3):208–13.

[111] Rothschild JM, Keohane CA, Cook EF, et al. A controlled trial of smart infusion pumps to improve medication safety in critically ill patients. Crit Care Med 2005;33(3):533–40.

[112] The Office of Generic Drugs. Available at: http://www.fda.gov/cder/drug/MedErrors/nameDiff.htm. Accessed September 29, 2007.

[113] Institute for Healthcare Improvement. Campaign Overview. Available at: http://www.ihi.org/IHI/Programs/Campaign/Campaign.htm?TabId=1. Accessed September 27, 2007.

[114] Fatal 1,000-fold overdoses can occur, particularly in neonates, by transposing mcg and mg. ISMP Medication Safety Alert! Acute Care Edition 2007;12:1–4. Available at: http://www.ismp.org/Newsletters/acutecare/articles/20070906.asp. Accessed September 29, 2007.

[115] Chuo J, Lambert G, Hicks RW. Intralipid medication errors in the neonatal intensive care unit. Jt Comm J Qual Patient Saf 2007;33(2):104–11.

[116] McCafferty MH, Polk HC Jr. Patient safety and quality in surgery. Surg Clin North Am 2007;87(4):867–81.

[117] Randolph AG, Pronovost P. Reorganizing the delivery of intensive care could improve efficiency and save lives. J Eval Clin Pract 2002;8(1):1–8.

[118] The Vermont Oxford Network. Available at: http://www.vtoxford.org/home.aspx. Accessed September 29, 2007.

[119] Horbar JD, Plsek PE, Leahy K. NIC/Q 2000: establishing habits for improvement in neonatal intensive care units. Pediatrics 2003;111:e397–410.

[120] Rinke ML, Zimmer KP, Lehmann CU, et al. Patient safety rounds in a pediatric tertiary care center. Jt Comm J Qual Patient Saf 2008;34:5–12.

[121] Executive rounding program improves communication, performance. Perform Improv Advis 2006;10(8):94–6, 85.

[122] Campbell DA, Thompson M. Patient safety rounds: description of an inexpensive but important strategy to improve the safety culture. Am J Med Qual 2007;22:26–33.

[123] Frankel A, Grillo SP, Baker EG, et al. Patient Safety leadership walkrounds at partners healthcare: learning from implementation. Jt Comm J Qual Patient Saf 2005;31(8):423–37.

ELSEVIER
SAUNDERS

CLINICS IN
PERINATOLOGY

Clin Perinatol 35 (2008) 163–181

Iatrogenic Environmental Hazards in the Neonatal Intensive Care Unit

Thomas T. Lai, MD*, Cynthia F. Bearer, MD, PhD

*Division of Neonatology, University Hospitals, Rainbow Babies and Childrens Hospital,
11100 Euclid Avenue, RBC Suite 3100 Cleveland, OH 44106-6010, USA*

Premature infants in the neonatal intensive care unit face many illnesses and complications. Another potential source of iatrogenic disease is the NICU environment. Research in this area, however, is limited. Patients in the neonatal intensive care unit (NICU) sustain a range of complex illnesses. Often, these patients are not only extremely premature and ill equipped to face the outside world but also face the potential for iatrogenic disease in the hospital. One such source of iatrogenic disease is their new surrounding environment. Light, sound, electromagnetic fields, radiation, inactive ingredients in medications, and chemicals are all potential sources of harm. When compared with older children and adults, premature neonates are particularly vulnerable due to still developing organ systems. This review attempts to discuss the major environmental dangers to neonates in the NICU and the recent literature available.

Light

The visual system of a newborn infant continues to develop well after birth until about 3 years of age. Preterm babies have the addition of light in their environment as opposed to the darkness in utero. All parts of the eye continue to develop—the retina, the neuronal connections, and even the eyelids [1]. Excessive light has been theorized to cause retinal damage, sleep pattern alterations, disturbance of circadian rhythms, and poor growth. The increased light in a NICU has the potential to impact visual development. In one study of a small group of premature infants born at 29 weeks' gestation or less, both eyes were covered for 23 hours a day until 32 weeks postmenstrual age to protect them from light. When pattern visual-evoked potentials were studied, there was no difference between the

---

* Corresponding author.
E-mail address: thomas.lai@uhhs.com (T.T. Lai).

covered and uncovered groups at term corrected age, 2 months corrected age, and 3 years corrected age [2].

Retinopathy of prematurity is a major cause of blindness in premature babies. Since the 1950s, the excessive use of oxygen has been known to increase the risk of retinopathy of prematurity. In the 1940s when the disease was first described, light was thought to be a contributor. Light when striking the retina is thought to increase the amount of energy in the eye, which, in turn, is thought to increase the number of free oxygen radicals in the retina. Various animal studies have demonstrated retinal injury from light; however, these studies have exposed the animals to extremely bright lights for prolonged periods of time, something not generally practiced in the NICU [3,4]. In one study, the incidence of retinopathy of prematurity decreased when isolettes were shielded with filters to reduce the amount of light by more than half to which the infants were exposed [5]. Other studies did not show similar results.

A study by Ackerman and colleagues [6] published in 1989 examined 161 infants, all of whom had blankets covering the top of their isolettes. They were compared with a historic control group of 129 infants. The blankets decreased the intensity of the light to one third of the normal uncovered intensity. There was no difference in the incidence of retinopathy of prematurity between both groups, even after breaking down the groups by gestational age. Reynolds and colleagues [7] conducted a multicenter prospective randomized trial (LIGHT-ROP) involving over 400 infants with a birth weight less than 1251 g and gestational age of less than 31 weeks. Infants' eyes were covered with goggles within the first 24 hours of life and kept covered until 31 weeks postmenstrual age or for a minimum of 4 weeks. The goggles decreased light exposure by 97% and UV exposure completely. There was no difference in rates of retinopathy of prematurity between the two groups even when broken down into subgroups of different birth weights, sexes, and races. When looking at infants whose eyes were covered within 6 hours of life versus those covered within 7 to 24 hours of life, there was no difference between controls and treated patients. A Cochrane review examined all of the studies regarding light reduction and the risk of retinopathy of prematurity published from 1949 to 1998. The review focused on five studies from 1952 to 1998 and found no difference in the incidence of retinopathy of prematurity if an infant's eyes were covered or left uncovered after birth [8].

Ambient light in the NICU has been thought to affect infant growth. Reduced lighting may confer advantages of improved sleep cycles and decreased stress. Several studies have examined these issues. The multicenter LIGHT-ROP study, which examined light reduction and retinopathy of prematurity, also examined infant growth. There was no difference between the group whose eyes were covered within 24 hours of birth and the group left uncovered. Both the unadjusted weight gain during the intervention as well as the weight gain adjusted for birth weight, gestational age, race, sex, and inborn status showed no significant difference between the treated and control groups. At the 34 week postmenstrual age and 6 month corrected age, both unadjusted and adjusted weights showed no significant difference between the treated and control groups [9].

The relationship between light and circadian rhythms has also been examined in infants. Circadian rhythms are typically 24-hour cycles based on an internal biologic clock. These rhythms affect the sleep-wake cycle and cyclic hormonal release that the human body experiences. In many animals, light can affect their circadian rhythms. In newborn primates, low intensity lighting can help regulate circadian rhythms. In term human infants, sleep cycles are not apparent until around 1 to 2 months of age, and hormone production cycles are first detected around 12 weeks of age. Preterm infants do not seem to have a specific circadian pattern; however, health care worker schedules may have a greater influence and mask any circadian rhythm [10]. Preterm infants at 32 to 34 weeks postmenstrual age were exposed to cycled light versus continuous dim lighting. Infants exposed to cycled light had significantly greater activity levels during the day immediately after discharge home. Similar activity level differences in the infants exposed to continuous dim lighting were not exhibited until 3 to 4 weeks after discharge home. No weight gain differences were noted [11]. Another study examined 40 preterm infants exposed to both cycled lighting and continuous dim lighting and found no difference in the sleep-wake cycles or temperatures of the infants. The infants did develop circadian rhythmicity regarding sleep cycles, but these findings were more related to their age and not environmental lighting [12].

Other researchers have focused on weight gain and cycled lighting as opposed to sleep cycles. In a prospective randomized controlled single center study involving 96 preterm babies, roughly half of the babies were exposed to continuous dim lighting and half to cycled lighting with lights on for 12 hours and lights off for 12 hours. When weight gain and the time it took for the infants to regain birth weight were examined, there was no significant difference between the two groups [13]. Other researchers have come to different conclusions. A study of 41 preterm infants showed that the 20 exposed to less noise and cycled light had better weight gain than those in the control nursery with no change in noise or light [14]. Another study of 62 infants found that premature infants exposed to cycled lighting from birth or from 32 weeks postconceptual age had better weight gain than infants exposed to only near darkness [15]. Studies regarding circadian rhythmicity and sleep and growth have thus far had conflicting results, and more research needs to be done to tease out the potential benefits of different lighting schemes in the NICU and when they need to be implemented.

Since 1831, light has also been used for diagnostic and procedural purposes [16]. Transillumination with high-intensity light is used to detect effusions, pneumothoraces, and other problems. It is also useful for venipuncture and arteriopuncture and placing peripheral intravenous and peripheral arterial catheters. Over time, the light source has changed from the sun to a candle to light bulbs to fiberoptic light sources. These devices can also cause burns when not used properly. Most contemporary devices have heat absorbing parts and cooling parts. With fiberoptic light sources, skin damage seems to occur at lower frequency wavelengths. By using a filter to block out light with a wavelength less than 570 nm, burns are minimized while still maintaining the effectiveness of a transilluminator [17]. Health care workers should take care to minimize the amount of time the transilluminator is in contact with the patient and should turn the device off when not using it to prevent it from getting too hot. Users should also check the transilluminator to make sure it appears intact, and they should test the light against their own skin to make sure it is not too hot [16,18].

Caregivers are also impacted by lighting in the NICU. Lights in this area need to be task appropriate. They should be flexible to provide more or less light given the circumstances. The Illuminating Engineering Society of North America recommends that light sources provide 1000 lux for critical visual tasks such as physical examination and procedures. The illuminance is the amount of light falling on a surface measured in lux or lumens per square meter. Lumens are measured in watts. A typical NICU has lighting ranging from 400 to 900 lux [19]. A typical office has lighting of 400 to 500 lux. These lights should not encroach upon other bed spaces. Medication stations and other slightly less critical areas should receive 500 lux. Direct light on patients should be avoided unless needed for specific tasks. Blankets or covers on the top of isolettes help to prevent unnecessary light exposure. Lighting, especially when used for hands-on care, should also have a high color-rendering index, which means that colors under lighting should appear as natural as possible [20].

Interior lighting of the NICU can also affect health care workers by impacting their circadian system and sleep-wake cycles. During the daytime, natural sunlight from windows and sky lights can help maintain the normal circadian rhythms of being awake during the day. North-facing windows in the Northern Hemisphere provide minimal glare and heat [21]. Windows facing other directions should be shaded to prevent glare and heat. At night, bright lights of about 2500 lux in break areas can cause an acute effect which can improve brain activity, cognitive performance, and feelings of alertness [20].

Light has many potential impacts on neonates in the NICU, both directly and indirectly. Ambient light does not increase the risk of retinopathy of prematurity, but more research is needed to determine whether cycled lighting affects circadian rhythms and growth in infants. Light can also cause burns in neonates during transillumination and can impact the levels of alertness of caregivers.

Sound and noise

Sound is a type of vibration that travels through the air or another medium and is sensed by the ear. As is true for the body of a premature baby, the auditory system continues to grow and develop. The outer ear, middle ear, and cochlea develop in parallel along with neural pathways during much of the time that an infant might spend in a NICU [22]. Noise refers to sound that is usually unpleasant or disturbing in nature. The hospital and especially the NICU can be a noisy place with the potential to affect a baby's hearing. Preterm babies are at particular risk of sensorineural hearing loss, with an incidence of 4% to 13% depending on size and age in comparison with a 2% incidence in all newborns [23]. The US Environmental Protection Agency (EPA) has suggested a day–night average sound level of less than or equal to 45 dB for indoor hospital areas to ensure adequate sleep, rest, and recovery of patients [24]. Incubators can produce noise and vibration up to 50 to 80 dB or greater, well above the recommended levels from the EPA [25,26]. Closing incubator doors, writing and tapping on incubators, talking near incubators, bumping equipment into walls and dropping it onto the floor, closing nearby drawers, and other loud noises can penetrate incubators.

In addition, medications such as diuretics and aminoglycosides have been thought to increase the risk of hearing loss. Furosemide is the diuretic most associated with the potential for hearing loss. The pathophysiology of how furosemide can cause hearing loss remains unknown. A case-control study looked at multiple factors involved with sensorineural hearing loss in neonates, including seizures, diuretics, and aminoglycosides. Only furosemide appeared to be significantly related to sensorineural hearing loss [27]. A later small retrospective chart review consisting of 264 neonates found no difference in the rate of sensorineural hearing loss in a group of neonates exposed to furosemide and one that was not exposed [28]. Animal studies on guinea pigs have demonstrated permanent cochlear changes with the administration of kanamycin while being exposed to the noise from incubators [29]. Studies in humans have shown conflicting results regarding the synergy of aminoglycosides and noise exposure [30].

Adults exposed to excessive noise and sound also develop noise-induced stimulation of the autonomic nervous system. Few studies have addressed this problem in premature neonates. Studies regarding noise-induced autonomic effects show that newborn term and preterm babies typically increase their heart rate with sudden sounds ranging from 55 to 100 dB [31]. Low birth weight infants have been shown to have increases in systolic and diastolic blood pressure to acoustic stimulation [32]. It is unknown whether acoustic stimulus can lead to chronic hypertension in neonates as it can in adults. Various studies have shown respiratory drive depression in premature infants with exposure to sound stimulus. In one case, a significant decrease in respiratory rate occurred upon exposure to 100 dB SPL (sound pressure level) stimuli [33]. In a second, sudden loud noises caused apnea and hypoxemic events [34].

Human preterm neonates showed differences on quantitative electroencephalography (qEEG) performed 2 weeks after the expected date of confinement when treated with environmental interventions including noise reduction, less opening and closing of incubator doors, and prolonged periods of quiet in a comparison with neonates who did not receive these interventions. The premature treated infants (30–34 weeks) who received environmental interventions had qEEG results similar to full-term control infants. Preterm control infants who did not receive any intervention had significantly different qEEG results, especially in the frontal region, further reinforcing the vulnerability of the premature infant [35].

Besides being detrimental to the patient directly, excessive noise in the NICU can impact caregivers. Excessive noise in general is a stressor. Excessive sound has been found in adults to cause hypertension, increased blood glucose, increased serum cholesterol, increased muscle tension, disturbed sleep, and altered immune function. Noise can also cause fatigue, irritability, annoyance, and decreased worker satisfaction [36]. With extra background noise, communication can be difficult at times and concentration can suffer. Work performance can also suffer [37]. Unfortunately, no studies have been performed specifically in relation to the NICU.

There are many angles from which to attack the problem of excessive noise in the NICU. Starting from outside to in, the location of the nursery in relation to a hospital's overall layout is important. Locating the nursery away from noisy streets or vehicular traffic, including helicopters and garbage collection, can decrease noise greatly. Sound proofing of the nursery can include special sound absorbent or reflective materials for windows, doors, walls, ceilings, and floors [38]. Individualized rooms or rooms with a small number of patients limit sound exposure. Locating work areas and major traffic pathways away from patient care areas will also limit noise exposure. Inside patient rooms, any noise producing equipment such as monitors, telephones, sinks, storage areas, and heating or cooling registers should be located away from the head of the bed [39]. Music has not been shown to have any significant benefit for neonates. A review of multiple studies showed that most investigations had problems with subject selection, sample size, or potential bias. Most of these studies also did not examine potential adverse outcomes [40]. Behavioral modification of staff members in the NICU can help to reduce noise levels but is difficult to maintain. Specific changes in behavior include not writing on incubator tops, responding quickly to alarms, removing water from ventilator tubing frequently, closing incubator doors quietly, and speaking softly around patients [41]. Other effective methods of decreasing noise exposure include earmuffs, covering incubators, and working with companies to develop quieter equipment. Padded drawers and doors and plastic bins instead of metal ones also help to decrease noise.

Electromagnetic fields

Every cell in the body has an electric potential. This electric potential can be manipulated via ion channels in the outer membrane. External sources of electricity and, in particular, electrical fields are also thought to have an impact on cells and possibly adversely affect the health of humans. In the NICU, premature neonates are still growing and developing and are surrounded by electrical equipment which has its own electromagnetic field.

Endogenous electromagnetic fields and currents are thought to help guide cell migration during development. Researchers have manipulated this internal electromagnetic current in chick embryos, leading to abnormalities in tail development. They have also produced limb bud and head developmental anomalies. The majority of tail abnormalities included neural tube defects [42]. In mammals, researchers have demonstrated that wounds in rat corneas have endogenous electromagnetic fields that affect the orientation of cell division. These electromagnetic fields also seem to affect the frequency of epithelial cell division. Medications that enhanced the endogenous electromagnetic field led to faster healing of the corneal wounds [43].

External electromagnetic fields are thought to be able to alter the normal development of animals and humans by interfering with endogenous electromagnetic fields associated with normal cell migration and development. Placing axolotl (a type of salamander) embryos in an exogenous electromagnetic field led to developmental abnormalities in the head and tail structures depending on the orientation of the embryos in the field. Defects included the absence of one or both eyes, misshapen heads, malformed tails, incomplete closure of neural folds, and irregular bodies [44]. Injecting *Xenopus laevis* (a type of frog) embryos with electromagnetic current has also led to developmental abnormalities including eye deformities, open neural tubes, and malformed heads [45]. Nevertheless, studies in mammals, specifically rats and mice, have shown conflicting results with few adverse outcomes. Some small skeletal anomalies have been seen, but these could not be attributed solely to electromagnetic fields [46]. Mammals overall have not shown the same susceptibility during embryologic development as have amphibians and birds.

In humans, besides prenatal development, the particular concern has been with the central nervous system. The central nervous system requires proper neuronal migration, apoptosis, and synaptogenesis. Development continues during childhood and adolescence. Given the evidence seen in vitro and in vivo in other animals, scientists have tried to tease out any potential effects of electromagnetic fields in humans. The majority of studies have been epidemiologic ones. Few people have looked at the effects of electromagnetic fields in the development and growth of children, and even fewer have examined whether neonates are at risk. There was no change in the rate of low birth weight babies and intrauterine growth retardation in women exposed to electromagnetic fields from using electric blankets in a comparison with women who did not use electric blankets [47]. Other studies have shown no relation between cleft defects, anencephaly, and spina bifida or other neural tube defects and electrically heated bed or blanket use [48,49].

The other main concern regarding electromagnetic fields is their potential to cause cancer. The International Agency for Research on Cancer, a part of the World Health Organization, has labeled these fields as a possible human carcinogen due to repeated epidemiologic data showing an association with childhood leukemia [50]; however, no causal relationship has been discovered. For neonates, the largest source of electromagnetic fields is the incubator. Premature babies spend a majority of their time in the NICU in incubators depending on their gestational age. The maximum electromagnetic field strength found in one study was 126 milligauss, with levels declining as the distance increased from the fan and heating unit [51]. Two case-control studies in Sweden looked at childhood leukemia and incubator use. The first study found a variety of factors associated with an increased risk of childhood myeloid leukemia, including maternal smoking, cesarean section, multiple birth, and maternal hypertension. Incubator use was found to have an increased risk, but when patients with Down's syndrome were excluded, the 95% confidence interval included the no-effect value [52]. A later study by some of the same researchers looking at only incubator use found no increased risk in relation to electromagnetic field or the duration of incubator use. They reported an electromagnetic field strength as high as 43.6 milligauss; however, the study looked only at durations of less than or greater than 30 days [53].

To date, despite the effect of electromagnetic fields on some animal models and the possibility of electromagnetic fields being carcinogenic for humans, there is little evidence to suggest that neonates are at increased risk while in the NICU. Nevertheless, shielding sources of electromagnetic fields would be an easy and inexpensive way to decrease any potential risk.

Electricity

Infants in the NICU are surrounded by electrical equipment and are dependent on it. Problems including malfunctioning, short circuits, sparks, and fires can arise if equipment is not maintained adequately. Normal and emergency back-up electrical outlets should be available to ensure a continual power source for life support equipment. Some organizations recommend at least 20 simultaneously accessible outlets at each bed spot [54]. Fire extinguishers should be easily accessible, and a fire safety plan should be in place in all NICUs.

Radiation

Radiation can both kill and modify cells. Both events can be detrimental to human life. Exposure to radiation has been linked to many forms of cancer. The major study describing the effects of exposure to radiation looked at the survivors of the atomic bombings at Hiroshima and Nagasaki, Japan. Fetal exposure to the radiation caused by the atomic bombs also led to mental retardation [55]. Humans are subject to natural radiation daily. Most of this radiation comes from cosmic rays and natural substances in the earth [56]. Babies in the NICU are exposed to radiation not only from natural sources but also from the x-ray studies performed on them and their neighbors.

The average annual dose of natural radiation humans are exposed to is 2.4 millisieverts (mSv) with a range of 1 to 10 mSv. The average annual dose from medically related radiation exposure is about 0.4 mSv with a range of 0.04 to 1 mSv. Life time doses of greater than 100 mSv are statistically significant as a risk for cancer when studying survivors of the atomic bombs in Japan [56]. The dose of radiation for a neonate from a two-view chest radiograph is around 25 to 60 μSv (mean, 40 μSv). About 25 two-view chest radiographs correspond to about 1 mSv, and about 75 two-view chest radiographs are equivalent to 1 year of natural background radiation [57]. Single-view abdominal films have a dose of 10 to 30 μSv, and single-view babygrams have a dose of 20 to 40 μSv [58]. The smallest, sickest, and most premature infants in the NICU tend to receive the greatest number of x-ray studies; therefore, they tend to have the greatest overall exposure. The median number of total chest, babygram, and abdominal radiographs was 31 in a study of 25 surviving infants with a birth weight of less than 750 g. The exposure from x-ray studies performed during a NICU stay for one of these infants using the highest dose would still be less than the average 1 year exposure from natural radiation. The increased risk of cancer from x-ray studies while in the NICU for a very low birth weight and extremely low birth weight infant is between 1 in 10,000 to 1 in 60,000 [58,59].

Despite the low risk of plain films in the NICU, health care workers should take steps to minimize the exposure of unnecessary areas to radiation. Extra parts of the patients were unnecessarily exposed to radiation in the majority of x-ray studies in five centers. For example, in 85% of all chest radiographs, the abdomen was also exposed. The thigh was irradiated along with the chest and abdomen in 62% of those films [60]. Proper x-ray beam collimation allows limiting radiation to only the requested area and avoiding unnecessary organ exposure. Genital shields can be used in larger infants during abdominal films to avoid irradiation of reproductive organs. Care should be taken to avoid repeated x-ray studies due to poor initial film quality. Technicians obtaining radiographs in the NICU should be trained in the proper use of these measures. Physicians can also help to minimize radiation by carefully evaluating each patient and their need for a film.

CT scans impart a much higher dose of radiation. They account for the major source of medical radiation despite comprising a small number of the procedures performed. In neonates, the most likely use of CT scan would be to check for abnormalities in the brain. According to the United Nations Scientific Committee on the Effects of Atomic Radiation, the calculated effective dose of radiation for a head CT scan is about 6 mSv and for an abdominal CT scan about 5.3 mSv [56]. Based on these numbers, a single

CT scan of the head carries a dose 200 times that of a single babygram and is about 2.5 times the natural radiation exposure in a year. Due to the high amount of radiation exposure from CT scans, physicians need to carefully consider possible alternatives to a CT scan for diagnosis. Both ultrasound and MRI have fewer known side effects when compared with a CT scan. If a CT scan is necessary, limiting the region of the body to be studied and using appropriate shielding when possible decreases the amount of radiation exposure. Specific pediatric parameters can also be designated by the radiologist or CT technologist to limit radiation.

Plasticizers

Polyvinyl chloride (PVC) is an extremely useful compound in everyday life. As a hard plastic, PVC is used for piping in water and sewage systems, as vinyl siding for houses and buildings, and as other hard plastics including car interiors and vinyl records. In the medical field, PVC is used mostly as a soft plastic. Potentially toxic plasticizers are added to PVC to give it flexibility and make it softer. Intravenous bags, catheters, and tubing, as well as chest tubes, Foley catheters, respiratory tubing, and extracorporeal membrane oxygenation (ECMO) and hemodialysis tubing are all made from PVC. The main plasticizer that is used is called diethylhexylphthalate (DEHP). DEHP does not bond with PVC and can leach, migrate, and evaporate from the PVC material. Lipophilic substances cause DEHP to leach out more readily. The main source of human DEHP exposure is from food that has been exposed, especially high fat foods. For babies, the main source of exposure is breast milk and infant formula. Pacifiers and bottle nipples can also contain DEHP; in the United States, this chemical has been removed [61].

DEHP is metabolized to monoethylhexylphthalate (MEHP) by lipases in the gut and then glucuronidated and excreted mainly in the urine. DEHP and its metabolites including MEHP are all toxic. MEHP is easily absorbed from the intestine. Inhaled DEHP is also absorbed and metabolized to MEHP. Parenteral DEHP is not as easily converted to MEHP, and higher levels are required to produce toxic effects. In neonates, glucuronidation is not mature; therefore, the half-life may be longer when compared with that in older children and adults. Also, because of their size and diet high in fatty foods, neonates may have a higher exposure per kilogram. Gastric lipase activity is higher in newborns. They may be able to metabolize DEHP to MEHP more easily than other patients but are then unable to metabolize MEHP and excrete it [62].

Most toxicology information is from animal studies, primarily in rodents. The LD_{50} (the dose that kills 50% of animals) of DEHP is around 25 g/kg in rats compared with an LD_{50} of 1.5 g/kg for MEHP [63]. Rats injected with large doses of MEHP experience hypotension and cardiac arrest [64]. Short-term oral exposure to DEHP has interfered with sperm formation in rodents. This effect was found to be reversible, but exposures before puberty also led to delayed sexual maturation. Long-term oral exposures in rodents seem to mainly affect the liver and male reproductive organs, even leading to liver cancer. Other studies have also shown effects in the thyroid, kidneys, and blood. The EPA has labeled DEHP as a "probable human carcinogen" [65]. Specifically, administration of DEHP to rats was found to cause apoptosis and necrosis of the germinal epithelium within the seminiferous tubules, leading to severe testicular atrophy. Exposed rats also had decreased overall weight gain when compared with controls [66]. Because the metabolism and excretion pathways in rodents are different than in primates, different species may be affected in different ways [61].

Both DEHP and its metabolites MEHP, MEHHP, and MEOHP have been found in the urine of neonates. In a study of six premature infants born at 23 to 26 weeks' gestation, a geometric mean of 100 ng/mL and a median of 129 ng/mL of MEHP were found in the urine [67]. These levels are much greater than the median concentration of 2.7 ng/mL used to calculate the DEHP exposure in the US adult population [68]. Another study looked at different exposure levels of three different groups of infants in the NICU. Low exposure infants were defined as receiving bottle or gavage feedings; medium exposure infants received continuous or gavage tube feedings, hyperalimentation by central venous access, or nasal continuous positive airway pressure (CPAP); and high exposure infants received mechanical ventilation via endotracheal intubation, hyperalimentation by central venous access, and stomach decompression via an indwelling naso- or orogastric tube. The median urinary MEHP concentrations were 25 ng/mL for low exposure infants, 40 ng/mL for medium exposure infants, and 89 ng/mL for high exposure infants [69]. Again, this study showed higher than average urinary concentrations in a comparison with the US population.

Few studies have addressed the potential adverse effects of DEHP in humans, and, to date, there is no publication showing an adverse effect on humans. The few studies regarding the potential adverse effects of DEHP on humans have focused on reproductive function and sexual organs. Researchers have examined specifically whether DEHP affects semen quality. In a study of men in the United States and Sweden, no association was found linking DEHP and its metabolites to reduced reproductive function or hormone levels [70,71]. In the NICU, one of the procedures associated with the highest exposure to DEHP is extracorporeal membrane oxygenation (ECMO). A 4-kg patient is exposed to between 42 and 140 mg/kg of DEHP when receiving 3 to 10 days of ECMO support. With blood transfusions, the same patient is exposed to about 0.5 mg/kg of DEHP [72]. Nevertheless, both short- and long-term adverse effects of this high DEHP exposure have not been seen. In one of the only studies looking at the follow-up of neonates exposed to DEHP, a small cohort of 19 adolescents who received ECMO in the NICU were examined. None of the 19 patients showed abnormal growth or abnormal thyroid, liver, or renal function.

Luteinizing hormone, follicle-stimulating hormone, testosterone, and estradiol levels were also normal, and all of the males showed normal testicular volume and phallus length [73]. The American Academy of Pediatrics statement from the Committee on Environmental Health concluded that more research needs to be done regarding more accurate levels of DEHP and its metabolites, the adverse effects related to exposure, toxicokinetics, and the exploration of possible safer substitutes [61].

Medications, transfusions, and intralipids

Many medications contain inactive ingredients, most of which are thought to be benign. A few of these chemicals have caused serious complications and illnesses in neonates. In 1982, two medical centers reported 16 neonatal deaths thought to be due to benzyl alcohol toxicity to the US Food and Drug Administration. At that time benzyl alcohol was commonly used in normal saline and sterile water as a preservative. Neonates were reported to have symptoms of metabolic acidosis, respiratory failure, gasping respirations, seizures, intracranial hemorrhage, hypotension, and death [74]. Other later findings included kernicterus, cerebral palsy, and developmental delay [75]. Infants with a birth weight less than 1250 g seemed to have the greatest morbidity and mortality [76]. In long-term studies, increased rates of cerebral palsy were noted [77]. Premature infants seem to have difficulty with detoxification of benzyl alcohol in their immature livers and kidneys when compared with adults [78]. Benzyl alcohol, which is no longer present in saline flushes and sterile water for use with neonates, is still present in many medications. Enalapril, lorazepam, pancuronium, dexamethasone, and even vitamin K all contain some benzyl alcohol [79]. Thus far, no further adverse effects from benzyl alcohol have been documented. It is also unclear whether benzyl alcohol has any more subtle effects on developing neonates and, in particular, on their developing central nervous system. No studies have been done examining any potential role smaller doses may have in developmental delay in premature neonates.

Propylene glycol is another inactive ingredient used as a drug solubilizer in medications that has been found to have adverse effects on neonates. These effects were first noted in a NICU after several small infants were noted to be hyperosmolar and have acute renal failure. The cause was traced back to an intravenous multivitamin containing propylene glycol [80]. An increased incidence of hyperbilirubinemia, seizures, and renal failure was noted during the period of time that the nursery used the intravenous multivitamin. Propylene glycol is found in many medications, including digoxin, sulfamethoxazole/trimethoprim, phenobarbital, phenytoin, diazepam, hydralazine, ergocalciferol, and nystatin ointment and cream. It has been reported to cause hemolysis, central nervous system depression, lactic acidosis, hyperosmolality and renal failure, respiratory depression, arrhythmia, hypotension, seizures, tachycardia, and hyperbilirubinemia. It is primarily metabolized into lactic acid and excreted in the urine. Neonates have a three times longer half-life when compared with adults [79,81]. As is true for benzyl alcohol, it is unclear whether smaller doses adversely affect developing neonates.

Blood transfusions have risks of reactions and potential blood-borne infections such as hepatitis and HIV. Along with these well-known risks, potential harmful contaminants in the blood can also be passed to the transfusion recipient. Concentrations of lead as high as 13 μg/dL with a median of 5 μg/dL were found in packed red blood cells that were transfused into premature infants. The investigators recommended using only packed red blood cells with a lead level less than 3.3 μg/dL for transfusions in premature infants or the administration of a total dose of less than 0.5 μg/kg of lead per transfusion [82]. Regional differences in exposure to the general population could lead to different levels of lead in donated blood; therefore, any kind of screening recommendations may need to be region specific [83]. Lead toxicity affects many organs, chief among them, the central nervous system. Cognitive injury can be irreversible if lead levels are high enough [84]. Donated blood can also contain other toxins and heavy metals, including cadmium, nickel, mercury, and arsenic.

Intralipid is another medication that has the potential to cause harm in patients. Intralipids are prepared from either soybean or safflower oil, and, depending on the process, pesticides on the crops used to produce these oils could be passed to patients. No studies have examined whether these chemicals are completely removed in the normal processing and manufacturing of these oils. Lipids can also harm patients by forming hydroperoxides, which are thought to cause a direct cytotoxic effect as an oxidant as well as potentially inhibiting the synthesis of prostaglandins and endothelium-derived relaxing factor. Via these oxidant effects, intralipids could potentially contribute to the development of bronchopulmonary dysplasia, retinopathy of prematurity, and necrotizing enterocolitis [85]. Helbock and colleagues [86] found average lipid hydroperoxide levels of 290 μmol/L, with levels as high as 655 μmol/L in bottles of unused intralipid. Plasma lipid hydroperoxide concentration is typically less than 30 nmol/L. Light seems to enhance lipid peroxidation. When syringes of intralipid were left in ambient light for 24 hours, lipid hydroperoxide levels increased threefold. Intralipid-filled tubing had levels that increased by more than a factor of seven. When exposed to a single phototherapy spot light, the levels of lipid hydroperoxides in intravenous tubing increased by a factor of 65. A similar increase was noted in the clinical setting but with slightly lower levels of lipid hydroperoxides found in the intravenous tubing, most likely owing to the continuous movement of intralipids through the tubing during the infusion. Covering the intravenous tubing and syringe with aluminum foil or adding sodium ascorbate before light exposure almost completely prevented the development of new lipid hydroperoxides [87].

Different means to stop or limit lipid hydroperoxide formation have been tested, such as various forms of tubing and different vitamin preparations. The multiple types of tubing (frosted, opaque white, amber, and dark brown) offered limited to no protection, but the multivitamin preparation when added before light exposure fully protected against the formation of lipid hydroperoxides. Adding separate preparations of water and fat-soluble vitamins also prevented peroxidation but was less effective than the single multivitamin preparation. When exposed to light, the multivitamin preparation added to the intralipid showed breakdown of riboflavin and ascorbic acid [88]. Although lipid hydroperoxides have the potential for harm in infants in the NICU, no randomized controlled trials have examined the benefits or harms from adding multivitamins to intralipids or covering intralipids with aluminum foil. Animal studies have shown some benefits of adding multivitamins to intralipids [89]. Other researchers have examined early versus late (after the fifth day of life) introduction of intralipids. By starting intralipids at a later time, infants would potentially be exposed to fewer lipid hydroperoxides. A Cochrane review in 2005 of five single-center studies found no statistically significant benefits or adverse effects in terms of nutritional and clinical outcomes in a comparison of early versus late intralipid use [90]. Currently, there is not enough research in neonates to suggest that adding multivitamins to intralipid preparations would prove harmful or beneficial. Aluminum foil covering can theoretically be used, but it may be too cumbersome in practice. Other forms of dark tubing also need to be studied further to assess both efficacy and cost-effectiveness.

Disinfectants

Many of the chemicals used in the NICU are potentially harmful to patients. The main chemical disinfectants used are bleach, ammonium compounds, and isopropyl alcohol. All of these substances are potentially toxic. Isopropyl alcohol can burn the skin of premature infants, especially if not diluted and left on the skin for a prolonged period of time [91,92]. If enough isopropyl alcohol is absorbed or ingested, patients could have gastrointestinal hemorrhage, hemolytic anemia, hypotension, or even more serious symptoms like coma, respiratory depression, and death. One reported death in a NICU stemmed from accidentally filling a ventilator humidifier with 70% isopropyl alcohol [93]. Bleach or sodium hypochlorite is another common disinfectant used in hospitals. It is an inexpensive germicide that is easy to use and has a broad antimicrobial spectrum. It does not leave any toxic residuals; however, sodium hypochlorite is a corrosive irritant to mucous membranes and can interact with certain chemicals (ammonia or acid) to form toxic chlorine gas. This gas can irritate mucous membranes and the respiratory tract, leading to possible pneumonitis or pulmonary edema [94]. Benzethonium chloride is often mixed with isopropyl alcohol for use as a detergent to sterilize equipment. It is also used in combination with other chemicals as a hand disinfectant and antiseptic. Benzethonium chloride can cause corrosive burns to mucous membranes, skin irritation, pulmonary edema, respiratory muscle paralysis, hypotension, seizures, metabolic acidosis, and, in rare cases, death [95]. All of these chemicals have the potential to harm patients in the NICU, but there have been no detailed studies examining what impact they may have on patients in the NICU and whether they contribute to their complex illnesses. After using these disinfectants, health care workers should allow adequate time for drying and appropriate ventilation of any fumes.

Summary

Information and research are scarce concerning many environmental hazards and their impact on neonates. As is true for many areas related to neonatology, more research needs to be done before caregivers can fully understand the relationship between the developing neonate and the surrounding environment. The available data are often obtained from a single center, and many studies show conflicting results. In the mean time, health care workers can take precautionary steps to minimize potential harm from several of these environmental hazards.

References

[1] Graven SN. Early neurosensory visual development of the fetus and newborn. Clin Perinatol 2004;31(2):199–216.
[2] Roy MS, Caramelli C, Orquin J, et al. Effects of early reduced light exposure on central visual development in preterm infants. Acta Paediatr 1999;88(4):459–61.
[3] Kuwabara T, Funahashi M. Light damage in the developing rat retina. Arch Ophthalmol 1976;94(8):1369–74.
[4] Messner KH, Maisels MJ, Leure-DuPree AE. Phototoxicity to the newborn primate retina. Invest Ophthalmol Vis Sci 1978;17(2):178–82.
[5] Glass P, Avery G, Subramanian K, et al. Effects of bright lights in the hospital nursery on the incidence of retinopathy of prematurity. N Engl J Med 1985;313(7):401–4.
[6] Ackerman B, Sherwonit E, Williams J. Reduced incidental light exposure: effect on the development of retinopathy of prematurity in low birth weight infants. Pediatrics 1989;83(6): 958–62.
[7] Reynolds JD, Hardy RJ, Kennedy KA, et al. Lack of efficacy of light reduction in preventing retinopathy of prematurity: Light Reduction in Retinopathy of Prematurity (LIGHT-ROP) Cooperative Group. N Engl J Med 1998;338(22):1572–6.
[8] Phelps DL, Watts JL. Early light reduction for preventing retinopathy of prematurity in very low birth weight infants. Cochrane Database Syst Rev 2001;1:CD000122.
[9] Kennedy KA, Fielder AR, Hardy RJ, et al. LIGHT-ROP Cooperative Group. Reduced lighting does not improve medical outcomes in very low birth weight infants. J Pediatr 2001;139(4):527–31.
[10] Rivkees SA. Emergence and influences of circadian rhythmicity in infants. Clin Perinatol 2004;31(2):217–28.

[11] Rivkees SA, Mayes L, Jacobs H, et al. Rest-activity patterns of premature infants are regulated by cycled lighting. Pediatrics 2004;113(4):833–9.

[12] Mirmiran M, Baldwin RB, Ariagno RL. Circadian and sleep development in preterm infants occurs independently from the influences of environmental lighting. Pediatr Res 2003;53(6): 933–8.

[13] Boo NY, Chee SC, Rohana J. Randomized controlled study of the effects of different durations of light exposure on weight gain by preterm infants in a neonatal intensive care unit. Acta Paediatr 2002;91(6):674–9.

[14] Mann NP, Haddow R, Stokes L, et al. Effect of night and day on preterm infants in a newborn nursery: randomized trial. Br Med J (Clin Res Ed) 1986;293(6557):1265–7.

[15] Brandon DH, Holditch-Davis D, Belyea M. Preterm infants born at less than 31 weeks' gestation have improved growth in cycled light compared with continuous near darkness. J Pediatr 2002;140(2):192–9.

[16] Mcartor RD, Saunders BS. Iatrogenic second-degree burn caused by a transilluminator. Pediatrics 1979;63(3):422–4.

[17] Uy J, Kuhns LR, Wall PM, et al. Light filtration during transillumination of the neonate: a method to reduce heat buildup in the skin. Pediatrics 1977;60(3):308–12.

[18] Kuhns LR, Wyman ML, Roloff DW, et al. A caution about using photoillumination devices. Pediatrics 1976;57(6):975–6.

[19] Lotas MJ. Effects of light and sound in the neonatal intensive care unit environment on the low-birth-weight infant. NAACOGS Clin Issu Perinat Womens Health Nurs 1992;3(1): 34–44.

[20] Rea M. Lighting for caregivers in the neonatal intensive care unit. Clin Perinatol 2004;31(2): 229–42.

[21] White RD. Lighting design in the neonatal intensive care unit: practical applications of scientific principles. Clin Perinatol 2004;31(2):323–30.

[22] Lasky RE, Williams AL. The development of the auditory system from conception to term. NeoReviews 2005;6(3):e141–52.

[23] Thiringer K, Kankkunen A, Liden G, et al. Perinatal risk factors in the aetiology of hearing loss in preschool children. Dev Med Child Neurol 1984;26(6):799–807.

[24] EPA, Office of Noise Abatement and Control. Information on levels of environmental noise requisite to protect public health and welfare with an adequate margin of safety [report no. 5509-74-004]. Washington, DC: Government Printing Office; 1974.

[25] Seleny FL, Streczyn M. Noise characteristics in the baby compartments of incubators. Am J Dis Child 1969;117(4):445–50.

[26] Blennow G, Svenningsen NW, Almquist B. Noise levels in infant incubators (adverse effects). Pediatrics 1974;53(1):29–32.

[27] Brown DR, Watchko JF, Sabo D. Neonatal sensorineural hearing loss associated with furosemide: a case-control study. Dev Med Child Neurol 1991;33(9):816–23.

[28] Rais-Bahrami K, Majd M, Veszelovszky E, et al. Use of furosemide and hearing loss in neonatal intensive care survivors. Am J Perinatol 2004;21(6):329–32.

[29] Dayal VS, Kokshanian A, Mitchell DP. Combined effects of noise and kanamycin. Ann Otol Rhinol Laryngol 1971;80(6):897–902.

[30] AAP: Committee on Environmental Health. Noise: a hazard for the fetus and newborn. Pediatrics 1997;100(4):724–7.

[31] Philbin MK, Klaas P. The full-term and premature newborn: evaluating studies of the behavioral effects of sound on newborns. J Perinatol 2000;20(8 Pt 2):S61–7.

[32] Jurkovicova J, Aghova L. Evaluations of the effects of noise exposure on various body functions in low birth weight newborns. Act Nerv Super (Praha) 1989;31(3):228–9.

[33] Wharrad HJ, Davis AC. Behavioral and autonomic responses to sound in pre-term and full-term babies. Br J Audiol 1997;31(5):315–29.

[34] Long JG, Lucey JF, Philip AG. Noise and hypoxemia in the intensive care nursery. Pediatrics 1980;65(1):143–5.

[35] Buehler DM, Als H, Duffy FH, et al. Effectiveness of individualized developmental care for low-risk preterm infants: behavioral and electrophysiologic evidence. Pediatrics 1995;96(5): 923–32.

[36] Thomas KA, Martin PA. The acoustic environment of hospital nurseries: NICU sound environment and the potential problems for caregivers. J Perinatol 2000;20(8 Pt 2): S94–9.

[37] Kjellberg A. Subjective, behavioral and psychophysiological effects of noise. Scand J Work Environ Health 1990;16(Suppl 1):29–38.

[38] Evans JB, Philbin MK. The acoustic environment of hospital nurseries: facility and operations planning for quiet hospital nurseries. J Perinatol 2000;20(8 Pt 2):S105–12.

[39] Philbin MK. Planning the acoustic environment of a neonatal intensive care unit. Clin Perinatol 2004;31(2):331–52.

[40] Philbin MK. The full-term and premature newborn: the influence of auditory experience on the behavior of preterm newborns. J Perinatol 2000;20(8 Pt 2):S77–87.

[41] Thomas KA. How the NICU environment sounds to a preterm infant. MCN Am J Matern Child Nurs 1989;14(4):249–51.

[42] Hotary KB, Robinson KR. Evidence of a role for endogenous electrical fields in chick embryo development. Development 1992;114(4):985–96.

[43] Song B, Zhao M, Forrester JV, et al. Electrical cues regulate the orientation and frequency of cell division and the rate of wound healing in vivo. Proc Natl Acad Sci U S A 2002;99(21): 13577–82.

[44] Metcalf MEM, Borgens RB. Weak applied voltages interfere with amphibian morphogenesis and pattern. J Exp Zool 1994;268:323–38.

[45] Hotary KB, Robinson KR. Endogenous electrical currents and voltage gradients in *Xenopus* embryos and the consequences of their disruption. Dev Biol 1994;166(2):789–800.

[46] Juutilainen J. Developmental effects of electromagnetic fields. Bioelectromagnetics 2005;7: S107–15.

[47] Bracken MB, Belanger K, Hellenbrand K, et al. Exposure to electromagnetic fields during pregnancy with emphasis on electrically heated beds: association with birth weight and intrauterine growth retardation. Epidemiology 1995;6(3):263–70.

[48] Dlugosz L, Vena J, Byers T, et al. Congenital defects and electric bed heating in New York State: a register-based case-control study. Am J Epidemiol 1992;135(9):1000–11.

[49] Milunsky A, Ulcickas M, Rothman KJ, et al. Maternal heat exposure and neural tube defects. JAMA 1992;268(7):882–5.

[50] International Agency for Research on Cancer. Non-ionizing radiation. Part 1. Static and extremely low-frequency electric and magnetic fields. IARC monographs on the evaluation of carcinogenic risk to humans. Lyons (France): International Agency for Research on Cancer; 2002. p. 80.

[51] Bearer CF. Electromagnetic fields and infant incubators. Arch Environ Health 1994;49(5): 352–4.

[52] Cnattingius S, Zack M, Ekbom A, et al. Prenatal and neonatal risk factors for childhood myeloid leukemia. Cancer Epidemiol Biomarkers Prev 1995;4(5):441–5.

[53] Söderberg KC, Naumburg E, Anger G, et al. Childhood leukemia and magnetic fields in infant incubators. Epidemiology 2002;13(1):45–9.

[54] White RD. Recommended standards for newborn ICU design. J Perinatol 2006;26:S2–18.

[55] AAP Committee on Environmental Health. Risk of ionizing radiation exposure to children: a subject review. Pediatrics 1998;101(4):717–9.

[56] United Nations Scientific Committee on the Effects of Atomic Radiation (UNSCEAR). Sources and effects of ionizing radiation. New York: United Nations; 2000.

[57] Arroe M. The risk of x-ray examinations of the lungs in neonates. Acta Paediatr Scand 1991; 80(5):489–93.

[58] Wilson-Costello D, Rao PS, Morrison S, et al. Radiation exposure from diagnostic radiographs in extremely low birth weight infants. Pediatrics 1996;97(3):369–74.

[59] Sutton PM, Arthur RJ, Taylor C, et al. Ionising radiation from diagnostic x-rays in very low birth weight babies. Arch Dis Child Fetal Neonatal Ed 1998;78(3):227–9.

[60] Bader D, Datz H, Bartal G, et al. Unintentional exposure of neonates to conventional radiography in the neonatal intensive care unit. J Perinatol 2007;27(9):579–85.

[61] Shea KM, American Academy of Pediatrics Committee on Environmental Health. Pediatric exposure and potential toxicity of phthalate plasticizers. Pediatrics 2003;111(6):1467–74.

[62] FDA. Safety assessment of di(2-ethylhexyl) phthalate (DEHP) released from PVC medical devices. Available at: www.fda.gov/cdrh/ost/dehp-pvc.pdf. Accessed September 17, 2007.

[63] Subotic U, Hannmann T, Kiss M, et al. Extraction of the plasticizers diethylhexylphthalate and polyadipate from polyvinylchloride nasogastric tubes through gastric juice and feeding solution. J Pediatr Gastroenterol Nutr 2007;44(1):71–6.

[64] Rock G, Labow RS, Franklin C, et al. Hypotension and cardiac arrest in rats after infusion of mono (2-ethylhexyl) phthalate (MEHP), a contaminant of stored blood. N Engl J Med 1987;316(19):1218–9.

[65] ATSDR. Toxicological profile for di(2-ethylhexyl) phthalate (DEHP). Available at: www.atsdr.cdc.gov. Accessed September 18, 2007.

[66] Park JD, Habeebu SS, Klaassen CD. Testicular toxicity of di-(2-ethylhexyl) phthalate in young Sprague-Dawley rats. Toxicology 2002;171(2–3):105–15.

[67] Calafat AM, Needham LL, Silva MJ, et al. Exposure to di(2-ethylhexyl) phthalate among premature neonates in a neonatal intensive care unit. Pediatrics 2004;113(5):e429–34.

[68] Kohn MC, Parham F, Masten SA, et al. Human exposure estimates for phthalates. Environ Health Perspect 2000;108(10):A440–2.

[69] Green R, Hauser R, Calafat AM, et al. Use of di(2-ethylhexyl) phthalate-containing medical products and urinary levels of mono(2-ethylhexyl) phthalate in neonatal intensive care unit infants. Environ Health Perspect 2005;113(9):1222–5.

[70] Hauser R, Meeker JD, Duty S, et al. Altered semen quality in relation to urinary concentrations of phthalate monoester and oxidative metabolites. Epidemiology 2006;17(6):682–91.

[71] Jonsson BAG, Richthoff J, Rylander L, et al. Urinary phthalate metabolites and biomarkers of reproductive function in young men. Epidemiology 2005;16(4):487–93.

[72] Schneider B, Schena J, Truog R, et al. Exposure to di(2-ethylhexyl) phthalate in infants receiving extracorporeal membrane oxygenation. N Engl J Med 1989;320(23):1563.

[73] Rais-Bahrami K, Nunez S, Revenis ME, et al. Follow-up study of adolescents exposed to di(2-ethylhexyl) phthalate (DEHP) as neonates on extracorporeal membrane oxygenation (ECMO) support. Environ Health Perspect 2004;112(13):1339–40.

[74] CDC. Neonatal deaths associated with use of benzyl alcohol—United States. MMWR Morb Mortal Wkly Rep 1982;31(22):290–1.

[75] Jardine DS, Rogers K. Relationship of benzyl alcohol to kernicterus, intraventricular hemorrhage, and mortality in preterm infants. Pediatrics 1989;83(2):153–60.

[76] Hiller JL, Benda GI, Rahatzad M, et al. Benzyl alcohol toxicity: impact on mortality and intraventricular hemorrhage among very low birth weight infants. Pediatrics 1986;77(4):500–6.

[77] Benda GI, Hiller JL, Reynolds JW. Benzyl alcohol toxicity: impact on neurologic handicaps among surviving very low birth weight infants. Pediatrics 1986;77(4):507–12.

[78] LeBel M, Ferron L, Masson M, et al. Benzyl alcohol metabolism and elimination in neonates. Dev Pharmacol Ther 1988;11(6):347–56.

[79] AAP Committee on Drugs. "Inactive" ingredients in pharmaceutical products: update. Pediatrics 1997;99(2):268–78.

[80] Glasgow AM, Boeckx RL, Miller MK, et al. Hyperosmolality in small infants due to propylene glycol. Pediatrics 1983;72(3):353–5.

[81] MacDonald MG, Getson PR, Glasgow AM, et al. Propylene glycol: increased incidence of seizures in low birth weight infants. Pediatrics 1987;79(4):622–5.

[82] Bearer CF, O'Riordan MA, Powers R. Lead exposure from blood transfusion to premature infants. J Pediatr 2000;137(4):549–54.

[83] Nakagawa M, Dempsey DA, Haller C, et al. Safe lead levels: blood transfusion of extremely low birth weight infants. Clin Pediatr 2004;43(7):681.

[84] Bellinger DC. Lead. Pediatrics 2004;113(4):1016–22.

[85] Krohn K, Koletzko B. Parenteral lipid emulsions in paediatrics. Curr Opin Clin Nutr Metab Care 2006;9(3):319–23.

[86] Helbock HJ, Motchnik PA, Ames BN. Toxic hydroperoxides in intravenous lipid emulsions used in preterm infants. Pediatrics 1993;91(1):83–7.

[87] Neuzil J, Darlow BA, Inder TE, et al. Oxidation of parenteral lipid emulsion by ambient and phototherapy lights: potential toxicity of routine parenteral feeding. J Pediatr 1995; 126(5 Pt 1):785–90.

[88] Silvers KM, Sluis KB, Darlow BA, et al. Limiting light-induced lipid peroxidation and vitamin loss in infant parenteral nutrition by adding multivitamin preparations to intralipid. Acta Paediatr 2001;90(3):242–9.

[89] Lavoie J-C, Rouleau T, Chessex P. Effect of coadministration of parenteral multivitamins with lipid emulsion on lung remodeling in an animal model of total parenteral nutrition. Pediatr Pulmonol 2005;40(1):53–6.

[90] Simmer K, Rao SC. Early introduction of lipids to parenterally fed preterm infants. Cochrane Database Syst Rev 2005;2:CD005256.

[91] Schick JB, Milstein JM. Burn hazard of isopropyl alcohol in the neonate. Pediatrics 1981; 68(4):587–8.

[92] Weintraub Z, Iancu TC. Isopropyl alcohol burns. Pediatrics 1982;69(4):506.

[93] Vicas IM, Beck R. Fatal inhalational isopropyl alcohol poisoning in a neonate. J Toxicol Clin Toxicol 1993;31(3):473–81.

[94] Rutala WA, Weber DJ. Uses of inorganic hypochlorite (bleach) in health care facilities. Clin Microbiol Rev 1997;10(4):597–610.

[95] NIH. Hazardous substances data bank: benzethonium chloride. Available at: http://www. toxnet.nlm.nih.gov. Accessed September 15, 2007.

ELSEVIER
SAUNDERS

CLINICS IN
PERINATOLOGY

Clin Perinatol 35 (2008) 183–197

Iatrogenic Hyperthermia and Hypothermia in the Neonate

Stephen Baumgart, MD

Children's National Medical Center, Department of Neonatology,
George Washington University, School of Medicine, 3W-600,
111 Michigan Avenue NW, Washington, DC 20010-2970, USA

The pregnant mother serves as a heat dispersal instrument removing heat from the incubating fetus across the placenta by a gradient in umbilical (arterial minus venous blood) temperature approaching 0.5°C [1–3]. Rather than "having a bun in the oven," the pregnant mother often feels too warm, taking measures to keep cool by shedding heavy clothing or adjusting the home's thermostat temperature downward. She either sweats or performs these complex behavioral and environmental adjustments to maintain her own "thermal comfort," unwittingly protecting the fetus from metabolic heat retention (estimated fetal metabolic rate between 33 and 47 kcal/kg/min [2.3–3.3 W/kg] [2,4]) potentially resulting in dangerous fetal hyperthermia. Pregnant mothers are advised to avoid hot tubs to prevent still births [5]. Maternal fevers with a temperature as low as 38.3°C early in pregnancy are associated with an increased risk of neural tube defects [6].

On parturition at term, the neonate becomes exposed to a more hostile extrauterine thermal environment. Ambient fluid temperature drops from 37°C to about 25°C as air replaces amniotic fluid near the skin, and evaporative heat loss begins at a rate of 0.58 kilocalories for each milliliter of water lost. Heat is also irradiated from the neonate's skin to the delivery room's cooler walls. The homeothermic response to a cold environment begins with the sensation of temperature. The newborn's sensation of cold by neonatal skin triggers an immediate cold-adaptive response followed by responses of the core sensors in the hypothalamus. Both sensors are integrated because the cold skin sensory response is inhibited by core sensor hyperthermia. Conversely, the skin sensor cold response is facilitated by hypothalamic cooling. Peripheral skin cold sensation is important, because early detection of heat loss from the skin aids in the infant's timely response

E-mail address: stbaumga@cnmc.org

doi:10.1016/j.clp.2007.11.002
perinatology.theclinics.com

for maintaining core temperature. Like all other mammalian species, term human neonates try to maintain a stable core temperature. The term human neonate exhibits a profound physiologic response to maintain a body temperature at or near 37.0°C (98.6°F).

The effector limb of the neonatal cold response is mediated by the sympathetic nervous system. The earliest maturing cold-specific response is vasoconstriction in dermal arterioles, resulting in a reduced flow of warm blood from the infant's core into the exposed skin's peripheral circulation. A reduction in skin blood flow also places a layer of insulating subcutaneous "white" fat between the core and the exposed skin in term infants.

Brown fat is the second sympathetic effector organ that provides a metabolic source of "non-shivering thermogenesis" [7]. Brown fat reservoirs are located in the axillary, mediastinal, paraspinal, perinephric, and interscapular regions of the newborn. Brown fat adipocyte membranes contain numerous norepinephrine and epinephrine receptor sites for sympathetically enervated and adrenal-mediated humoral stimulation. With cold stress, sympathetic receptors activate lipoprotein lipase activity (cyclic AMP mediated). Thyroid hormone is permissive to this effect, and a thyroid surge occurs at birth in neonates [8–10]. Electron microscopy demonstrates an abundance of mitochondria in brown fat adipocytes to hydrolyze and re-esterify triglycerides and oxidize free fatty acids [10]. In the term infants, these reactions are exothermic and increase the metabolic rate temporarily by twofold or more. The visible appearance of brown fat is produced by blood vessels that conduct the heat produced by brown fat into the core circulation, providing feedback to the hypothalamus. Infant behavior may also contribute to heat production. An irritable baby generates heat and commands the mother to intervene in heat loss through drying, cuddling, and swaddling the baby. Without intervention, rapid environmental cooling results in the body temperature dropping at a rate of 0.2 to 1.0°C/min at birth despite a homeothermic response. Indeed, astute parents and caregivers perceive an infant's thermal discomfort and intervene to prevent extreme heat loss.

Prematurity and functional poikilothermy

In contrast to the term infant's vigorous homeothermic response, premature and low birth weight infants have a far less robust response. On preterm birth, skin and core temperatures may diminish even more precipitously when compared with that of larger term neonates. Nevertheless, premature neonates remain temperature sensitive, manifesting vasoconstriction and an increased metabolic rate despite limited amounts of brown (metabolic) and white subcutaneous (insulating) fat. The premature neonate will also manifest behavioral irritability when cold stimulated, triggering caretaker intervention (through incubation) to promote survival [11–16].

Without intervention, the preterm neonate is functionally poikilothermic, is unable to maintain body temperature above environmental temperature, and succumbs to hypothermia eventually extinguishing heart and metabolic rates.

Prematurity and survival studies and kangaroo care

The obstetrician Tarnier first applied the principle of incubation to human premature neonates in Paris in 1830 using a covered incubator (*couveuse*). Tarnier's students, Budin and Auvard, modified Tarnier's device by adding a thermometer to alert the infant's attendant of deviations in environmental temperature [17–19]. Over the next 60 years, Tarnier's and Budin's incubation and feeding techniques resulted in a survival rate increasing from 38% to 66% for premature infants weighing less than 2000 g at birth [19]. In 1958, Silverman and colleagues [14] suggested using higher air temperatures instead of humidity to avoid bacterial contamination within incubator chambers. Incubator temperatures in Silverman's dry incubators ranged from 29°C to 31°C. These investigators demonstrated significantly improved survival rates using these higher temperatures. In these survival studies, incubator air and wall temperatures remained less than the premature neonate's skin surface and core temperatures. Conventional convection warmed incubators (like the mother during fetal life) dissipate heat waste from the baby's metabolic processes while permitting the infant to maintain homeothermy between 36.5°C and 37°C using non-metabolic processes (vasoconstriction and dilation, discussed later in the section on thermal neutral temperature).

Kangaroo care

The term *Kangaroo care* [20] connotes neonatal warming by skin-to-skin contact with the mother or father in which premature infants are held naked between the axillary folds or the breasts, mimicking a kangaroo's pouch. These regions of the adult body are close to the core temperature of 37°C, in contrast to the ambient adult-comfort environment near 25°C. First implemented in Bogotá, Columbia, this method was popularized for non-intubated premature infants in cooler Scandinavian and European countries in the 1980s. Kangaroo care has been shown to promote a thermal neutral metabolic response and temperature stability in stable growing premature infants nurtured in non-equatorial regions. Early studies have suggested a significant reduction in early mortality and morbidity, enhanced mother–infant attachment, increased infant alertness, more stable sleep patterns, better weight gain, and earlier hospital discharge. Moreover, during kangaroo care, infants with bronchopulmonary dysplasia have improved oxygenation with less periodic breathing and reduced apnea. In the contemporary nursery, kangaroo care may be initiated even during mechanical ventilation in stable infants.

Infant should be covered with a blanket to avoid outward convective and evaporative heat losses, and sessions (initially limited to 0.5 to 1 hour) can be increased successively up to 4 hours. This author is aware of no documented adverse reports of kangaroo care. Its use in neonatal intensive care units (NICUs) has increased dramatically in recent years.

Minimal metabolic cost and the thermal neutral temperature

Cross and Hill in London in 1959 first proposed the thermal neutral temperature range when caring for human neonates in incubators [21,22]. The thermal neutral temperature for premature newborn infants is analogous to the adult thermal comfort zone at which adults (at rest in a single layer of clothing) remain comfortable without metabolic cost in a thermal adaptive response (shivering). By 1962, Bruck in Germany had demonstrated a minimal observed metabolic rate of oxygen consumption as an indication of thermal neutral temperature in newborn infants maintained within specific narrow ranges of environmental temperature within incubators [11–13]. Glass and colleagues in 1968 investigated the deleterious effects in premature infants nurtured in dry ambient air environments of either 35°C or 36.5°C in the first few days of life [15]. Significant increases in weight gain were demonstrated in the infants in the warmer environment, achieving better growth. Rectal temperatures assessed in both groups of infants were normal. It follows that the thermogenic response in the infants in the slightly cooler environment was sufficient to consume calories which otherwise might have been used for growth. These investigators subsequently noted that graded temperature regulation within incubators (to promote a thermal neutral environment) was essential not only to the survival of preterm infants but also to reduce their morbidity and achieve optimal growth following premature birth. By 1969, Sir Edmund Hey and coworkers in England described thermal neutral environments for premature infants [23,24] and developed the Hey and Katz nomograms for incubator temperature regulation. Ultimately, Sir Edmond Hey was knighted for his contributions to neonatal medicine.

The thermal neutral environment is demonstrated in Fig. 1 in which environmental temperature is plotted against the infant's metabolic rate of heat production (indicated indirectly by measuring their rate of oxygen consumption) [25]. Fig. 1 suggests that, although newborn infants (in particular premature babies) can neither shiver nor use abundant brown fat, they respond to environmental cooling by increasing the metabolic rate of heat production with "non-shivering thermogenesis." Within a narrow range of environmental temperatures (bordered by a low critical temperature on the left and a high critical temperature on the right), the infant may control body temperature near normal using mechanisms of physical regulation alone (eg, vasoconstriction) without necessitating an increase in metabolic

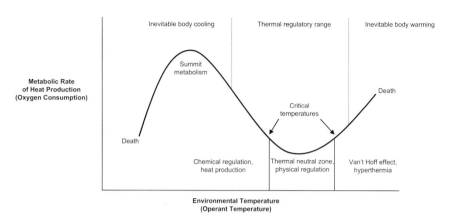

Fig. 1. Thermal neutral temperature. (*From* Baumgart S. Incubation of the human newborn infant. In: Pommerance J, Richardson CJ, editors. Issues in clinical neonatology. Norwalk (CT): Appleton & Lange; 1992. p. 140; with permission.)

rate. The region bounded between the low and high critical temperatures defines the relatively narrow thermal neutral temperature zone. Below the critical temperature of the thermal neutral zone, infant metabolic rate increases dramatically.

Body temperature may be maintained outside the thermal neutral zone temporarily by an increased metabolic rate of heat production. Because core temperature is maintained at the expense of metabolic energy expenditure, simply monitoring the core body temperature (either rectal or axillary) is insufficient to detect whether an infant resides within the thermal neutral zone of environmental temperature (determined by measuring incubator ambient air temperature and humidity combined with incubator wall temperature). Once the environmental temperature has decreased past a maximal or "summit" metabolism, inevitable body cooling occurs resulting in deepening hypothermia. If pursued to an extreme, the infant may succumb to death by hypothermic exposure.

In contrast, incubation at an inappropriately high environmental temperature results in inevitable body heating (Fig. 1). Beyond the infant's ability to dissipate body heat (by vasodilation and transepidermal evaporation), the van't Hoff-Arrhenius effect occurs with inevitable body warming (an increase in temperature will cause an increase in the rate of an endothermic reaction). Like boiling chemicals in a crucible, the metabolic rate accelerates, resulting in excess metabolic heat production without sufficient heat elimination. Body temperature rises to the point at which infants denature brain protein, suffer seizures, and die. Thermal regulation for neonates is a complex process; maintenance of both physical and physiologic parameters is required to maintain a noncompromised homeothermic state characteristic of mammalian physiology.

Iatrogenic hypothermia

Inappropriate incubation

By far the most common cause of neonatal hypothermia is surface cooling of the skin with inappropriate incubation due to naiveté, ignorance, or incubator mishap. As the World Health Organization has suggested (http://www.who.int/reproductive-health/publications/MSM_94_12/MSM_94_12_chapter7.en.html), neonatal hypothermia is a leading cause of infant mortality in non-industrialized nations, particularly with preterm births. Provision of maternal-fetal and neonatal care must include education of thermal support for prospective parents, midwives, emergency transport, and hospital personnel. Appropriate diagnosis of clinical hypothermia in the infant requires recognition of the following signs: irritability, excessive motor activity and crying, tachy- or bradyarrhythmias, and a vasoconstricted appearance of the skin with mottling, pallor, or cyanosis.

Appropriate temperature assessment

Use of a mercury-in-glass thermometer was first proposed by Berthod in 1887 [19]. This recommendation has recently been revisited, with normal axillary temperature measured between 36.5°C and 37.4°C [26]. To avoid a false diagnosis of hypothermia, Mayfield and colleagues [26] recommended obtaining axillary temperature by sampling for at least 5 minutes (mercury-in-glass only) or performing deep rectal monitoring with a calibrated electronic thermistor. Recent incubator manufacturing has excluded mercury-in-glass measurements to avoid environmental mercury exposure mishaps (personal communication, Scientific Advisor to the American Academy of Pediatrics, Taskforce on Standards for Infant Incubators, 1983, Washington, DC).

Gunn and Gunn [27] have proposed the following degrees of hypothermia: mild, 1 to 3°C below normal (ie, down to about 34°C); moderate, 4 to 6°C below normal down to 31°C; severe, 8 to 10°C below normal down to 27°C; and profound, more than 15 to 20°C below normal to as low as 15°C performed with deep hypothermic circulatory arrest during surgical repair of complex congenital heart disease. These researchers acknowledged differences among species and opinions. Day [28] has written, "Close attention to the incubator during the initial warming up period is required, either by a doctor or a nurse familiar with the problems....The [incubator] apparatus is satisfactory once it is understood." Day also states, "If the wire to the abdominal thermistor breaks or falls off, more heat is called for." Continuous monitoring of anterior abdominal wall skin temperature by the thermistor is recommended, with corroboration by a second core temperature assessment (either axillary or rectal). An initial skin control set point of 36.5°C provides safe re-warming from mild hypothermia [26]. Re-warming from more severe hypothermia should proceed at about

+0.5°C per hour by adjusting the temperature controller more slowly to avoid tachycardia, dangerous electrolyte shifts, and hyperthermic overshoot [29].

Hypothermia for cerebral protection

Recently, therapeutic hypothermia has been introduced for a highly selected population of near-term or term neonates with hypoxic-ischemic insults after birth [29–31]. Two recent studies suggest that cerebral cooling with whole body cooling (to a 33.5°C core esophageal temperature, that is, moderate hypothermia) or selective head cooling (10°C along with mild whole body cooling to 34°C) reduces the risk for death or moderate-to-severe neurologic sequelae from 60% or more to less than 50% (Fig. 2) [29,30]. The National Institutes of Health's Institute of Child Health and Human Development (NICHD) Experts Panel Workshop held in May 2005 emphasized the need to use standardized protocols for hypothermia treatment and to provide continual follow-up until school age to develop, refine, and optimize new therapies for hypoxic-ischemic injury [31].

The author's center has adopted the NICHD's Neonatal Network protocol for providing whole body hypothermia. Additionally, we provide continuous electroencephalographic (EEG) neuro-monitoring as part of our hypothermia protocol. A full montage video-EEG (modified International 10–20 system for newborns) is recorded by computer for about 96 hours to include cooling and recovery periods. Amplitude-integrated EEG

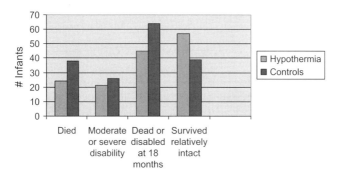

Fig. 2. Results of the Neonatal Network hypothermia trial. (*Data from* Shankaran S, Laptook AR, Ehrenkkranz RA, et al, for the NICHHD, Neonatal Research Network. Whole-body hypothermia for neonates with hypoxic-ischemic encephalopathy. N Engl J Med 2005;353:1581). These researchers reported that 64 of 106 control infants were dead or seriously disabled at 18 to 22 months of age. Of these infants, 38 had died (ie, 64−38), leaving 26 seriously disabled survivors. In a study population of 106 control infants, 68 survived (ie, 68−26 disabled), leaving 42 survivors relatively intact. A total of 45 of 102 hypothermic infants were dead or disabled at 18 to 22 months, with 24 having died, leaving 21 seriously disabled subjects. Of 102 treated infants, 78 survived (ie, 78−21), leaving 57 survivors relatively intact. Primary outcome data were available for only 205 of the 208 infants enrolled. The three subjects lost to follow-up may have favorably biased the survival-intact estimates shown in this figure.

(aEEG) is also reviewed for characterization of the background pattern and detection of seizures. Seizure detection is confirmed on raw EEG.

To receive cooling therapy, infants must be 36 weeks or more of completed gestation, must arrive for treatment within 6 hours of birth, and must have experienced a hypoxic-ischemic insult. Evidence of hypoxic-ischemic injury includes resuscitation at delivery, an umbilical vessel blood gas pH of less than or equal to 7.00, or a significant base deficit of at least −16. Also qualifying for therapy are infants with blood gas disturbances within the first hour of life with a pH of 7.01 to 7.15 and a base deficit between −10 to −15.9 along with an ominous perinatal history (fetal heart rate decelerations, umbilical cord prolapse or rupture, uterine rupture, severe maternal trauma preceding birth and abruption of the placenta, or any life-threatening event requiring cardiopulmonary resuscitation experienced by the expectant mother). Signs of a moderate-to-severe encephalopathy must also be present (an infant who is lethargic or completely stuporous or who has diminished or completely absent activity and muscle tone, weak or absent sucking and Moro reflexes, fixed-constricted or unresponsive dilated pupils, fixed flexion or extension posturing of extremities, or a clinically observed seizure). Without hypothermic intervention, infants with such symptoms persisting for several days have about a 60% risk for death before hospital discharge. The majority of survivors experience moderate-to-severe, life-long neurologic-developmental disabilities (cerebral palsy, deafness, blindness, mental retardation, or recurrent seizure disorder).

Infants meeting these criteria at admission are placed before 6 hours of age supine onto a water-filled cooling blanket pre-cooled to 5°C (41°F, similar to a household refrigerator box temperature, eg, 37°F). The author and his colleagues use a Blanketrol II Hyper-Hypothermia System (Cincinnati Sub-Zero, Cincinnati, Ohio), a device familiar to our emergency department and available in the operating suite where it is used to reduce high fevers in young children. An esophageal temperature probe is positioned in the distal third of the esophagus, and the thermostatic controller of the water mattress cooling unit is immediately set to 33.5°C. A second larger pediatric-size blanket is attached parallel into the cooling system. Water circulates through both blankets, with the larger blanket hung on an intravenous rack at bedside serving as a capacitor to diminish fluctuations in the esophageal temperature to less than ± 1.0°C. Although we use a warmer bed platform as a crib of convenience, the overhead warmer is not used during the cooling period.

Abdominal wall skin temperature is monitored with a surface probe available with the warmer bed (monitoring mode only, warmer off). Esophageal, skin, and axillary temperatures are monitored and recorded every 15 minutes for the first 4 hours of cooling, every hour for the next 8 hours, and every 4 hours during the remaining 72-hour period of hypothermia. After 72 hours, the set point of the automatic controller on the cooling system is increased by 0.5°C per hour. After 6 hours, the esophageal probe and cooling blankets are removed, and anterior abdominal wall skin temperature is regulated using the radiant warmer's servomechanism set at 36.5°C (warmer on). The purpose of re-warming slowly is to avoid rapid shifts in critical electrolytes (calcium and potassium), cardiac arrhythmias, and re-warming overshoot. Infants otherwise receive routine clinical care, including the continuous monitoring of vital signs (mild bradycardia of 80 to 90 bpm and a small decrease in blood pressure <10 mm Hg are commonly observed and treated rarely) and frequent surveillance of blood samples to detect a disturbance in glucose metabolism, coagulopathy, and other major organ dysfunction (eg, liver enzymes and renal function). Above all, hyperthermia greater than a 37.5°C axillary temperature is avoided, because fever in this setting contributes to brain injury [32].

Our clinical experience over 15 months with more than 40 infants meeting strict criteria for therapeutic hypothermia was commensurate with that reported from the Neonatal Network. We achieved a target esophageal temperature of 33.5 ± 1.0°C within 30 to 40 minutes without major circulatory mishap. Continuous EEG monitoring has been instructive for intervening seizure activity (observed in almost half of the infants), and we have generally observed improvements in background voltages and patterns during hypothermia. Specifically, an improvement of background activity, the appearance of sleep–wake cycling, and the disappearance of seizures have been observed at the time of re-warming [33]. The disappearance of seizures during re-warming is in contrast to the observations of the Neonatal Network study in which seizures emerged more frequently upon re-warming, leading to our caution in re-warming more slowly [29]. We presently are acquiring and reviewing infant neurologic and developmental follow-up data.

An additional clinical observation was that the water mattress felt warm to touch during most of the cooling period [34]. The median ambient temperature in our NICU ($T_{ambient}$) was 23.1°C (range, 20.9–25.4°C) (Table 1). This temperature was usually less than both the blanket water and baby temperatures. No infant had acidemia during cooling. The temperature gradients suggest that whole body cooling is achieved more through surface heat loss from skin exposed to the ambient environment and not predominantly through heat loss to the water blanket. Except in

Table 1
Temperature gradients during cooling therapy in 18 neonates with hypoxic-ischemic encephalopathy

°C	30 min	1 h	6 h	12 h	24 h	48 h	72 h
1. T_{water}	15.8 ± 16	37.6 ± 9.6	33.4 ± 4.4	35 ± 2	31.9 ± 6.3	32.1 ± 4.1	36.1 ± 3.3
2. T_{esoph}	33.1 ± 1	32.6 ± 0.5	33.4 ± 0.2	33.3 ± 0.1	33.3 ± 0.2	33.5 ± 0.2	33.4 ± 0.3
3. T_{axilla}	32.1 ± 0.6	32.3 ± 1	32.7 ± 0.4	32.5 ± 0.6	32.5 ± 1.2	32.9 ± 0.7	33.1 ± 0.5
$^\Delta$1–2	−6.9	+4.9	+0.1	+1.7	−1.5	−1.4	+2.7
$^\Delta$1–3	−5.9	+0.5	+0.8	+2.5	−0.7	−0.8	+3.0

Data from Baumgart S, Massaro A, Chang T, et al. Whole body cooling therapy: is it really a cooling mattress [abstract]. Toronto: Society for Pediatric Research; 2007.

the first 30 minutes, the blanket more often provided warmth to maintain the $T_{esophageal}$ at 33.5°C. Theoretically, whole body cooling might also be provided by regulating an incubator air temperature or a radiant heater's output to maintain the desired $T_{esophageal}$.

Hyperthermia

Inappropriate incubation

The most common cause of neonatal hyperthermia is inappropriate incubation (high ambient air temperature and humidity). Metabolic heat production is a waste product that should be eliminated through appropriate incubation in an adult comfortable environment. For a term neonate, after drying and clothing the infant in a single layer of clothing or a receiving blanket (usually cotton), the mother's axilla and breast are the most common sense locations for management of neonatal temperature. A term infant probably does not require a convection-warmed human incubator and is likely to become hyperthermic if managed in one set at greater than adult comfort temperature.

Radiant warmers

There is a fundamental difference between how a convection-warmed incubator and radiant warmers provide a thermal neutral temperature [35]. The author and his colleagues performed partitional calorimetry [35] in a small series of premature neonates with a birth weight ranging from about 700 to 2000 g while they nurtured under radiant warmers servocontrolled to maintain an anterior abdominal wall skin temperature at 36.5°C (previously identified as the thermal neutral temperature [16]). Results from this study are shown in Fig. 3.

There were large heat losses to convection and evaporation in the NICU environment set to maintain adult thermal comfort. When combined, these heat losses are much larger than the infant's metabolic rate of heat production and can only be balanced by a negative net radiant heat loss (ie, heat gain). The radiant warmer is the only human incubator (including the gravid mother) that actually injects heat into the baby to maintain thermal equilibrium. As such, the American Academy of Pediatrics has published the following warning statement [36]: "The use of infant radiant warmers poses a hazard of neonatal hyperthermia. Serious overheating can result from mechanical failure of the controls, from dislodgment of the sensor probe, or from manual operation without careful monitoring. Deaths have been associated with hyperthermia induced by radiant warmers."

Malignant hyperthermia of anesthesia

A rare cause of hyperthermia that involves the release of calcium within skeletal muscles and tetany is the use of halogenated inhalation anesthetic

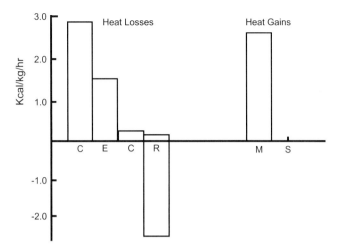

Fig. 3. Partitional calorimetry for premature infants nurtured naked and supine on a radiant warmer bed servocontrolled to maintain an abdominal skin temperature between 36.5 and 37.2°C. Equilibrium is achieved when radiant heat delivered from the warmer balances large convective (C), evaporative (E), and radiant (R) heat losses. The metabolic rate of heat production (M) and heat storage (S = 0 at equilibrium) are relatively small when compared with the magnitude of physical heat exchanges with the surrounding environment. (*Adapted from* Baumgart S. Radiant heat loss vs. radiant heat gain in premature neonates under radiant warmers. Biol Neonate 1990;57:15; with permission.)

agents. The disorder is autosomal dominantly inherited and may be delayed in onset for several hours after recovery from anesthesia. Core temperature rises rapidly to 41 to 45°C, resulting in tachyarrhythmias, tissue hypoxia, lactic acidosis, and hyperkalemia with rhabdomyolysis and disseminated intravascular coagulation [37]. The author is unaware of reported neonatal cases. Rather than inhalational anesthetics, our preferred anesthetic management for neonates is an opioid plus a muscle relaxant.

Neonatal fever

Craig [38–40] defines neonatal pyrexia as a rectal (core body) temperature greater than 37.4°C. The author uses a 37.5°C axillary temperature as a threshold to intervene while re-warming asphyxiated neonates, slowing the process at a lower servocontrol set point temperature of 36.2 to 36.5°C or even less on the radiant warmer; however, other investigators accept normal temperatures up to cores of 37.8°C [15]. Between 1% and 2.5% of all newborns admitted to the nursery experience a fever as judged by rectal or axillary temperatures, depending on the limits chosen. Sepsis is unlikely but is the most feared cause of neonatal fever in the term nursery. Fever is an infrequent sign of sepsis, with fewer than 10% of febrile neonates having culture proven sepsis, and temperature elevation may be seen with several other clinical entities as described in the next section.

Mechanisms producing neonatal fever

Mechanisms producing neonatal fever are not well understood. Fever most commonly results from disturbances in the complex interactions between central heat conservation and heat dissipation integrated at the hypothalamic level, which may be caused by various immunogenic pyrogens (commonly PGE_2). In contrast to different homeothermic mammalian species, human neonates react in peculiar ways to known pyrogens; human newborns may sustain documented bacterial infections without fever and more commonly present in the emergency setting with hypothermia.

In addition, exposure to excess environmental heat (poor incubator monitoring, summer heat wave without air conditioning) or insulation (excessive swaddling) can quickly increase the core temperature of newborn infants due to poor heat dissipation (absence of sweating). Such overheating commonly occurs when term babies are nursed in uncontrolled incubators or under radiant warmers. Temperature elevation may also occur with an increased infant metabolic rate, such as with skeletal muscle rigidity syndrome [41] and status epilepticus (particularly in asphyxiated hypoxic-ischemic brain injury) [29,30]. Another cause of temperature elevation is occasionally observed in well breastfeeding newborn infants on the third to fourth day of life and is thought to result from dehydration owing to insufficient milk production [42,43]. Rehydration alone resolves these fevers and reassures the diagnosis. There are more recent reports of an increased incidence of neonatal fever in infants of mothers receiving epidural analgesia. The mechanisms for temperature elevation in these latter two situations are unknown.

Determining the cause of fever

Sepsis is an uncommon but treatable cause of high fever, especially with temperatures greater than 38 to 39°C. Paradoxically, septic neonates more frequently present with hypothermia as the metabolic rate drops in the later phase of illness. Most neonatal febrile episodes are noted in the first day of life (54% in one series); however, any fever occurring at or beyond the third day of life, or any fever with a temperature greater than 39°C has been correlated with a significantly higher chance of bacterial or viral infection [44]. Herpes simplex encephalitis should be considered in such neonates [44].

Hyperthermia due to overheating has been reported in term or preterm infants as a complication of improper use of shielding devices (swaddling premature infants in plastic wrap) or excessive environment heating, particularly in equatorial and tropical countries with the routine use of incubators for larger preterm infants. Dehydration fever is infrequently recognized in the newborn period, usually occurring in healthy breastfed term infants between the third and fourth day of life. Temperature may range between 37.8 and 40°C. Rehydration leads to resolution of fever and is key to the diagnosis of this entity [42,43]. In two recent reports, fever was more commonly observed in neonates born to mothers receiving epidural analgesia during labor when compared with infants born to those without epidural analgesia (7.5% versus 2.5%; 14.5% versus 1%) [39,40]. With the increasing use of epidural analgesia during labor, the recognition of epidural neonatal fever is an important consideration.

Unusual and uncommon causes of neonatal fever include neonatal typhoid fever, congenital malaria (third world countries), and hepatitis B vaccination. In addition, temperature elevations may be seen with central nervous system malformations, subarachnoid or other intracranial hemorrhages, and, on rare occasions, neonatal spinal neurenteric cysts (especially in the presence of prolonged fever of more than 3 weeks with myelopathy).

Crisponi syndrome is evident at birth and is characterized by a marked muscular contraction facial grimace in response to tactile external stimuli or during crying, with trismus and abundant salivation as in a myotonic tetany. The contractions disappear as the infant calms down. It has been described in 18 patients from Sardinian (Italian) families. There is also opisthotonos. In some infants, generalized seizures have occurred. The clinical course is characterized by the appearance of fever at about 38°C, with peaks of hyperthermia over 42°C, with onset ranging from birth to a few weeks. Crisponi syndrome is probably transmitted as an autosomal recessive trait. In most cases, death occurs in the first few months and coincides with a fever of about 42°C.

Management

Although fever may be the only sign of severe bacterial disease, the relevant perinatal history should be evaluated for risk factors before pursuing an extensive laboratory evaluation and presumptive treatment to rule out an unlikely infection. Furthermore, physical signs suggestive of sepsis (diminished activity, irritability, seizures) should be assessed. All neonates with fever should be evaluated for dehydration and weight loss. They should be examined carefully for foci of infection (cellulitis, septic arthritis, osteomyelitis, omphalitis, mastitis, and the presence of colonized foreign bodies [eg, a central venous or arterial line]). Febrile neonates without a clinical history or signs of infection present a challenge, with insufficient data in the literature on appropriate management.

The infant's environment should be examined for overheating and temperature-monitoring thermistors checked or replaced. Dehydration fever should be considered in breastfeeding infants with fever at 3 to 4 days and excessive weight loss. Mothers receiving epidural analgesia often manifest shivering with their temperature rise and experience a rapid defervescence after discontinuation of the epidural infusion. Recognition of this pattern may avoid unnecessary sepsis evaluations in neonates with fever in the first (hours) day of life after maternal epidural analgesia.

Cooling a neonate with fever should be accomplished by unswaddling the overwrapped infant and returning him or her to an appropriately thermal neutral environment (in an incubator only after the equipment has been checked). The author does not usually prescribe acetaminophen or other pyrolytic agents during the neonatal period, preferring environmental intervention. Except in the setting of hypoxic-ischemic encephalopathy, the author does not recommend using a cooling device specifically. Surface cooling is passive, rapid, and safe.

References

[1] Morishima HO, Yeh MN, Niemann WH, et al. Temperature gradient between fetus and mother as an index for assessing intrauterine fetal condition. Am J Obstet Gynecol 1977; 129:443.
[2] Power GG, et al. Temperature responses following ventilation of the fetal sheep in utero. J Dev Physiol 1986;8:477.
[3] Schroder H, Gilbert RD, Power GG. Computer model of fetal-maternal heat exchange in sheep. J Appl Physiol 1988;65(1):460.
[4] Ryser G, Jequier E. Study by direct calorimetry of thermal balance on the first day of life. Eur J Clin Invest 1972;2:176.
[5] Li DK, Janevic T, Odouli R, et al. Hot tub use during pregnancy and the risk of miscarriage. Am J Epidemiol 2003;158(10):931–7.
[6] Milunsky A, Ulcickas M, Rothman KJ, et al. Maternal heat exposure and neural tube defects. JAMA 1992;268(7):882–5.
[7] Alexander G, Williams D. Shivering and non-shivering thermal genesis during summit metabolism in young lambs. J Physiol (Lond) 1968;198:251.
[8] Bray GA, Goodman HM. Studies on the early effects of thyroid hormones. Endocrinology 1965;76:323.
[9] Klein AH, Reviczky A, Padbury JF. Thyroid hormones augment catecholamine-stimulated brown adipose tissue thermal genesis in the ovine fetus. Endocrinology 1984;114:1065.
[10] Silva JE, Larsen PR. Adrenergic activation of triiodothyronine production in brown adipose tissue. Nature 1983;305:712.
[11] Bruck K, Parmelee AH, Bruck M. Neutral temperature range and range of "thermal comfort" in premature infants. Biol Neonate 1962;4:32.
[12] Bruck K. Heat production and temperature regulation. In: Stave U, editor. Perinatal physiology. New York: Plenum Publishing; 1978. p. 455–98.
[13] Bruck K. Temperature regulation in the newborn infant. Biol Neonate 1961;3:65.
[14] Silverman WA, Fertig JW, Berger AP. The influence of the thermal environment upon the survival of the newly born premature infant. Pediatrics 1958;22:876–86.
[15] Glass L, Silverman WA, Sinclair JC. Effect of the thermal environment on cold resistance and growth of small infants after the first week of life. Pediatrics 1968;41:1033–46.
[16] Malin S, Baumgart S. Optimal thermal management for low birth weight infants nursed under high-power radiant warmers. Pediatrics 1987;79:47–54.
[17] Southwick GR. The care of weak or prematurely born infants. New England Medical Gazette 1890;25:310.
[18] Marx S. Incubation and incubators. American Medical and Surgical Bulletin 1896;9:311.
[19] Berthod P. La Couveuse et le Gavage a la Maternite de Paris [thesis]. Maternite de Paris. Paris: G. Rougier, 1887 [French].
[20] Anderson GC. Current knowledge about skin-to-skin (kangaroo care) for preterm infants. J Perinatol 1991;11:216–26.
[21] Hill JR. The oxygen consumption of newborn and adult mammals: its dependence on the oxygen tension in the inspired air and on the environmental temperature. J Physiol 1959; 149:346.

[22] Hill JR, Rahimtulla KA. Heat balance and the metabolic rate of newborn babies in relation to environmental temperature, and the effect of age and of weight on basal metabolic rate. J Physiol 1965;180:239.

[23] Hey EN, Katz G. The optimum thermal environment for naked babies. Arch Dis Child 1970; 45:328–34.

[24] Hey EN. The relation between environmental temperature and oxygen consumption in the newborn baby. J Physiol 1969;200:589.

[25] Baumgart S. Incubation of the human newborn infant. In: Pommerance J, Richardson CJ, editors. Issues in clinical neonatology. Norwalk (CT): Appleton & Lange; 1992. p. 139–50.

[26] Mayfield SR, Bhatia J, Nakamura KT, et al. Temperature measurement in term and preterm neonates. J Pediatr 1984;104:271–5.

[27] Gunn AJ, Gunn TR. The 'pharmacology' of neuronal rescue with cerebral hypothermia. Early Hum Dev 1998;53:19–35.

[28] Day RL. Maintenance of body temperature of premature infants. Pediatrics 1963;31:717–8.

[29] Shankaran S, Laptook AR, Ehrenkranz RA, et al, for the NICHHD, Neonatal Research Network. Whole-body hypothermia for neonates with hypoxic-ischemic encephalopathy. N Engl J Med 2005;353:1574–84.

[30] Gluckman PD, Wyatt JS, Azzopardi D, et al. CoolCap study group. Selective head-cooling with mild systemic hypothermia after neonatal encephalopathy: multi-center randomized trial. Lancet 2005;365–70.

[31] Higgins RD, et al. Hypothermia and perinatal asphyxia: executive summary of the National Institute of Child Health and Human Development workshop. J Pediatr 2006;148:170–5.

[32] Yager JY, Armstrong EA, Jaharus C, et al. Preventing hyperthermia decreases brain damage following neonatal hypoxic-ischemic seizures. Brain Res 2004;48–57.

[33] El-Dib M, Massaro AN, Baumgart S, et al. Amplitude integrated electroencephalogram (aEEG) background changes and seizures during therapeutic whole-body hypothermia [abstract]. Presented at the Society for Pediatric Research, Toronto, May 2007.

[34] Baumgart S, Massaro A, Chang T, et al. Whole body cooling therapy: is it really a cooling mattress [abstract]. Toronto: Society for Pediatric Research; 2007.

[35] Baumgart S. Radiant heat loss vs. radiant heat gain in premature neonates under radiant warmers. Biol Neonate 1990;57:10–20.

[36] Committee on Environmental Hazards, Committee on Fetus and Newborn, Committee on Accident and Poison Prevention. Hyperthermia from malfunctioning radiant heaters. Pediatrics 1977;59(6 Pt 2):1041–2.

[37] Simon HB. Hyperthermia. N Engl J Med 1993;329:483–7.

[38] Craig WS. The early detection of pyrexia in the newborn. Arch Dis Child 1963;41:448–50.

[39] Lieberman E, Lan JM, Frigoletto F Jr, et al. Epidural analgesia, intrapartum fever, and neonatal sepsis evaluation. Pediatrics 1997;99:415–9.

[40] Pleasure JR, Stahl GE. Do epidural anesthesia-related maternal fevers alter neonatal care? Pediatr Res 1990;27:221A.

[41] Shum-Tim D, Nagashima M, Shinoka T, et al. Postischemic hyperthermia exacerbates neurologic injury after deep hypothermic circulatory arrest. J Thorac Cardiovasc Surg 1998;116: 780–92.

[42] Tiker F, Gurakan B, Kilicdag H, et al. Dehydration: the main cause of fever during the first week of life. Arch Dis Child Fetal Neonatal Ed 2004;89(4):F373–4.

[43] Manzar S. Fever in the neonatal period. Arch Dis Child Fetal Neonatal Ed 2004;89(3):F282.

[44] Caroline M, Rudnick CS, Hoekzema GS. Neonatal herpes simplex virus infections. Am Fam Physician 2002;65:1138–42, 1143.

ELSEVIER
SAUNDERS

CLINICS IN
PERINATOLOGY

Clin Perinatol 35 (2008) 199–222

Complications of Vascular Catheters in the Neonatal Intensive Care Unit

Jayashree Ramasethu, MD, FAAP

Division of Neonatology, Georgetown University Hospital, 3800 Reservoir Road, NW Suite M 3400, Washington, DC 20007, USA

Vascular catheters are considered "life lines," indispensable in neonatal intensive care. Insertion of an intravascular catheter is the most common invasive procedure in the neonatal ICU (NICU). With every passing decade, technological innovations in catheter materials and sizes have allowed vascular access in infants who are smaller and sicker, for purposes of blood pressure monitoring, blood sampling, and infusion of intravenous fluids and medications. On the other hand, there is growing recognition of potential risks to life and limb associated with the use of intravascular catheters. Medical literature is now replete with isolated case reports of complications succinctly described by Garden and Laussen [1] as "An unending supply of 'unusual' complications from central venous catheters" (CVCs).

This article reviews complications of venous and arterial catheters in the NICU and also discusses treatment approaches and methods to prevent such complications, based on current evidence.

Venous catheters used in the NICU include short peripheral catheters or cannulas placed in superficial veins and longer CVCs placed in larger deep veins. These include umbilical venous catheters, percutaneously placed CVCs (also known as peripherally placed central catheters, PICCs), which are soft, flexible catheters inserted into peripheral veins and threaded into the central venous system, and surgically inserted external tunnelled central catheters such as Broviac or Hickman catheters. Indwelling arterial catheters in the NICU include peripheral arterial catheters and umbilical arterial catheters (UACs). Carotid arterial catheterization is performed in the NICU for extracorporeal membrane oxygenation, and the femoral artery frequently is used for cardiac catheterization; complications from these procedures are similar to those of indwelling arterial catheters.

E-mail address: jr65@gunet.georgetown.edu

0095-5108/08/$ - see front matter © 2008 Elsevier Inc. All rights reserved.
doi:10.1016/j.clp.2007.11.007 *perinatology.theclinics.com*

Peripheral venous catheters

Complications of peripheral venous catheters include thrombophlebitis, infection, and extravasation or inadvertent infiltration of intravenously administered solutions into subcutaneous tissue. Thrombophlebitis from peripheral venous catheters is an uncommon complication in NICU, probably because the average dwell time for such catheters is relatively short, ranging from 9 to 133 hours [2]. Thrombophlebitis can be relatively benign, with redness and tenderness over the course of the vein resolving with discontinuation of the intravenous fluids, or a more serious suppurative complication, which is a source of continuous bacteremia, with metastatic foci of infection [3].

The prevalence of extravasation injury resulting in skin necrosis in NICUs is reported to be approximately 4%, with 70% of these injuries occurring in infants of 26 weeks' gestation or less [4]. Fragility of the skin, particularly in the first 2 weeks of life, and the lack of subcutaneous tissue in preterm neonates makes them uniquely susceptible to injury and skin loss, resulting in a range of sequelae from minor scarring to loss of limb structure and function [4,5]. The degree of cellular injury is determined by the volume of the infiltrating solution and physicochemical characteristics, such as pH, osmolarity, and degree of dissociability (pKa). Infiltration of vasopressors such as dopamine and epinephrine produces intense local vasoconstriction and tissue ischemia [6], but parenteral alimentation fluids, antibiotics, calcium, potassium, and sodium bicarbonate solutions also have the potential to cause severe tissue necrosis [4,7].

Extravasation of intravenous fluids is marked initially by pain and swelling, which then progresses to blanching, blistering, and discoloration of the skin. Fussiness, crying, and withdrawal of the limb on flushing the intravenous cannula are early warning signs, but these signs may be absent in infants who are sedated or critically ill. Persistent induration often progresses to a dry black eschar in 1 or 2 weeks, which then usually sloughs to reveal an ulcer. Objective staging of extravasations is useful for quality improvement purposes and for deciding the degree of intervention required [8].

Treatment is determined by the stage of extravasation, the nature of the infiltrating solution, and the availability of specific antidotes. In all cases of infiltration, the intravenous infusion should be stopped promptly, and any constricting bands or tapes should be removed. Treatment protocols for severe extravasations vary from conservative to aggressive management of the acute injury [4,5,9,10], with additional variations in wound management [7,11,12]. Local injections of hyaluronidase increase permeability and reduce tissue damage in neonates with infiltrations of solutions containing high concentrations of dextrose, calcium, or sodium bicarbonate and nafcillin [13–15]. Chandavasu and colleagues [16] advocate multiple punctures of the tense skin to allow free drainage of the infiltrating solution and to decrease the swelling. Some centers have had good results using a saline flushout technique to remove or dilute the extravasated material after injecting hyaluronidase subcutaneously, even with infiltrations of vasoconstrictive agents [5,10,17,18]. Phentolamine and nitroglycerine have been used to reverse the vasoconstrictive effects of catecholamine extravasations [6,19]. Comparison of the different strategies of treatment is confounded by heterogeneity in the severity of injuries, the nature of the infiltrating fluids, and factors such as gestational age and medical condition of the infants [10,20]. Wound-care regimens also differ among different institutions. Practices vary from exposing the wound to air to occlusive dressings with hydrocolloids or hydrogels or nonocclusive saline or other dressings [4,7,11,20]. The goal of wound management in neonates who have partial or full-thickness skin loss is to achieve primary or secondary healing while avoiding contractures.

Measures to prevent extravasation include careful insertion of peripheral venous cannulae in neonates, flushing with sterile saline to ensure patency, and suitable taping to prevent movement, without obscuring possible swelling or erythema. Regular inspection of the site and regulated delivery of intravenous fluids from continuous infusion pumps (usually limited to an hour at a time) may prevent the inadvertent infiltration of a large amount of fluid before detection. Although occlusion alarms on infusion pumps may be set to the lowest limit possible, increased pressure is not always registered [21]. Hyperosmolar fluids, acidic or alkaline solutions, or infusates with irritant or vesicant properties should be given through central venous lines, if possible, or should be diluted or neutralized appropriately. The addition of heparin either to flush solutions or to continuous infusions has not been shown to prolong peripheral catheter patency or to reduce the incidence of infiltration or extravasations conclusively [22].

Central venous catheters

CVCs provide stable intravenous access to infants who need long-term parenteral alimentation or medications [23]. In the NICU, CVCs may be in the form of umbilical venous catheters or percutaneous CVCs, also known as PICCs. PICCs have become much more prevalent than cut-downs or open surgical techniques, because the procedure is simpler to perform, relatively rapid, less expensive, and requires only mild sedation or pain relief. The catheters, made of silicone, polyurethane, or polyethylene, are widely available in sizes as small as 1.2 Fr, facilitating insertion in micropremies weighing less than 500 g to 700 g. Surgically inserted catheters, such as Broviac catheters, remain invaluable when peripheral access is unavailable. Surgical techniques permit insertion of larger silicone catheters (3–7 Fr), and access to jugular and other veins generally not approached by the percutaneous route. Direct catheterization of the subclavian or femoral veins is resorted to in NICUs only in exceptional circumstances [24].

Complications from CVCs include injury to other vessels or organs during insertion, catheter migration or malposition with extravasation from the malpositioned catheter causing further problems, infection, thromboembolism (TE), catheter breakage, and dysfunction.

Injury to other vessels and organs during insertion

Injury to vessels, nerves, and other organs is uncommon when the vein is superficial and visible during insertion of the catheter (eg, with placement of a PICC), as opposed to blind placement in relation to surface landmarks (eg, when subclavian catheters are placed without sonographic guidance). Bleeding, hematomas, arterial puncture, brachial plexus injury, pneumothorax, and pneumomediastinum are all potential complications during subclavian venous catheterization [25].

Catheter tip position

A discussion of the appropriate position of the tip of CVCs is germane to this discussion, because the most serious complications of CVCs are related to the position of the catheter. The "central" position of the tip of CVCs is determined by the need for rapid hemodilution of the infusate, and hence the tip typically is positioned in as large a vein as possible, usually the inferior vena cava (IVC) or superior vena cava, close to the heart (Fig. 1A, B). Although recommendations for the correct placement of the CVC tip vary, there is general agreement that the tip should not be in the right atrium

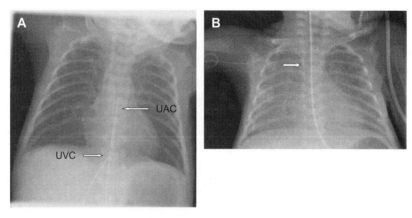

Fig. 1. (A) Umbilical venous catheter (UVC) and umbilical arterial catheter (UAC) in appropriate positions. The UVC tip is at the inferior vena cava/right atrial junction, and the UAC is at the level of the T7 vertebra. (B) Peripherally inserted central venous catheter tip (arrow) in superior vena cava.

(Fig. 2) because of the risk of pericardial effusions [26–30]. Although one large, retrospective audit of 2186 catheters showed that catheters with tips in the right atrium and not coiled were not associated with pericardial effusions [31], other authors insist that the catheter tip should remain outside the pericardial reflection, a distance estimated to be about 1 cm outside the cardiac silhouette in preterm neonates and 2 cm outside the cardiac silhouette in term neonates [26]. When inserted from a lower extremity or for umbilical venous catheters, the tip of the catheter should be at the junction of the IVC and right atrium [32,33]. It also has been suggested that the catheter should be parallel with the long axis of the vein so that the tip does not abut the vein or heart wall [32].

Malposition

Because insertion lengths of PICCs in the NICU are estimated from surface landmarks, the tip of the catheter may reach deep inside the cardiac chambers, fall short of the caval veins and end in the brachiocephalic or subclavian vein, or migrate through venous tributaries to entirely unexpected locations. Sites of misplacement of PICCs include the cardiac chambers, internal jugular veins, the contralateral subclavian vein, the ascending lumbar vein, and superficial abdominal and renal veins [26,28–30,33–36]. Extravasation of fluid from the catheters in each of these positions has led to serious, and occasionally lethal, complications.

Spontaneous correction of malpositioned lines within 24 hours of placement in upper extremity veins has been demonstrated in a few cases when the tip of the catheter initially was looped into the internal jugular vein or in the contralateral brachiocephalic vein but subsequently "flipped back" toward the right atrium, probably secondary to the direction of venous blood flow [37,38].

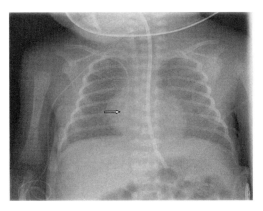

Fig. 2. Peripherally inserted catheter tip (*arrow*) in right atrium.

Appropriate initial placement does not always ensure that the catheter will stay in place, because secondary catheter migration has also been described, possibly as a consequence of poor catheter fixation at the skin surface or movements at joints. Arm movements have been shown to have a significant effect on the position of the tip of PICCs [39]. Catheters placed in the basilic or cephalic veins below the level of the elbow are likely to move toward the heart when the elbow is flexed. Catheters placed in the basilic or axillary veins migrate toward the heart with adduction of the arm, and catheters placed in the cephalic vein move away from the heart with adduction of the arm. In fact, simultaneous shoulder adduction and elbow flexion has caused the tips of catheters placed in the basilic vein to move as much as 15.11 ± 1.22 mm. Knowledge of the effect of arm movements on the position of catheter tips has been used to correct malpositions in a few cases [39]. Umbilical venous catheters can migrate inwards with retraction and mummification of the cord remnant in the first few days of life [40].

Central venous catheters in noncentral positions

Although PICCs are intended to be placed in central veins, occasionally they cannot be advanced to an ideal position, and the tip remains in a noncentral location within the brachiocephalic or subclavian vein. Thiagarajan and colleagues [41], in a study of 587 PICCs placed in neonates and older children, showed that complication rates between the noncentral and central catheters were similar (32% versus 27%), but in this study catheter tip placement in the subclavian vein was considered "central," and almost half the "central" catheters were in the subclavian vein. A later study of 1266 PICCs showed that true central placement of the catheter tip results in fewer complications. There were 42 complications in 1096 centrally placed catheters (3.8%) versus 49 complications in 170 noncentral catheters (28.8%) [42]. The major complications were phlebitis, leaking, and occlusion. It has been postulated that when the catheter tip is in a noncentral location, venous tortuosity, valves, and decreased venous size increase the possibility of the tip's impinging on the vessel wall and disrupting the endothelium, triggering the coagulation cascade or perforating the wall.

Pericardial effusion/cardiac tamponade

There now are a large number of reports of pericardial effusion and cardiac tamponade associated with CVCs in neonates. The incidence of this life-threatening complication is estimated to range from 0.76% to 1.8% of catheters placed in neonates, but the true incidence is probably higher, because the complication may not be recognized until autopsy is performed [26,29,33,36]. The most common clinical presentation is sudden cardiovascular collapse. Unexplained or subacute cardiorespiratory instability and a sudden requirement for inotropic or respiratory support is present in about a third of patients. Pericardial rub and jugular venous distension have not been noted in most case reports, and pulsus paradoxus has been detected only occasionally. Cardiomegaly may be detected on the chest radiograph. Schulman and colleagues [43] described unexpected resistance to sternal compression when associated with sudden cardiovascular collapse unresponsive to the usual resuscitative measures and negative thoracic transillumination leading to a working diagnosis of pericardial tamponade and life-saving therapeutic pericardiocentesis. Urgent echocardiography remains the mainstay of diagnosis, and immediate pericardiocentesis is the only life-saving therapy. In a large series of 61 CVC-related pericardial effusions in infants, mortality was reported to be 8% in patients who had pericardiocentesis and 75% in patients who did not [26]. Attempts to remove the pericardial fluid by aspirating through the misplaced catheter have not been successful [26,44]. Although most centers immediately stop infusing fluids through the CVC when pericardial effusion is suspected, there are reports of successful continued use of the catheter after it has been withdrawn so that the tip is in a more appropriate position, a considerable advantage in a sick baby with limited venous access [26].

Over and over again, most reports emphasize that the tip of the catheter was in the right atrium (see Fig. 2) at the time the pericardial effusion was noted [26,29,33,36,40,43], with only rare reports of pericardial effusions occurring with the umbilical venous catheter tips in the "correct" location at the junction of the IVC and right atrium [44,45]. The physical and biochemical characteristics of the pericardial fluid obtained by pericardiocentesis or noted at autopsy have been consistent with the infusate. Perforation with or without myocardial necrosis/thrombosis has been noted on autopsy, but in some cases no perforation has been detected. In view of this finding, and because the pericardial effusion is not bloody, it is postulated that constant abrasion of the endocardial wall by the tip of the catheter in the thin-walled right atrium leads to inflammation and then necrosis or thrombosis with perforation that may self-seal or that there is transmural diffusion of hyperosmolar fluid across the injured endocardium and myocardium [26]. An increased angle of incidence between the catheter tip and the cardiac/vessel wall or angulation of the catheter tip has been associated with perforation [29]. Although one may assume that perforation and cardiac tamponade are more likely with stiffer polyurethane and polyethylene catheters, this complication has been described with all types of catheters, including the very pliant silicone or silicone rubber catheters [26,29,43].

Pleural effusion

Pleural effusions caused by extravasation of parenteral alimentation fluid are a common complication of CVCs in the newborn, although the actual incidence is not known. Respiratory distress resulting from pleural effusions may arise within a few hours or several days after placement of the catheter

[46–48]. Although some effusions may be caused by actual erosion or perforation of the intrathoracic veins, in other cases migration of the catheter into
the pulmonary artery (from the right atrium to the right ventricle to the pulmonary artery, to become wedged in one of the branches) or pulmonary vein
(from the right atrium, through the foramen ovale, to the left atrium and
thence into a pulmonary vein) has been described [49,50]. In these cases,
the effusions have been attributed to increased vascular permeability secondary to endothelial damage by hyperosmolar infusates or to increased hydro-
static pressure [50].

Neurologic complications

At least 10 cases of neurologic complications have been reported in neonates caused by the inadvertent malposition of CVCs in the ascending
lumbar vein, after placement of the catheter in a vein in the lower extremity
[51–60]. In all cases, initial placement of the CVC was considered satisfactory, based on standard anteroposterior views of abdominal radiographs
showing the catheter apparently to be in the iliac vein or IVC. The interval
between placement of the catheter and appearance of symptoms ranged
from 1 to 11 days. In some infants, symptoms were nonspecific and con-
sisted of lethargy and oxygen desaturation, prompting a "sepsis workup."
Some infants had tonic-clonic or myoclonic seizures, mainly of the lower extremities. Lumbar puncture revealed "milky" spinal fluid, with very elevated
glucose or triglyceride levels, consistent with the composition of parenteral
alimentation fluid. Cerebrospinal fluid white cell counts also were elevated
in some cases. Although most infants recovered when the administration
of parenteral alimentation fluids was stopped and the catheter was removed,
some suffered permanent neurologic damage, including flaccid paraplegia
and neurogenic bladder.

The ascending lumbar vein drains the vertebral venous plexus into the
common iliac vein and is accessed easily by femoral or saphenous vein catheterization, particularly on the left side, because the angle formed by the left
ascending lumbar vein with the left common iliac vein is less acute than the
angle on the right side (Fig. 3). This explains the relative preponderance of
malposition of catheters into the left ascending vein when placed in the left
leg. Lavandosky and colleagues [60] described three warning signs: (1) absence of blood on aspiration of the catheter, (2) lateral deviation or
a "hump" of the catheter at the level of L4 and L5 on frontal abdominal
radiographs when catheters were placed from the left side, and (3) a catheter
path directly over the vertebral column rather than to the right of the midline for an IVC catheter. Schoonakker and Hardig [61] described a loop or
bend in the catheter visible in the region of the iliofemoral vein, particularly
on the left side, when the ascending lumbar vein is catheterized inadvertently. These findings are quite subtle and could be missed easily by inexpe-
rienced practitioners. Cross-table lateral radiographs will reveal the catheter

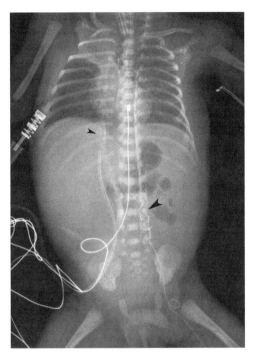

Fig. 3. The PICC tip in ascending lumbar vein. Note contrast medium dispersing via the left ascending lumbar vein into the vertebral venous plexus (*large arrowhead*) and crossing midline into the IVC (*small arrowhead*). IVC inferior vena cava; PICC peripherally inserted central catheter. (*From* Filan PM, Salek-Haddadi Y, Nolan I, et al. An under-recognized malposition of neonatal long lines. Eur J Pediatr 2005;164 (8):470; with permission.)

to be anterior to the spinal column if the catheter is in the IVC. Catheter positions superimposed on the spinal canal or deviating posteriorly at the level of L4–L5 vertebra indicate that the catheter is misplaced in the ascending lumbar vein and must be removed (Fig. 4A, B) [57–60,62].

Catheter-related sepsis

Catheter-related sepsis is the most common complication of CVCs with rates ranging from 0 to 29% of catheters placed, and from 2 to 49 per 1000 catheter days, with the smallest and most immature infants being at the greatest risk [31,63–68]. Contamination of the catheter hub and exit site has been postulated as the portal of entry for intraluminal bacterial colonization of CVCs, with adherence properties of certain organisms allowing persistence of infection and preventing eradication [65,66]. The rate of infections varies significantly among different neonatal units, secondary to differences in patient population, practice styles, and reporting variances [63,64,66–68]. The recent National Health Care Safety Network Report update of the National Nosocomial Infections Surveillance System showed the

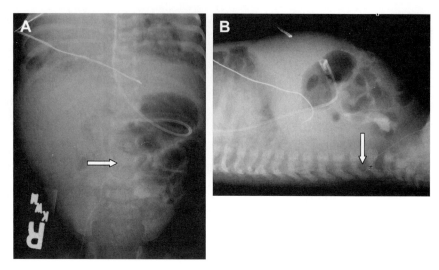

Fig. 4. (*A*) Anteroposterior view of abdomen revealing central venous catheter tip in the midline (*arrow*). (*B*) Lateral view of abdomen demonstrating the central venous catheter (*arrow*) within the lumbar spine (*From* Perry MS, Billars L. Extravasation of hyperalimentation into the spinal epidural space from a central venous line. Neurology 2006;67(4):715; with permission.)

average incidence of central line–related blood stream infections in level 3 NICUS was 6.4 per 1000 catheter days for infants weighing 750 g or less (median, 5.2; tenth to ninetieth percentile, 0–15.6), decreasing to 3.1 per 1000 catheter days for infants weighing more than 2500 g. The rates of umbilical catheter–associated blood stream infections also were high in babies weighing 750 g or less (pooled mean, 6.9; median, 2.9; ninetieth percentile, 19.1) but were much lower in babies weighing more than 2500 g (ninetieth percentile, 1.7) [64].

Coagulase-negative staphylococci are the most frequent cause of bacteremia associated with CVCs in the NICU, but *Staphylococcus aureus*, gram-negative bacteria, and Candida also may cause catheter-related sepsis. An accurate diagnosis of catheter-related sepsis caused by coagulase-negative staphylococci may be difficult to make, because false-positive cultures may be caused by contamination from the skin. Repeatedly positive blood cultures, positive cultures from more than one site, or the association of positive blood cultures with clinical and hematologic signs of sepsis are regarded as evidence of infection.

Removal of the foreign body (ie, the central line) is crucial to eradicate the infection but is not always possible in small and sick infants. The outcome for infants in whom the catheter is not removed within 24 hours after the organism is identified is significantly worse (odds ratio, 9.8), than it is for those whose catheters are removed promptly, with increased risk of end-organ damage or death [69]. Prompt removal of the CVC is recommended for catheter-related sepsis caused by *S aureus*, non-enteric gram-negative bacteria, and Candida [69,70]. Treatment with appropriate antibiotics without removal of the CVC may be attempted for coagulase-negative staphylococcal bacteremia, but removal of the line is essential if the blood cultures are repeatedly positive [69,71].

Prevention of catheter-related sepsis is at the top of the agenda of most hospitals because of potential reductions in mortality, morbidity, and cost. Data from randomized, controlled trials have shown that the risk of infections can be minimized with simple interventions [72]. These precautions include the use of maximal barrier precautions (long-sleeved gown, sterile gloves, mask, cap, and a large, sterile sheet drape) during insertion of the catheter [73], the use of chlorhexidine-containing antiseptics rather than povidone iodine for preparing the catheter insertion site [74], the use of chlorhexidine-impregnated dressings over the CVC insertion site for patients other than very low birth weight neonates [75], decreased manipulations of the CVC [76], and application of a closed medication system to prevent repeated entries into the CVC [68]. Strict protocols for central line care and education of physicians and nurses, with a methodology of surveillance and data feedback, have been shown to reduce infection rates [66,68,77,78]. The risk of infection increases with the duration of catheterization; daily assessment for the continued need for CVCs is necessary, so that catheters are removed as soon as they are no longer essential for patient care.

Thromboembolism

With the exception of renal vein thrombosis, almost all (approximately 90%) of venous TEs in neonates are associated with CVCs [79]. Thrombosis has been detected in 20% to 30% of neonates who have CVCs, even with the continuous infusion of heparin [80–82]. Neonates are particularly susceptible to TE because of the small caliber of blood vessels, quantitative and qualitative immaturity of thrombolytic and fibrinolytic systems, and disturbances of the hemostatic balance by complications such as perinatal asphyxia, hypovolemia, septicemia, dehydration, polycythemia, or congenital heart disease [83]. Nowak-Gottl and colleagues [84] demonstrated an increased incidence of congenital prothrombotic disorders in neonates who had catheter-related thrombosis, but other authors have not found congenital prothrombotic disorders to be a significant risk factor in neonates [82,85].

Catheter-related venous TE can be asymptomatic or can result in severe complications such as deep vein thrombosis, portal vein thrombosis, superior vena cava syndrome, intracardiac thrombosis, or pulmonary embolism [82,86]. Clinical manifestations of symptomatic catheter-related thrombosis in neonates depend on the site of the thrombosis. Catheter dysfunction, thrombocytopenia, or persistent bacteremia may be associated with vascular thrombosis at any site. Apart from the loss of venous access from catheter-related thrombosis, there is potential danger of injury to vital organs secondary to thrombus propagation, embolization, or infection.

The incidence of TE disease in the newborn depends on the zeal with which surveillance is performed, the timing and frequency of monitoring, and the diagnostic method used. In one study, no signs or symptoms were present in 32 of 37 neonates in whom catheter-related thrombosis was diagnosed by echocardiography before removal of the central venous line or was discovered coincidentally during investigations for other reasons, such as cardiac evaluation [79]. Roy and colleagues [81] showed that the overall sensitivity of Doppler echocardiography for the detection of asymptomatic thrombosis is poor, but asymptomatic thrombi could be detected by contrast venography in 30% of patients who had umbilical venous catheters. Kim and colleagues [87] found clinically silent portal venous thrombosis in 43 of 100 neonates who had serial sonograms, with complete or partial resolution in 20 of 36 babies who were followed up for 2 to 73 days. On the other hand, Schwartz and colleagues [88] detected portal venous thrombosis by color Doppler sonography in only 1 of 100 neonates. The low incidence of portal venous thrombosis in this study may have resulted from the shorter duration of umbilical venous catheterization in some patients as well as from the resolution of thrombi with time.

The management of catheter-related venous TE in neonates is controversial. A full discussion of anticoagulants and thrombolytics is beyond the scope of this article but can be found in other reviews [89,90]. The guidelines published by the Seventh American College of Chest Physicians Conference on Antithrombotic and Thrombolytic Therapy in Children are currently the most authoritative but are likely to change as new data become available [90]. Treatment in each neonate should be individualized with consideration of the risk/benefit ratio. Treatment with either unfractionated heparin or low molecular weight heparin is recommended, with close monitoring of anticoagulation and clot resolution. Thrombolytic therapy with recombinant urokinase or recombinant tissue type plasminogen activator is not recommended for treatment of venous TE in neonates unless a major vessel occlusion is causing a critical compromise of organs or limbs. In general, central venous lines or umbilical lines should be removed if thrombosis is detected. Consultation with a pediatric hematologist and vascular/plastic surgeon is appropriate. A free consultative service, maintained 24 hours a day for physicians caring for children who have TE disease, provides current management protocols and links to the network and its services. The toll-free number in the United States is 1- 800-NO-CLOTS. Infants who have TE disease should be managed in a suitably staffed and equipped neonatal center, where anticoagulant or thrombolytic therapy can be administered and monitored appropriately and where laboratory, blood bank, and surgical support is readily available.

Long-term complications of venous TE in infants include the development of collateral circulation in the skin over the chest, back, neck, and face, superior vena cava syndrome, and loss of venous access. Infants and children who have extensive IVC thrombosis are at risk for persisting venous disease and postthrombotic syndrome, including exanthema, leg edema, phlebothrombosis of lower extremity veins, and leg ulcers [91]. Portal vein thrombosis secondary to umbilical venous catheterization is a common cause of portal hypertension in childhood [92]. A recent 5-year study of the outcome of portal vein thrombosis in infants showed that portal hypertension or atrophy of the left lobe of the liver was diagnosed in 27% of infants and was significantly more common in those who had inappropriately placed umbilical venous catheters or severe grades of thrombosis [93].

Other complications

Obstruction of CVCs, characterized by inability to infuse fluids or withdraw blood or by increased infusion pump pressures, often is caused by thrombosis but also may be secondary to malposition, thrombosis, or precipitates caused by minerals, drugs, or lipids [94]. The catheter position should be checked radiographically. If malposition is ruled out, dissolving the clot or precipitate may be attempted only if salvaging the catheter is vital. A review of the drugs or fluids administered through the catheter may provide clues to the probable cause of the obstruction. Recombinant tissue plasminogen activator or recombinant urokinase has been effective in clearing fibrin deposits or blood clots [94,95]. Sodium bicarbonate has been used for alkaline medications, hydrochloric acid for calcium salts and acidic medications, and ethanol for lipid deposits, with special techniques to clear the line without infusing these solutions into the infant [96].

Catheters may be severed by the introducer needle (during insertion of a PICC), may snap because of excessive tension on the external portion of the catheter, or may rupture because of excessive pressure, application of constricting clamps, or constricting sutures. The intravascular portion of the broken catheter may migrate into the heart and require endovascular removal [97,98].

There may be difficulty in removing CVCs that have been in place for a long time, because of the formation of a fibrin sheath or secondary to *Malassezia furfur* infection. If the tethered catheters cannot be removed with gentle traction, thrombolytic therapy or surgical incision may be required [96,99].

Arterial catheters

Indwelling radial or ulnar arterial catheters (peripheral arterial line catheters) or UAC are placed in newborn infants for monitoring purposes, whereas carotid artery catheterization is performed for extracorporeal membrane oxygenation, and the femoral artery frequently is used for cardiac catheterization. Temporal artery catheterization is not recommended, because of potential neurologic complications. Injury to adjacent structures during insertion is a potential complication of peripheral and femoral arterial lines, and infection is a possibility with any indwelling catheter; however, the most common complications of arterial catheterization are vascular spasm and TE. The predisposing factors for arterial TE in the newborn are the same as for venous TE, with the presence of intravascular catheters being the most important risk factor.

Vascular spasm

Vascular spasm is temporary, reversible arterial constriction, often triggered by arterial blood sampling or catheterization, and is characterized by transient pallor or cyanosis of the involved extremity with diminished pulses or perfusion. The clinical effects of vascular spasm usually last less than 4 hours from onset, but it may be difficult to differentiate vasospasm from more serious TE. The diagnosis of vasospasm is generally made retrospectively, after documentation of the transient nature of signs and complete recovery of perfusion within a few minutes or hours. If mild cyanosis of the fingers or toes is noted after placement of an arterial catheter, but peripheral pulses are still palpable, a trial of reflex vasodilatation by warming the contralateral extremity is reasonable, with close observation, because vascular spasm may resolve. The benefits of keeping the catheter versus the risk of further ischemia should be evaluated continually. A white or blanched-appearing extremity is an indication for immediate removal of the catheter. Topical application of 2% nitroglycerine ointment at a dose of 4 mm/kg body weight, applied as a thin film over the affected areas, and repeated after 8 hours, if necessary, has been shown to reverse peripheral ischemia in very low birth weight infants [100–102].

Umbilical arterial catheters

Position of the catheter

UACs usually are placed with the catheter tip in one of two positions: a high position at a level between thoracic vertebrae 6 and 9 (see Fig. 1A), which positions the tip above the origin of the celiac axis, and a low position at the level of lumbar vertebra 3 or 4, which positions the tip just above the aortic bifurcation but below major aortic branches [103]. Meta-analysis of five randomized, controlled trials and one alternate assignment study showed that high-placed UACs with the tip above the diaphragm have a lower incidence of clinical vascular complications than those placed in the low position [104]. Infusion of glucose into high-placed UACs has been associated with hypoglycemia secondary to streaming of glucose to the celiac and superior mesenteric arteries [105].

Malpositions of the UAC into the femoral, gluteal, or renal arteries and into the celiac plexus have been described, with severe complications in some cases [106–108]. More than 100 cases of gluteoperineal necrosis associated with sciatic nerve palsy secondary to thrombosis of the inferior gluteal artery have been recorded, and although many have been attributed to the injection of hypertonic or alkaline medications through the UAC, some have occurred even when the catheter was in an appropriate position and infused only with heparinized saline [107,108]. Similarly, cases of acute and irreversible paraplegia following umbilical arterial catheterization have been attributed to infarction of the spinal cord following vasospasm or thromboembolic phenomena involving the artery of Adamkiewicz, the large anterior radiculomedullary artery that supplies the anterior spinal artery [109–112].

Thromboembolism

UACs may be associated with TE complications involving the aorta, iliac, renal, mesenteric, or other vessels. Symptoms of arterial TE include pallor or coldness of the lower extremities with diminished or absent pulses and systemic hypertension, with or without renal failure if the renal arteries are affected. In a large systematic study of UAC-associated thrombosis, Boo and colleagues [113] detected abdominal aortic thrombi by two-dimensional abdominal sonography in 32% of 99 infants upon removal of umbilical arterial catheters. Although some of the thrombi extended through the length of the aorta and even into one of the common iliac arteries, the diameter of the thrombi was less than half that of the aorta, and none of the thrombi occluded the aorta completely. After controlling for confounding variables, Boo and colleagues estimated that the probability of developing aortic thrombosis in an infant with an UAC in situ for 1 day was approximately 16%, increasing progressively to 32% at 7 days, 57% at 14 days, and 78% at 21 days. Coleman and colleagues [114] detected only one of case of thrombosis in 33 infants who had a UAC in place, but only 13 of the infants had catheters in place for up to 5 days.

The effect of catheter materials and design in the generation of thrombosis also is important. No clinically relevant difference has been noted in outcomes between the use of polyvinyl chloride catheters and other materials, although one nonrandomized study suggested that silicone rubber catheters may be less thrombogenic [115]. End-hole catheters are associated with a lower risk of thrombosis than side-hole catheters [116]. Most institutions use heparinized fluid in UACs; this measure has been shown to decrease the incidence of catheter occlusion but does not seem to affect the frequency of aortic thrombosis [117].

Treatment of UAC-associated TE is similar to the treatment of venous TE [89,90]. Treatment is highly individualized and is determined by the extent of thrombosis and the degree to which diminished perfusion to the limb or organ affects function. Management may involve supportive care with correction of volume depletion, blood pressure, electrolyte abnormalities, anemia, and thrombocytopenia in addition to specific anticoagulation, fibrinolytic therapy, or surgical intervention.

Although 50% of UAC-related thrombi disappear before discharge from the hospital, the long-term consequences of persistent thrombosis have not been studied systematically. UAC-associated TE has been linked to hypertension, abnormalities in renal function and in leg growth, abdominal aortic aneurysm, and acquired aortic coarctation, sometimes years after apparent resolution of the thrombosis [118–121]. Mycotic aneurysms of the aorta have been noted in infants, particularly in association with S aureus infection [122,123].

Peripheral artery catheterization

For more than 30 years many authors have advocated percutaneous catheterization of peripheral arteries (eg, the radial, ulnar, and posterior tibial arteries) as being a safer alternative to umbilical arterial catheterization [124–127]. In the NICU, the radial and posterior tibial arteries are the primary sites for cannulation. Because of potential risk of ischemic injury to the entire hand or arm, the ulnar, brachial, and axillary arteries generally are used for cannulation only if arterial access at the primary sites is unsuccessful [128–130]. The radial artery contributes the major blood supply to the thumb and index finger and anastomoses with the deep branch of the ulnar artery system. The predominant blood supply to the hand is usually from the ulnar artery, but multiple variations are possible [131]. Hack and colleagues [132] demonstrated by repeated Doppler flow measurements that the radial artery was completely occluded in 63% of infants who had radial artery catherization and that blood flow to the site distal to the cannulation site was dependent on the existence of an adequate collateral circulation. Nevertheless, blood flow in the radial artery resumed within 1 to 29 days after catheter removal in all infants. The modified Allen test has long been advocated to assess adequacy of the collateral circulation of the hand before radial artery catheterization, but the test is inaccurate and suffers from poor interobserver reliability [133].

Although there are multiple case reports of ischemic injury [100–102,134], and there are very limited data in extremely low birth weight infants, the overall risk of ischemic injury secondary to radial or ulnar artery catheterization seems to be approximately 5% [124,128,135]. Because peripheral ischemia may be recognized immediately (Fig. 5), and appropriate action taken, gangrene and permanent loss of the digits may be avoided in some, but not all, cases [100–102,134,136]. Topical nitroglycerine has been found to be effective in restoring perfusion in a few cases in which radial artery catherization resulted in cold, cyanotic, and stiff hands with absent radial pulses [100–102].

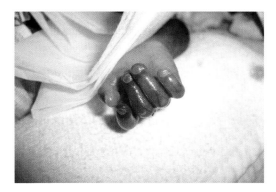

Fig. 5. Ischemic changes in fingers of extremely preterm infant following an attempt at radial artery catherization.

Nonischemic complications of arterial catheterization, or even of repeated attempts at catheterization, include bleeding, pseudoaneurysms, arteriovenous fistulae, median nerve palsy, carpal tunnel syndrome, and injury to the tendon sheaths [137–139].

Box 1. Guidelines to reduce risk of complications from central venous catheters

1. Use strict aseptic precautions for insertion and maintenance of the catheter, including dressing changes, tubing connections, and medication administration.
2. Ensure that blood can be aspirated freely into the catheter when it is inserted before it is taped into position. Confirm the location of the catheter tip radiographically (using radio-opaque contrast if necessary) on initial insertion. Repeat radiographs if there is any question of catheter movement or malfunction. Scrutinize radiographs obtained for any reason for appropriate catheter position.
3. The tip of the CVC should be just above the superior vena cava/right atrium junction for insertions from the upper extremity and at the IVC/right atrium junction for insertions from the lower extremity or the umbilical venous catheter.
4. Inspect the insertion site daily. Transparent dressings should be changed every 7 days except when the risk of dislodging the catheter outweighs the benefit of changing the dressing. Replace all damp, loose, or soiled dressings.
5. Add 0.5 to 1.0 mL of heparin per mL of intravenous fluids being infused.
6. Remove catheter as soon as medically feasible if it is obstructed or if there is evidence of thrombosis or infection.

Box 2. Guidelines to reduce risk of complications from arterial catheters

1. Use strict aseptic precautions for insertion and maintenance of the catheter, including dressing changes and tubing connections.
2. Monitor extremities for signs of vascular compromise frequently: examine tips of fingers or toes for peripheral catheters, the lower extremities including buttocks for UACs.
3. Infuse catheters with heparinized saline continuously. Avoid the administration of any other medication, fluid, or blood transfusions through the arterial catheter.
4. Remove catheters as soon as medically feasible or if there are signs of vascular compromise or suspicion of thrombosis.

Summary

Arterial and venous catheters remain indispensable in neonatal intensive care despite the risk of numerous complications, with short- and long-term implications. Although catheter materials and designs continue to improve, simple precautions taken during the insertion and vigilance in the maintenance of catheters may help reduce complication rates. Boxes 1 and 2 provide basic guidelines for prevention of complications, based on currently available evidence.

References

[1] Garden AL, Laussen PC. An unending supply of "unusual" complications from central venous catheters. Paediatr Anaesth 2004;14(11):905–9.
[2] Franck LS, Hummel D, Connell K, et al. The safety and efficacy of peripheral intravenous catheters in ill neonates. Neonatal Netw 2001;20(5):33–7.
[3] Khan EA, Correa AG, Baker CJ. Suppurative thrombophlebitis in children: a ten year experience. Pediatr Infect Dis J 1997;16(1):63–7.
[4] Wilkins CE, Emmerson AJB. Extravasation injuries in regional neonatal units. Arch Dis Child Fetal Neonatal Ed 2004;89(3):F274–5.
[5] Casanova D, Bardot J, Magalon G. Emergency treatment of accidental infusion leakage in the newborn: report of 14 cases. Br J Plast Surg 2001;54(5):396–9.
[6] Subhani M, Sridhar S, DeCristofaro JD. Phentolamine use in a neonate for the prevention of dermal necrosis caused by dopamine: a case report. J Perinatol 2001;21(5):324–6.
[7] Brown AS, Hoelzer DJ, Piercy SA. Skin necrosis from extravasation of intravenous fluids in children. Plast Reconstr Surg 1979;64(2):145–50.
[8] Montgomery LA, Otto A, Hanrahan K, et al. Guideline for IV infiltrations in pediatric patients. Pediatr Nurs 1999;25(2):167–80.
[9] Kumar RJ, Pegg SP, Kimble RM. Management of extravasation injuries. ANZ J Surg 2001; 71(5):285–9.

[10] Harris PA, Bradley S, Moss ALH. Limiting the damage of iatrogenic extravasation injury in neonates. Plast Reconstr Surg 2001;107(3):893–4.

[11] Friedman J. Plastic surgical problems in the neonatal intensive care unit. Clin Plast Surg 1998;25(4):599–617.

[12] Falcone PA, Barrall DT, Jeyarajah DR, et al. Nonoperative management of full- thickness intravenous extravasation injuries in premature neonates using enzymatic debridement. Ann Plast Surg 1989;22(2):146–9.

[13] Laurie SWS, Wilson KL, Kernahan DA, et al. Intravenous extravasation injuries: the effectiveness of hyaluronidase in their treatment. Ann Plast Surg 1984;13(3):191–4.

[14] Raszka WV Jr, Keuser TK, Smith FR, et al. The use of hyaluronidase in the treatment of intravenous extravasation injuries. J Perinatol 1990;10(2):146–9.

[15] Zenk KE, Dungy CI, Greene GR. Nafcillin extravasation injury. Use of hyaluronidase as an antidote. Am J Dis Child 1981;135(12):1113–4.

[16] Chandavasu O, Garrow E, Valda V, et al. A new method for the prevention of skin sloughs and necrosis secondary to intravenous infiltration. Am J Perinatol 1986;3(1):4–5.

[17] Gault DT. Extravasation injuries. Br J Plast Surg 1993;46(2):91–6.

[18] Davies J, Gault D, Buchdahl R. Preventing the scars of neonatal intensive care. Arch Dis Child 1994;70(1):F50–1.

[19] Denkler KA, Cohen BE. Reversal of dopamine extravasation injury with topical nitroglycerine ointment. Plast Reconstr Surg 1989;84(5):811–3.

[20] Ramasethu J. Prevention and management of extravasation injuries in neonates. NeoReviews 2004;5:e1–7.

[21] Phelps SJ, Helms RA. Risk factors affecting infiltration of peripheral venous lines in infants. J Pediatr 1987;111(3):384–9.

[22] Shah PS, Ng E, Sinha SK. Heparin for prolonging peripheral intravenous catheter use in neonates. Cochrane Database Syst Rev 2005;4:CD002774.

[23] Ainsworth SB, Clerihew L, McGuire W. Percutaneous central venous catheters versus peripheral cannulae for delivery of parenteral nutrition in neonates. Cochrane Database Syst Rev 2007;3:CD004219. DOI:10.1002/14651858.CD004219.pub3.

[24] Wardle SP, Kelsall AWR, Yoxall CW, et al. Percutaneous femoral arterial and venous catheterization during neonatal intensive care. Arch Dis Child Fetal Neonatal Ed 2001;85(2): F119–22.

[25] Citak A, Karabocuoglu M, Ucsel R, et al. Central venous catheters in pediatric patients— subclavian approach as the first choice. Pediatr Int 2002;44(1):83–6.

[26] Nowlen TT, Rosenthal GL, Johnson GL, et al. Pericardial effusion and tamponade in infants with central catheters. Pediatrics 2002;110(1):137–42.

[27] Beardsall K, White DK, Pinto EM, et al. Pericardial effusion and cardiac tamponade as complications of neonatal long lines: are they really a problem? Arch Dis Child Fetal Neonatal Ed 2003;88(4):292–5.

[28] Jouvencel P, Tourneux P, Perez T, et al. Central catheters and pericardial effusion: results of a multicentric retrospective study. Arch Pediatr 2005;12(10):1456–61.

[29] Darling JC, Newell SJ, Mohamdee O, et al. Central venous catheter tip in the right atrium: a risk factor for neonatal cardiac tamponade. J Perinatol 2001;21(7):461–4.

[30] Nadroo AM, Lin J, Green RS, et al. Death as a complication of peripherally inserted central catheters in neonates. J Pediatr 2001;138(4):599–601.

[31] Cartwright DW. Central venous lines in neonates: a study of 2186 catheters. Arch Dis Child Fetal Neonatal Ed 2004;89(6):504–8.

[32] Fletcher SJ, Bodenham AR. Safe placement of central venous catheters: where should the tip of the catheter lie? Br J Anaesth 2000;85(2):188–91.

[33] Pezzati M, Filippi L, Chiti G, et al. Central venous catheters and cardiac tamponade in preterm infants. Intensive Care Med 2004;30(12):2253–6.

[34] Perry MS, Billars L. Extravasation of hyperalimentation into the spinal epidural space from a central venous line. Neurology 2006;67(4):715.

[35] Baker J, Imong S. A rare complication of neonatal central venous access. Arch Dis Child Fetal Neonatal Ed 2002;86(1):F61–2.

[36] Nadroo AM, al-Sowailem AM. Extravasation of parenteral alimentation fluid into the renal pelvis—a complication of central venous catheter in a neonate. J Perinatol 2001;21(7): 465–6.

[37] Rastogi S, Bhutada A, Sahni R, et al. Spontaneous correction of the malpositioned percutaneous central venous line in infants. Pediatr Radiol 1998;28(9):694–6.

[38] Al Tawil K, Eldemerdash A, Al Hathlol K, et al. Peripherally inserted central venous catheters in newborn infants: malpositioning and spontaneous correction of catheter tips. Am J Perinatol 2006;23(1):37–40.

[39] Nadroo AM, Glass RB, Lin J, et al. Changes in upper extremity position causes migration of peripherally inserted central catheters in neonates. Pediatrics 2002;110(1):131–6.

[40] Traen M, Schepens E, Laroche S, et al. Cardiac tamponade and pericardial effusion due to venous umbilical catheterization. Acta Paediatr 2005;94(5):626–33.

[41] Thiagarajan RR, Bratton SL, Gettmann T, et al. Efficacy of peripherally inserted central venous catheters placed in noncentral veins. Arch Pediatr Adolesc Med 1998;152(5):436–9.

[42] Racadio JM, Doellman DA, Johnson ND, et al. Pediatric peripherally inserted central catheters; complication rates related to catheter tip location. Pediatrics 2001;107(2):e28.

[43] Schulman J, Munshi UK, Eastman ML, et al. Unexpected resistance to external cardiac compression may signal cardiac tamponade. J Perinatol 2002;22(8):679–81.

[44] Sehgal A, Cook V, Dunn M. Pericardial effusion associated with an appropriately placed umbilical venous catheter. J Perinatol 2007;27(5):317–9.

[45] Onal EE, Saygili A, Koc E, et al. Cardiac tamponade in a newborn because of umbilical venous catheterization: is a correct position safe? Paediatr Anaesth 2004;14(11):953–6.

[46] Keeney SE, Richardson CJ. Extravascular extravasation of fluid as a complication of central venous lines in the neonate. J Perinatol 1995;15(4):284–8.

[47] Leipala J, Petaja J, Fellman V. Perforation complications of percutaneous central venous catheters in very low birthweight infants. J Paediatr Child Health 2001;37(2):168–71.

[48] Seguin JH. Right sided hydrothorax and central venous catheters in extremely low birth weight infants. Am J Perinatol 1992;9(3):154–8.

[49] Pigna A, Bachiocco V, Fae M, et al. Peripherally inserted central venous catheters in preterm newborns: two unusual complications. Paediatr Anaesth 2004;14(2):184–7.

[50] Madhavi P, Jameson R, Robinson MJ. Unilateral pleural effusion complicating central venous catheterization. Arch Dis Child Fetal Neonatal Ed 2000;82(3):F248–9.

[51] Knobel RB, Meetze W, Cummings J. Case report: total parenteral nutrition extravasation associated with spinal cord compression and necrosis. J Perinatol 2001;21(1):68–71.

[52] Rajan V, Waffarn F. Focal neurological manifestations following aberrant central venous catheter placement. J Perinatol 1999;19(6):447–9.

[53] Bass WT, Lewis DW. Neonatal segmental myoclonus associated with hyperglycorrachia. Pediatr Neurol 1995;13(1):77–9.

[54] Mitsufuji N, Matsuo K, Kakita S, et al. Extravascular collection of fluid around the vertebra resulting from malpositioning of a peripherally inserted central venous catheter in extremely low birth weight infants. J Perinat Med 2002;30(4):341–4.

[55] Filan PM, Salek- Haddadi Y, Nolan I, et al. An under-recognized malposition of neonatal long lines. Eur J Pediatr 2005;164(8):469–71.

[56] Zenker M, Rupprecht T, Hofbeck M, et al. Paravertebral and intraspinal malposition of transfemoral central venous catheters in newborn. J Pediatr 2000;136(6):837–40.

[57] Clarke P, Wadhawan R, Smyth J, et al. Parenteral nutrition solution retrieved by lumbar puncture following left saphenous vein catheterization. J Paediatr Child Health 2003; 39(5):386–9.

[58] Chen CC, Tsao PN, Yau KIT. Paraplegia: complication of percutaneous central venous line malposition. Pediatr Neurol 2001;23(5):65–8.

[59] Bergman KA, Doedens R, Akker EV, et al. Displacement and extravascular position of a saphenous vein catheter: a serious complication. Eur J Pediatr 1999;158(10):868–9.

[60] Lavandosky G, Gomez R, Montes J. Potentially lethal misplacement of femoral central venous catheters. Crit Care Med 1996;24(5):893–7.

[61] Schoonakker BC, Harding D. Radiological sign of a long line in the ascending lumbar vein. Arch Dis Child 2005;90(9):982.

[62] Coit AK, Kamitsuka MD, Pediatrix Medical Group. Peripherally inserted central catheter using the saphenous vein: importance of two view radiographs to determine the tip location. J Perinatol 2005;25(10):674–6.

[63] Perlman SE, Saiman L, Larson EL. Risk factors for late onset health care–associated blood stream infections in patients in neonatal intensive care units. Am J Infect Control 2007; 35(3):177–82.

[64] Edwards JR, Peterson KD, Andrus ML, et al. National Healthcare Safety Network (NHSN) report, data summary for 2006, issued June 2007. Am J Infect Control 2007; 35(5):290–301.

[65] Mahieu LM, De Dooy JJ, De Muynck AO, et al. Microbiology and risk factors for catheter exit site and hub colonization in neonatal intensive care unit patients. Infect Control Hosp Epidemiol 2001;22(6):357–62.

[66] US Department of Health and Human Services. Centers for Disease Control and Prevention. Guideline for prevention of intravascular device-related infection. MMWR Recomm Rep 2002;51(RR-10):1–36.

[67] Chien L, Macnab Y, Aziz K, et al. Variations in central venous catheter-related infection risks among Canadian neonatal intensive care units. Pediatr Infect Dis J 2002;21(6):505–11.

[68] Aly H, Herson V, Duncan A, et al. Is bloodstream infection preventable among premature infants? A tale of two cities. Pediatrics 2005;115(6):1513–8.

[69] Benjamin DK, Miller W, Garges H, et al. Bacteremia, central catheters and neonates: when to pull the line. Pediatrics 2001;107(6):1272–6.

[70] Karlowicz MG, Hashimoto LN, Kelly RE, et al. Should central venous catheters be removed as soon as candidemia is detected in neonates? Pediatrics 2000;106(5):e63.

[71] Karlowicz MG, Furigay PJ, Croitoru DP, et al. Central venous catheter removal versus in situ treatment in neonates with coagulase-negative staphylococcal bacteremia. Pediatr Infect Dis J 2002;21(1):22–7.

[72] Mermeel LA. Prevention of central venous catheter–related infections: what works other than impregnated or coated catheters? J Hosp Infect 2007;65(S2):30–3.

[73] Raad II, Hohn DC, Gilbreath BJ, et al. Prevention of central venous catheter related infections by using maximal sterile barrier precautions during insertion. Infect Control Hosp Epidemiol 1994;15(4 Pt1):231–8.

[74] Chaiyakunapruk N, Veenstra DL, Lipsky BA, et al. Chlorhexidine compared with povidone iodine solution for vascular site care: a meta- analysis. Ann Intern Med 2002; 136(11):792–801.

[75] Garland JS, Alex CP, Mueller CD, et al. A randomized trial comparing povidone iodine to a chlorhexidine gluconate impregnated dressing for prevention of central venous catheter infections in neonates. Pediatrics 2001;107(6):1431–6.

[76] Mahieu LM, De Dooy JJ, Lenaerts AE, et al. Catheter manipulations and the risk of catheter-associated bloodstream infection in neonatal intensive care unit patients. J Hosp Infect 2001;48(1):20–6.

[77] Schelonka RL, Scruggs S, Nichols K, et al. Sustained reductions in neonatal nosocomial infection rates following a comprehensive infection control intervention. J Perinatol 2006;26(3):141–3.

[78] Anderson C, Hart J, Vemgal P, et al. Prospective evaluation of a multifactorial prevention strategy on the impact of nosocomial infection in very low birth weight infants. J Hosp Infect 2005;61(2):162–7.

[79] Van Ommen CH, Heijboer H, Buller HR, et al. Venous thromboembolism in childhood: a prospective two year registry in the Netherlands. J Pediatr 2001;139(5):676–81.

[80] Shah PS, Kalyn A, Satodia P, et al. A randomized, controlled trial of heparin versus placebo infusion to prolong the usability of peripherally placed percutaneous central venous catheters (PCVCs) in neonates: the HIP (Heparin Infusion for PCVC) study. Pediatrics 2007; 119(1):e284–91.

[81] Roy M, Turner-Gomes S, Gill G, et al. Accuracy of Doppler ultrasonography for the diagnosis of thrombosis associated with umbilical venous catheters. J Pediatr 2002;140(1): 131–4.

[82] Salonvaara M, Riikonen P, Kekomaki R, et al. Clinically symptomatic central venous catheter related deep venous thrombosis in newborns. Acta Paediatr 1999;88(6):642–6.

[83] Kuhle S, Male C, Mitchell L. Developmental hemostasis: pro- and anticoagulant systems during childhood. Semin Thromb Hemost 2003;29(4):329–37.

[84] Nowak-Gottl U, von Kreiss R, Gobel U, et al. Neonatal symptomatic thromboembolism in Germany: a two year survey. Arch Dis Child Fetal Neonatal Ed 1997;76(3):F163–7.

[85] Albisetti M, Moeller A, Waldvogel K, et al. Congenital prothrombotic disorders in children with peripheral venous and arterial thrombosis. Acta Haematol 2007;117(3):149–55.

[86] Ferrari F, Vagnarelli F, Gargano G, et al. Early intracardiac thrombosis in preterm infants and thrombolysis with recombinant tissue type plasminogen activator. Arch Dis Child Fetal Neonatal Ed 2001;85(1):F66–72.

[87] Kim JH, Lee YSL, Kim SH, et al. Does umbilical vein catheterization lead to portal venous thrombosis? Prospective evaluation of 100 neonates. Radiology 2001;219(3):645–50.

[88] Schwartz DS, Gettner PA, Konstantino MM, et al. Umbilical venous catheterization and the risk of portal vein thrombosis. J Pediatr 1997;131(5):760–2.

[89] Ramasethu J. Management of vascular thrombosis and spasm in the newborn. NeoReviews 2005;6:e298–311.

[90] Monagle P, Chan A, Massicote P, et al. Antithrombotic therapy in children. The seventh ACCP conference on antithrombotic and thrombolytic therapy. Chest 2004;126(Suppl 3): 645S–87S.

[91] Hausler M, Hubner D, Delhaas T, et al. Long term complications of inferior vena cava thrombosis. Arch Dis Child 2001;85(3):228–33.

[92] Alvarez F, Bernard O, Brunelle F, et al. Portal obstruction in children. I. Clinical investigation and hemorrhage risk. J Pediatr 1983;103(5):696–702.

[93] Morag I, Epelman M, Daneman A, et al. Portal vein thrombosis in the neonate: risk factors, course and outcome. J Pediatr 2006;148(6):735–9.

[94] Kerner JA, Garcia-Careaga MG, Fisher AA. Treatment of catheter occlusion in pediatric patients. JPEN J Parenter Enteral Nutr 2006;30(Suppl 1):S73–81.

[95] Svoboda P, Barton RP, Barbarash OL, et al. Recombinant urokinase is safe and effective in restoring catheter patency to occluded central venous devices: a multicenter, international trial. Crit Care Med 2004;32(10):1990–6.

[96] Massin M, Lombet J, Rigo J. Percutaneous retrieval of broken Silastic catheter from the left atrium in a critically ill premature infant. Cathet Cardiovasc Diagn 1997;42(4): 409–11.

[97] Ochikubo CG, O'Brien LA, Kanakriyeh M, et al. Silicone rubber catheter fracture and embolization in a very low birth weight infant. J Perinatol 1996;16(1):50–2.

[98] Serrano M, Garcia-Alix A, Lopez JC, et al. Retained central venous lines in the newborn: report of one case and systematic review of the literature. Neonatal Netw 2007;26(2): 105–10.

[99] Nguyen ST, Lund CH, Durand DJ. Thrombolytic therapy for adhesions of percutaneous central venous catheters to vein intima associated with Malassezia furfur infection. J Perinatol 2001;21(5):331–3.

[100] Wong AF, McCulloch LM, Sola A. Treatment of peripheral tissue ischemia with topical nitroglycerine ointment in neonates. J Pediatr 1992;121(6):980–3.

[101] Vasquez P, Burd A, Mehta R, et al. Resolution of peripheral artery catheter induced ischemic injury following prolonged treatment with topical nitroglycerine ointment in a newborn: a case report. J Perinatol 2003;23(4):348–50.

[102] Baserga MC, Puri A, Sola A. The use of topical nitroglycerine ointment to treat peripheral tissue ischemia secondary to arterial line complications in neonates. J Perinatol 2002;22(5): 416–9.

[103] Narla LD, Hom M, Lofland GK, et al. Evaluation of umbilical catheter and tube placement in premature infants. Radiographics 1991;11(5):849–63.

[104] Barrington KJ. Umbilical catheters in the newborn: effects of position of the catheter tip. Cochrane Database Syst Rev 2000;2:CD00505.

[105] Carey BE, Zeilinger TC. Hypoglycemia due to high positioning of umbilical artery catheters. J Perinatol 1989;9(4):407–10.

[106] Beluffi G, Perotti G. Where has the umbilical arterial catheter gone? An unusual position. Pediatr Radiol 2007;37(4):403.

[107] Giannakopoulou C, Korakaki E, Hatzidaki E, et al. Peroneal nerve palsy: a complication of umbilical artery catheterization in the full term newborn of a mother with diabetes. Pediatrics 2002;109(4):e66.

[108] de Sanctis N, Cardillo G, Rega AN. Gluteoperineal gangrene and sciatic nerve palsy after umbilical vessel injection. Clin Orthop Relat Res 1995;316:180–4.

[109] Munoz ME, Roche C, Escriba R, et al. Flaccid paraplegia as complication of umbilical artery catheterization. Pediatr Neurol 1993;9(5):401–3.

[110] Haldeman S, Fowler GW, Ashwal S, et al. Acute flaccid neonatal paraplegia: a case report. Neurology 1983;33(1):93–5.

[111] Brown MS, Phibbs RH. Spinal cord injury in newborns from use of umbilical artery catheters: report of two cases and a review of literature. J Perinatol 1988;8(2):105–10.

[112] Lemke RP, Idiong N, al- Saedi S, et al. Spinal cord infarct after arterial switch associated with an umbilical arterial catheter. Ann Thorac Surg 1996;62(5):1532–4.

[113] Boo NY, Wong NC, Sulkifli SS, et al. Risk factors associated with umbilical vascular catheter associated thrombosis in newborn infants. J Paediatr Child Health 1999;35(5):460–5.

[114] Coleman MM, Spear ML, Finkelstein M, et al. Short term use of umbilical arterial catheters may not be associated with increased incidence of thrombosis. Pediatrics 2004;113(4): 770–4.

[115] Barrington KJ. Umbilical artery catheters in the newborn: effects of catheter materials. Cochrane Database Syst Rev 2000;2:CD000949.

[116] Wesstrom G, Finnstrom O, Stenport G. Umbilical artery catheterization in newborns.1. Thrombosis in relation to catheter type and position. Acta Paediatr Scand 1979;68(4): 575–81.

[117] Barrington KJ. Umbilical artery catheters in the newborn: effects of heparin. Cochrane Database Syst Rev 2000;2:CD000507.

[118] Seibert JJ, Northington FJ, Miers JF, et al. Aortic thrombosis after umbilical artery catheterization in neonates: prevalence of complications on long term follow-up. AJR Am J Roentgenol 1991;156(3):567–9.

[119] Adelman RD. Abdominal aortic aneurysm 18 years after apparent resolution of an umbilical catheter-associated aortic thrombosis. J Pediatr 1998;132(5):874–5.

[120] Starc TJ, Abramson SJ, Bierman FZ, et al. Acquired coarctation of the aorta. Pediatr Cardiol 1992;13(1):33–6.

[121] Adelman RD, Morrell RE. Coarctation of the abdominal aorta and renal artery stenosis related to an umbilical artery catheter placement in a neonate. Pediatrics 2000;106(3):e36.

[122] Rabin E, Vye MV, Farrell EE. Umbilical artery catheterization complicated by multiple mycotic aneurysms. Arch Pathol Lab Med 1986;110(5):442–4.

[123] Deliege R, Cneude F, Barbier C, et al. Ruptured mycotic aneurysm with hemoperitoneum: an unusual septic complication of umbilical arterial catheter. Arch Pediatr 2003;10(8): 716–8.

[124] Adams JM, Rudolph AJ. The use of indwelling radial artery catheters in neonates. Pediatrics 1975;55(2):261–5.

[125] Todres ID, Rogers MC, Shannon DC, et al. Percutaneous catheterization of the radial artery in the critically ill neonate. J Pediatr 1975;87(2):273–5.

[126] Randel SN, Tsang BH, Wung JT, et al. Experience with percutaneous indwelling peripheral arterial catheterization in neonates. Am J Dis Child 1987;141(8):848–51.

[127] Sellden H, Nilsson K, Larrson LE, et al. Radial arterial catheters in children and neonates: a prospective study. Crit Care Med 1987;15(12):1106–9.

[128] Kahler AC, Mirza F. Alternative arterial catheterization site using the ulnar artery in critically ill pediatric patients. Pediatr Crit Care Med 2002;3(4):370–4.

[129] Piotrowski A, Kawczynski P. Cannulation of the axillary artery in critically ill newborn infants. Eur J Pediatr 1995;154(1):57–9.

[130] Schindler E, Kowald B, Suess H, et al. Catheterization of the radial or brachial artery in neonates and infants. Paediatr Anaesth 2005;15(8):677–82.

[131] Wallach SG. Cannulation of the radial artery: diagnosis and treatment algorithm. Am J Crit Care 2004;13(4):315–9.

[132] Hack WW, Vos A, van der lei J, et al. Incidence and duration of total occlusion of the radial artery in newborn infants after catheter removal. Eur J Pediatr 1990;149(4):275–7.

[133] Barone JE, Madlinger RV. Should an Allen test be performed before radial artery cannulation? J Trauma 2006;61(2):468–70.

[134] Lemke RP, al-Saedi SA, Belik J, et al. Use of tolazoline to counteract vasospasm in peripheral arterial catheters in neonates. Acta Paediatr 1996;85(12):1497–8.

[135] Hack WW, Vos A, Okken A. Incidence of forehand and hand ischemia related to radial artery cannulation in newborn infants. Intensive Care Med 1990;16(11):50–3.

[136] Coombs CJ, Richardson PW, Dowling GJ. Brachial artery thrombosis in infants: an algorithm for limb salvage. Plast Reconstr Surg 2006;117:1481–8.

[137] Dzepina I, Unusic J, Mijatovic D, et al. Pseudoaneurysms of the brachial artery following venipuncture in infants. Pediatr Surg Int 2004;20(8):594–7.

[138] Pape KE, Armstrong DL, Fitzhardinge PM. Peripheral median nerve damage secondary to brachial arterial blood gas sampling. J Pediatr 1978;93(5):852–6.

[139] Skoglund RR, Giles EE. The false cortical thumb. Am J Dis Child 1986;140(4):375–6.

ELSEVIER
SAUNDERS

CLINICS IN
PERINATOLOGY

Clin Perinatol 35 (2008) 223–249

Hospital-Acquired Infections in the NICU: Epidemiology for the New Millennium

Alison J. Carey, MD[a],*, Lisa Saiman, MD, MPH[b,c], Richard A. Polin, MD[a]

[a]Division of Neonatology, Columbia University Medical Center, New York-Presbyterian Hospital, 3959 Broadway, CHC-115, New York, NY 10032, USA
[b]Division of Pediatric Infectious Disease, Columbia University Medical Center, New York-Presbyterian Hospital, 650 West 168th St., PH 4-470, New York, NY 10032, USA
[c]Department of Hospital Epidemiology, Columbia University Medical Center, New York-Presbyterian Hospital, 650 West 168th Street, PH 4-470, New York, NY 10032, USA

More than 150 years ago, Ignac Philipp Semmelweis (1818–1865) recommended disinfection of the hands of health care professionals as a way to prevent puerperal ("childbed") fever in women giving birth [1]. As a young assistant professor of obstetrics and gynecology, Semmelweis recognized that cadaverous particles adhering to the hands of examiners (including himself) were being transmitted to the genital tracts of women in labor. Although Semmelweis did not know the cadaverous particles were bacteria, the practice of examining women in labor with hands that had not been disinfected resulted in increased mortality in those women and their newborn infants. Interestingly, the mortality rate for women delivering on "the street" was strikingly lower.

Unfortunately, the lessons of Semmelweis (published in 1860–1861) were ignored by his peers, and he died at the age of 47 years in the Lower Austrian Mental Home after displaying signs of psychosis. A few years after Semmelweis' death, the bacterial nature of disease (and wound infections) was elucidated by Pasteur and Lister, and in 1879, Pasteur identified hemolytic streptococcus as the cause of childbed fever.

* Corresponding author. Division of Neonatology, Columbia University Medical Center, 3959 Broadway, CHC 12N-1201, New York, NY 10032.
E-mail address: alc7007@nyp.org (A.J. Carey).

0095-5108/08/$ - see front matter © 2008 Elsevier Inc. All rights reserved.
doi:10.1016/j.clp.2007.11.014 *perinatology.theclinics.com*

It is estimated that there are more than 2 million nosocomial infections and 48,600 catheter-associated blood stream infections in children and adults in the United States annually. Furthermore, recent data suggest that 17,000 deaths are directly attributable to catheter-associated infections (Fig. 1) [2]. The resulting extended lengths of hospital stay and treatment for infection-related illnesses add $17 billion to $29 billion to health care costs each year [3,4].

The subset of infants who remain in the neonatal intensive care unit (NICU) for extended periods of time are at increased risk for a hospital-acquired infection. The distribution of common pathogens in the first episode of neonatal late-onset sepsis is shown in Table 1. Hospital-acquired infections in the NICU are associated with increased morbidity and mortality, prolonged hospitalization, and increased hospital costs [3,4]. Although it may not be possible to completely prevent hospital-acquired infections in the NICU, recent data suggest that collaborative quality improvement initiatives can substantially reduce the incidence of catheter-related infections [5,6]. This review focuses on two of the most common pathogens for

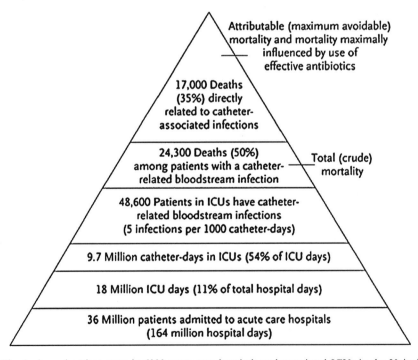

Fig. 1. Annual patient stays in 6000 acute care hospitals and associated ICUs in the United States. (*From* Wenzel RP, Edmond MB. Team-based prevention of catheter-related infections. N Engl J Med 2006;355(26):2781; with permission.)

Table 1
Distribution of pathogens associated with the first episode of late-onset sepsis: NICHD
Neonatal Research Network, September 1, 1998, through August 31, 2000

Organism	Number	Percentage
Gram-positive organisms	922	70.2
Staphylococcus (coagulase-negative)	629	47.9
Staphylococcus aureus	103	7.8
Enterococcus sp	43	3.3
Group B streptococcus	30	2.3
Other	117	8.9
Gram-negative organisms	231	17.6
Escherichia coli	64	4.9
Klebsiella	52	4.0
Pseudomonas	35	2.7
Enterobacter	33	2.5
Serratia	29	2.2
Other	18	1.4
Fungi	160	12.2
Candida albicans	76	5.8
Candida parapsilosis	54	4.1
Other	30	2.3
Total	1313	100

Data from Stoll BJ, Hansen N, Fanaroff AA, et al. Late-onset sepsis in very low birth
weight neonates: the experience of the NICHD Neonatal Research Network. Pediatrics
2002;110(2 Pt 1):285–91.

hospital-acquired infections in the NICU, *Candida* and methicillin-resistant
Staphylococcus aureus (MRSA), and discusses the importance of meningitis
as an associated complication.

Meningitis complicating nosocomial sepsis

Neonatal meningitis is associated with a high risk of morbidity and
mortality. Recent data indicate that infants with meningitis have a 1.6- to
2.2-fold increased risk of neurocognitive impairment when compared with
infants of similar gestational age who are uninfected [4]. Sicker infants
(with coma, seizures, and a need for inotropic support) are at higher risk
for adverse outcomes [7]. Unfortunately, the diagnosis of meningitis in a hospitalized preterm infant may be difficult to determine because signs attributable to meningitis are often absent and may be obscured by those associated
with other disease processes. For many years, most neonatologists assumed
that meningitis was a rare event in hospitalized neonates; therefore, there
was a reluctance to perform a lumbar puncture in an unstable infant with
a suspected hospital-acquired infection unless bacteremia or fungemia was
documented.

Recent information indicates that the incidence of nosocomial meningitis
is more common than previously appreciated [8]. In a retrospective study
from the National Institute of Child Health and Human Development

(NICHD) Neonatal Research Network, 134 infants with meningitis were identified among 2877 infants who had at least one lumbar puncture, which represented 5% of patients evaluated with a cerebrospinal fluid (CSF) culture; however, depending on the gestational age of the infant, only half of the infants in whom late-onset sepsis was suspected actually received a lumbar puncture. Surprisingly, even in infants with a positive blood culture, a lumbar puncture was performed only 66% of the time; therefore, the incidence of meningitis in infants with suspected hospital-acquired sepsis is likely to be substantially higher than 5%. Importantly, one third of the infants with meningitis had a positive CSF culture without an associated positive blood culture. When cases of meningitis due to coagulase-negative staphylococci (a common skin contaminant) were excluded from the analysis, the percentage of infants with meningitis (*Enterococcus* sp, *Staphylococcus aureus,* Group B streptococcus, *Escherichia coli, Klebsiella, Serratia,* and *Candida* sp) without a positive blood culture was 47%. In a recent prospective study of neonatal candidiasis [9], approximately 8% of infants had fungal meningitis; however, only 51% of infants in this study had a lumbar puncture as part of the sepsis evaluation, and 48% of those with a positive CSF culture had a negative blood culture. Meningitis significantly increases the risk of mortality (23% of meningitis cases versus 9% of infants with negative cultures) [8]. The mortality rate is higher for gram-negative meningitis (41%) and fungal meningitis (33%) than for meningitis due to gram-positive organisms (9%). The major conclusion of these studies is that late-onset meningitis is probably underdiagnosed in preterm infants.

A major area of controversy is centered on the interpretation of diagnostic studies of the CSF. In 1976, Sarff and coworkers published reference values for cell counts, protein, and glucose in CSF [10]. CSF values from infants with "clinical signs" of a viral illness and those with a grossly bloody tap were excluded from analysis. In that study, CSF cell counts ranged from 0 to 32 cells/mm^3 (mean, 8.4 with 60% neutrophils), and protein concentrations ranged from 20 to 170 mg/dL in term infants and 65 to 150 mg/dL in preterm infants. The mean CSF glucose value was 81% of the glucose value in the blood in term infants and 74% of that in preterm infants. There was considerable overlap in CSF values in infants with and without meningitis, but only one infant (of 32) with a positive CSF culture had completely normal CSF values. Although the study by Sarff and colleagues was quoted for many years as the gold standard, more recent studies in which viral testing was included and infants with intraventricular hemorrhage or traumatic taps were excluded have demonstrated different norms [11–14]. These studies suggest the following normal values:

1) Mean CSF cell counts in term and preterm infants generally range from 4 to 8 cells/mm^3. Although the range of cell counts is wide, it is unusual to have a CSF cell count greater than 20 cells/mm^3 in an atraumatic tap. The percentage of neutrophils is less than 20%.

2) In healthy term infants, CSF protein concentrations should be less than 100 mg/dL. Values in preterm infants may be considerably higher and vary inversely with gestational age.
3) The range of normal glucose values is as previously reported, that is, 81% and 74% of the glucose value of the blood in term and preterm infants, respectively.

The data from Sarff and colleagues [10] suggest that when CSF protein concentrations, cell counts, and glucose concentrations are evaluated, all three values are rarely normal in the neonate with meningitis; however, these data were collected during an era when intrapartum prophylaxis was almost never used, and antibiotics were often delayed until a lumbar puncture could be done. Because antibiotic pretreatment often occurs, it is uncertain whether a lumbar puncture with normal cell counts, protein, and glucose concentrations can be used as reassurance that meningitis is not present. Using a database from the Pediatrix medical group, Garges and colleagues [11] evaluated the accuracy of current clinical diagnostic strategies in the identification of meningitis among term and preterm neonates. Twenty-three percent of the infants had a lumbar puncture after day 3 of life. Ninety-five infants (out of 9111 lumbar punctures) grew a potential CSF pathogen. Cultures with a mixture of bacterial organisms or skin flora (including coagulase-negative staphylococci) were excluded from further analysis; therefore, infants with late-onset bacterial meningitis in this study were more likely to have meningitis due to *Staphylococcus aureus*, *Enterococcus* sp, or gram-negative organisms. The blood culture was positive in 62% of the infants with a positive CSF culture. In infants with meningitis, the median white blood cell count was 477 cells/mm^3 (versus 6 cells/mm^3 in infants without meningitis), although 15% had counts of 0 to 3 cells/mm^3 (Table 2). Using 21 cells/mm^3 as the cutoff value for white blood cells, the sensitivity of the lumbar puncture for the diagnosis of meningitis was 79% and the specificity 81% (Table 3). The median glucose value in infants with bacterial meningitis was 20 mg/dL and the median protein concentration 273 mg/dL. CSF glucose values were less sensitive but had higher specificities than white blood cell counts for the diagnosis of meningitis. Protein concentrations greater than 120 mg/dL had a sensitivity of 76% and a specificity of 63%. These data indicate that no single CSF value can be used to exclude meningitis and further support the inclusion of a CSF culture in a sepsis evaluation. In addition, adjunct laboratory tests (eg, white blood cell counts) are not helpful in identifying infants with meningitis [11]. Cytokine determinations on CSF may be useful in identifying infants with bacterial meningitis; however, the data are limited in the neonatal population [12,13].

Based on these data, several recommendations can be made. Any infant with a positive blood culture or in whom sepsis is highly suspected should have a lumbar puncture. This procedure is especially important in the infant with a negative blood culture who does not respond quickly to antimicrobial

Table 2
CSF parameters by culture results showing test parameters and positive (+) and negative (−) likelihood ratios

Variable	Negative (n = 8912)	Positive (n = 95)[a]	Sensitivity, % (95% CI)	Specificity, % (95% CI)	LR+	LR−
WBC count, mm³						
0	506	2	—	—	—	—
1–8	2293	8	97 (88–99)	11 (10–12)	1.09	0.92
9–21	891	2	83 (71–91)	61 (60–63)	2.13	0.47
22–100	591	8	79 (67–89)	81 (80–82)	4.16	0.24
>100	285	38	66 (52–78)	94 (93–95)	11	0.09
Unknown	4346	37	—	—	—	—
Glucose, mg/dL						
<20	25	24	44 (30–58)	98 (97–99)	22	0.05
20–60	3504	25	89 (78–96)	20 (18–21)	1.11	0.90
>60	860	6	—	—	—	—
Unknown	4523	40	—	—	—	—
Protein, mg/dL						
0–40	83	0	—	—	—	—
41–90	1616	9	100 (84–100)	2 (1–3)	1.02	0.98
90–120	1073	4	84 (71–92)	28 (27–29)	1.17	0.86
>120	1624	42	76 (63–87)	63 (62–64)	2.05	0.49
Unknown	4516	40	—	—	—	—

Abbreviations: CI, confidence interval; LR, likelihood ratio; WBC, white blood cell.
[a] Coagulase-negative staphylococci and known skin flora are excluded here.
Data from Garges HP, Moody MA, Cotten CM, et al. Neonatal meningitis: what is the correlation among cerebrospinal fluid cultures, blood cultures, and cerebrospinal fluid parameters? Pediatrics 2006;117(4):1094–100.

Table 3
Parameters of 12 neonates with meningitis and normal CSF white blood cell counts[a]

Organism	CSF WBCs, cells/mm³	CSF glucose, mg/dL	CSF protein, mg/dL	Blood culture	CSF Gram stain	Bacterial antigen	Gestational age, wk	Day of life at CSF culture
Acinetobacter	3	—	—	—	—	—	39	26
Escherichia coli	1	58	56	Positive	—	—	40	3
Enterobacter	5	52	81	Negative	—	Negative	36	0
Enterococcus	3	59	216	Negative	—	—	36	0
Enterococcus	0	45	41	Negative	Negative	—	39	6
Gram-positive cocci	3	49	126	Negative	—	—	40	1
Gram-positive cocci	1	52	43	Negative	—	—	40	17
Gram-positive cocci	3	74	167	Positive	Negative	—	34	1
Group B streptococcus	15	—	—	Negative	—	—	37	3
Pseudomonas aeruginosa	2	60	102	Negative	—	—	35	1
Pseudomonas aeruginosa	13	60	159	Negative	—	—	38	0
Staphylococcus aureus	0	51	110	Negative	—	—	42	1

Abbreviation: WBC, white blood cell.

[a] Coagulase-negative staphylococci and known skin flora are excluded here.

Data from Garges HP, Moody MA, Cotten CM, et al. Neonatal meningitis: what is the correlation among cerebrospinal fluid cultures, blood cultures, and cerebrospinal fluid parameters? Pediatrics 2006;117(4):1094–100.

therapy. When the index of suspicion for sepsis is low and the infant recovers quickly (<12 hours), meningitis is unlikely. In those infants, a lumbar puncture is probably not required. Lumbar punctures should only be obtained when the infant is clinically stable.

Methicillin-resistant *Staphylococcus aureus* in the neonatal intensive care unit

Since the 1970s, MRSA has been a major pathogen in hospital-acquired infections [14]. Neonates are particularly susceptible to infection because of abnormalities of the immune system [15] and extrinsic risk factors, such as the use of central venous catheters and surgical procedures [16]. Nosocomial infection rates in the NICU range from 15% to 20%, which is significantly higher than in the pediatric ICU population [17,18]. Treatment options are limited for MRSA in the NICU population; therefore, preventative strategies offer the greatest opportunity to decrease the frequency of infection.

Epidemiology

Different areas of the world have different rates of MRSA which reflect, in part, different infection control policies. Northern European countries such as the Netherlands have been able to maintain prevalence levels of nosocomial MRSA infections at less than 1% [19] with a stringent protocol of "search and destroy." In this strategy, high-risk patients (ie, previously identified MRSA carriers or those transferred from endemic settings) are screened for MRSA and put on contact isolation until screening cultures are negative. In contrast, Southern European countries and the United States have prevalence rates of 40% to 50% among hospitalized patients.

To the authors' knowledge, specific rates of MRSA in the NICU have not been published, as most literature describes outbreaks of MRSA. The NICHD Neonatal Research Network maintains a prospective registry of early- and late-onset infections among very low birth weight (VLBW) infants. *S aureus* is a rare cause of early-onset sepsis in these infants. In an evaluation of 5447 VLBW infants, 84 patients had early-onset sepsis of which only one patient was infected with *S aureus* [20]. In contrast, 7.8% of all first episodes of late-onset sepsis were due to *S aureus* [21]. In these reports, it was not noted whether the isolated pathogens were methicillin sensitive or resistant.

Molecular typing: the move from hospital-acquired to community-acquired MRSA

In past years, MRSA infections were relegated to patients with direct contact with the health care system; however, this pattern has changed dramatically, and serious infections with MRSA in previously healthy children and adults have become more commonplace [22,23]. Molecular epidemiology has demonstrated that the majority of these community-acquired infections are caused by the USA300 clone [24]. Besides clonality, community-acquired strains have other molecular markers. Different staphylococcal chromosome cassette (SCC) *mec* types are associated with hospital-acquired (HA)-MRSA (SCC *mecA* I-III) and community-acquired (CA)-MRSA (type SCC *mecA* IV-V). HA-MRSA is more resistant to antibiotics because the SCC harbors more resistant determinants. In contrast, CA-MRSA is usually susceptible to more non-lactam antibiotics, such as trimethoprim-sulfamethoxazole, clindamycin, and quinolone agents.

By following *mec* types and the presence or absence of Panton-Valentine leukocidin (PVL), one can track how the epidemiology of MRSA infections has changed. MRSA is now causing outbreaks in the community among sports teams and in schools, as well as in higher risk groups in close quarters such as prison inmates [25], homosexual men [26], and personnel in military barracks [27]. Lowy and colleagues [25] found that 10.5% of inmates were colonized with MRSA in two New York State prisons, and among inmates with invasive infection caused by *S aureus*, 48.3% of strains were MRSA. In addition, there have been reports of MRSA outbreaks in the well-newborn nursery [28], a hospital area that is often overcrowded and understaffed.

Recent reports have also described the potential for vaginal carriage and vertical transmission of MRSA. In 2002, Morel and colleagues [29] published a report of a mother colonized with MRSA in the nares that was linked to MRSA infections in three of her four quadruplet babies. Additionally, Saiman and colleagues [30] reported on eight postpartum women who presented with serious skin and soft tissue infections, including mastitis with abscess and surgical wound infections, an average of 23 days after delivery. Molecular typing demonstrated that the outbreak strain was indistinguishable from a common CA-MRSA strain, MW2. Of note, MW2 is a strain that originated in the Midwest, and this was the first report of a hospital-acquired and transmitted CA-MRSA strain. Chen and colleagues [31] investigated the rates of vaginal colonization among pregnant women and found that 2.8% were colonized with CA-MRSA. These women could potentially act as reservoirs of MRSA and transmit this pathogen to their infants at the time of delivery. Previous studies have shown vertical transmission of MRSA through contaminated breast milk [32,33].

Colonization as a risk factor

No prospective cohort study has investigated the link between colonization and invasive clinical disease with MRSA in the neonatal population, but it has been demonstrated that the vast majority of *S aureus* blood infections are preceded by colonization in the adult population [34]. There is literature demonstrating that colonization with potential pathogens is a risk factor for invasive disease in neonates with *Candida* sp [35] and gram-negative bacilli [36]. Furthermore, some data from outbreak investigations in the NICU show that an infection ultimately develops in a high percentage of infants colonized with MRSA [37]. Saiman and colleagues [37] showed that an infection developed in 4 of 14 (28.5%) MRSA-colonized infants during an outbreak in 2001.

Virulence factors and pathophysiology

MRSA has specific virulence factors that help the pathogen make the leap from colonization to invasive disease. The SCC *mecA* has the genes that encode antibiotic resistance, including *mecA*, which encodes for the penicillin-binding protein 2A (PBP 2A). PBP 2A has a much lower affinity for beta-lactam antibiotics, a property that interrupts the mechanism by which the beta-lactams block cell wall synthesis [38].

Some strains of MRSA express PVL and staphylococcal enterotoxins, which have been implicated as potential virulence factors in skin and soft tissue infections [30]. PVL genes lead to the production of cytotoxins that form pores in the cellular membrane and cause tissue necrosis and cell lysis [38]. This mode of toxicity may lead to furunculosis and severe necrotizing pneumonia often seen in CA-MRSA. In a study of national rates of MRSA colonization, only 8% of isolates were positive for PVL [39]. In contrast, investigators have found that SCC *mec* type IV clones have a 42% rate of PVL [40], and others have found that the omnipresent USA300 clone has rates as high as 78% [41]. The exact role of PVL as a virulence factor has not been completely elucidated. To directly test whether PVL is critical for the pathogenesis of CA-MRSA, Saïd-Salim and colleagues [42] evaluated the lysis of human polymorphonuclear leukocytes during phagocytic interaction with PVL-positive and PVL-negative CA-MRSA strains. Surprisingly, they found that there was no difference in the lysis of polymorphonuclear leukocytes, which interacted with either PVL-positive or negative MRSA strains; therefore, it was concluded that other virulence factors must have a role in the pathogenicity of MRSA.

Another troubling virulence factor is the emergence of increasing resistance of MRSA to vancomycin. The early development of resistance can be seen in several studies reporting an increase in the mean inhibitory concentrations (MIC) to vancomycin [43,44]. Steinkraus and colleagues [43] reported a significant increase in the MIC of MRSA for oxacillin, vancomycin, and linezolid. Simply looking at categorical results of resistance or susceptibility, one would not have been able to detect this relative decline in susceptibility, so-called "MIC creep." In addition, within a given clinical specimen, some isolates are highly resistant, whereas others are susceptible to vancomycin. This phenomenon has been shown to be associated with a higher rate of treatment failure [45]. There are increasing reports of vancomycin-intermediate *S aureus* (VISA) and vancomycin-resistant *S aureus*

(VRSA) around the world [46,47]. Thus far, these reports have involved adults with complex comorbid conditions.

Clinical presentations

The following sections describe the most common presentations of MRSA infection, although there are relatively few studies describing the clinical presentations of MRSA infections in the NICU population.

Blood stream infections

The gold standard for diagnosing a blood stream infection is a positive blood culture. Chuang and colleagues [48] investigated a case series of 90 infants in their Taiwanese NICU with MRSA bacteremia. Taiwan has high rates of MRSA, with more than half of S aureus isolates being methicillin resistant. In their series, the predominant presentation of bacteremia was a catheter-related blood stream infection, accounting for 54% of all episodes of bacteremia [48]. Some of the most common clinical signs were nonspecific and included apnea or hypoxia, fever, elevated C-reactive protein (>10 mg/L), and leukocytosis ($>15,000/mm^3$). Although these signs and symptoms were each present in at least 45% of the infants with MRSA bacteremia, they certainly were not diagnostic for MRSA infection.

Septic arthritis/osteomyelitis

S aureus is the primary cause of septic arthritis and acute osteomyelitis in the neonate. Risk factors coincide with those for bacteremia and include umbilical artery catheterization, respiratory distress syndrome, and prematurity [49], but there have been case reports of MRSA osteomyelitis in healthy term neonates [50]. Diagnosing acute osteomyelitis in the neonate can be challenging because the presentation can be nonspecific, such as poor feeding or increased irritability. Soft tissue swelling and erythema may be the only useful clinical signs. Septic arthritis is a frequent complication of acute osteomyelitis and can lead to long-term sequelae, such as limitation of motion, limping gait, and abnormalities of bone growth [51]. These signs coupled with a positive blood, joint aspirate, or bone culture and characteristic radiographic changes confirm the diagnosis.

Endocarditis

Neonates with congenital heart disease and percutaneous central catheters are at higher risk for endocarditis [52,53]. S aureus is an important cause of pediatric endocarditis. Saiman and colleagues [52] found that 39% of pediatric patients with endocarditis were infected with S aureus, although only a small percentage was methicillin resistant. In contrast, another study found that 65% of hospital-acquired endocarditis in children due to S aureus was methicillin resistant [54]. Endocarditis may be more prevalent than reported because clinicians may not have a high index of suspicion and may not obtain echocardiograms in patients who are persistently bacteremic. As evidence, one case series reported a 12% rate of infective endocarditis in a pediatric population with *S aureus* bacteremia [53]. Similarly, Friedland and colleagues [54] found clinically silent endocarditis in 4 (11%) of 36 hospitalized children with staphylococcal bacteremia who underwent echocardiographic examination despite an obvious focus of infection, such as a catheter-related blood stream infection. Echocardiography is strongly recommended in infants with more than one positive blood culture for *S aureus*, even if a central venous catheter is in place [53,55].

Surgical site infections

Neonates are at increased risk for surgical site infections when compared with the pediatric and adult populations [56]. Risk factors include increased incision length, increased duration of surgery, and contamination of the operative site. Davenport and Doig [56] reported that *S aureus* was the most frequent cause of surgical wound infection in their neonatal surgical unit during a 13-year period, comprising 37% of the infections. In their review, the only clinical presentation indicating a surgical wound infection was the expression of pus from the surgical site.

Skin and soft tissue infections

S aureus is the most common pathogen causing pustulosis and cellulitis in the neonate. As discussed previously, CA-MRSA has virulence factors such as PVL which are thought to contribute to the pathogen's ability to cause skin and soft tissue infections. This factor coupled with the preterm neonate's underdeveloped epidermis and frequent breeches in the skin integrity (eg, due to peripheral and central intravenous catheters or blood draws and heel sticks) places the preterm neonate at risk for localized skin infections.

Meningitis

S aureus meningitis is rare in the neonate despite a steady increase in the number of *S aureus* infections [57]. Krcméry and colleagues [58] reported 12 cases of neonatal meningitis, four of which were attributed to *S aureus*. All four cases occurred in patients 3 to 6 months of age following insertion or removal of ventriculoperitoneal shunts.

Eradication of colonization with MRSA and treatment of invasive disease

Using molecular methods, Von Eiff and colleagues demonstrated that 86% of adult patients in the ICU and general ward had the same clone causing *S aureus* colonization and bacteremia, thereby showing that *S aureus* bacteremia most likely had an endogenous source [43]. They concluded that interrupting this cycle by eradicating colonization could reduce infections. In fact, the rate of *S aureus* infections has been reduced in perioperative cardiothoracic surgery patients [59] and hemodialysis patients [60] by treating them with intranasal mupirocin for 5 days. Similarly, Sandri and colleagues [61] demonstrated that by identifying patients in their ICU with MRSA colonization and using a combination of 5 days of intranasal mupirocin and three daily chlorhexidine baths, MRSA infections were reduced. Although there are no studies demonstrating a reduction in MRSA infections among colonized neonates, there have been reports of mupirocin effectively controlling an outbreak of MRSA in a NICU by treating a colonized health care worker [37,62]. The universal use of mupirocin for 1 month in colonized and un-colonized patients ended a 14-month MRSA outbreak [63]. Many NICUs are using mupirocin routinely to eradicate endemic MRSA. Lower eradication rates have been observed in infants who are nasotracheally intubated or receiving nasal continuous positive airway pressure [63].

Mupirocin-resistant MRSA has been reported in the adult population [64,65]. Jones and colleagues [65] found an 8.6% rate of high resistance to mupirocin in MRSA isolates from the nares of surgical intensive care patients upon admission, despite a low rate of mupirocin use. As discussed previously, MRSA is developing some resistance to many common treatment options. It is likely that MRSA is not more virulent than methicillin-sensitive *S aureus* (MSSA); rather, infections with MRSA often occur in patients with comorbid conditions which can become overwhelming if inappropriate antibiotic therapy is used [45]. Before the advent of penicillin in the 1940s, staphylococcal bacteremia had an 80% mortality rate; therefore, the judicious use of antibiotics is of paramount importance, especially in light of the MIC creep described earlier.

Vancomycin remains the first-line therapy for MRSA, and many NICUs with endemic MRSA use vancomycin as empiric therapy for late-onset sepsis while awaiting culture results. Peak concentrations of vancomycin reach 20 to 40 µg/mL, and trough levels are maintained between 5 and 10 µg/mL [66]. Trough levels must be carefully monitored, particularly in infants with renal insufficiency or receiving concomitant nephrotoxic drugs; serious adverse effects such as ototoxicity and nephrotoxicity can occur at levels greater than 10 µg/mL [67]. Standard dosing for vancomycin is 15 mg/kg every 24 hours for neonates less than 28 weeks' postconceptual age (PCA), with decreasing intervals as PCA increases. By 40 to 45 weeks' PCA, the dose interval is comparable to that used in older children, that is, every 8 hours [68]. These dosing recommendations are simply guidelines, because levels vary widely even within a given PCA.

In cases in which the clinician is faced with VISA or vancomycin allergy, linezolid remains an effective and relatively safe [69,70] alternative for the treatment of MRSA and other multidrug resistant gram-positive organisms. Unfortunately, currently, linezolid is the last line of defense.

Kearns and colleagues [69] investigated the clearance rate of linezolid in neonates of different gestational and postnatal ages and observed a significant difference between infants who were less than 8 days old and those who were 8 days of age or older. The clearance rate among the younger babies was 50% less than among the older babies. There was no precise physiologic explanation for these differences, but the researchers hypothesized developmentally related alterations in the enzymes that metabolize linezolid; 65% of linezolid is cleared through nonrenal pathways. Interestingly, no differences in the pharmacokinetic properties of linezolid were found among infants whose gestational age was less than 34 weeks in a comparison with those 34 weeks or older; therefore, based on the pharmacokinetics of linezolid in the neonate and the necessary drug concentrations to accomplish a therapeutic MIC, the recommended dose is 10 mg/kg every 8 hours for those infants with a PNA 8 days or older, and 10 mg/kg every 12 hours for those infants who are less than 8 days old [69].

Treatment duration is dependent on the specific infection. For skin and soft tissue infections and bacteremia, a 7- to 10-day course is generally appropriate; however, as discussed previously, S aureus has a high propensity for metastatic disease such as endocarditis and osteomyelitis. In these cases, a minimum of 4 weeks of treatment is necessary, and many specialists recommend 6 to 8 weeks of therapy depending on the clinical course. Patients with metastatic disease with persistently positive blood cultures despite therapeutic doses of vancomycin, or infants with VISA or heterogeneous resistant MRSA may not clear infection with monotherapy. In these cases, both rifampin and gentamicin can be used for synergy [52,71].

Prevention

Published data show that the excess cost associated with a MRSA infection versus no infection or infection with MSSA is between $9275 and $27,000 [72,73]. In light of the high cost associated with MRSA infection, implementation of infection control procedures has been found to be cost effective [73,74]. The Centers for Disease Control and Prevention recommend using an alcohol-based hand sanitizer before patient contact and only washing hands with soap and water when the hands are physically soiled. Hand hygiene should be performed before touching patients, after touching patients, after removing gloves, and after touching the patient care environment and equipment due to the ability of MRSA to survive on inanimate objects. Alcohol-based hand sanitizers have been shown to improve compliance with appropriate hand hygiene as well as improve the skin integrity of health care workers [75]; however, prevention of MRSA goes far beyond basic hand hygiene practices.

It is difficult to determine which measures are the most effective at containing MRSA because, during an outbreak, many measures are instituted concurrently. In 2006, Gerber and colleagues [76] released a consensus statement from the Chicago Department of Public Health on management of outbreaks of MRSA in a NICU. Their recommendations included an alcohol-based rub for hand hygiene, isolation and cohorting of MRSA-colonized infants, and regular neonatal surveillance cultures. They also emphasized the use of molecular typing as an integral part of control because it can determine the ongoing transmission of a particular clone. They did not make a recommendation for decontamination with mupirocin; this intervention was left to the discretion of the primary clinical care team because the efficacy of this strategy is still uncertain.

Molecular typing by pulsed field gel electrophoresis (PFGE) is used to monitor the success of infection control strategies, including targeted surveillance. If ongoing transmission of a dominant clone persists despite infection control interventions, additional measures can be implemented to help halt transmission. MRSA isolates are genotyped by PFGE using the restriction endonuclease *Sma*I [77]. This genotyping can be a powerful tool in alerting the clinical team to the route of transmission. For example, in January of 2001, there was an increase in the number of infants infected with MRSA in the authors' NICU. Basic infection control methods were ineffective at halting the outbreak. PFGE typing showed the epidemiology team that the predominant clone was one that had been prevalent in our adult facility from January 1999 to November 2000 [37]. Three health care workers, two of whom rotated through the adult facility, were also found to be colonized with the predominant clone. The outbreak was contained by furloughing these health care workers until they had demonstrated clearance of MRSA colonization.

The practice of obtaining regular surveillance cultures is growing in popularity in NICUs as MRSA becomes more prevalent. As described previously, some countries with a low MRSA prevalence (1%–2%) advocate a search and destroy protocol. Such countries identify a high-risk patient as an individual previously identified as a MRSA carrier or transferred from an endemic area. All patients, as well as health care workers, are cultured on a unit if an incident case of MRSA occurs in a previously low-risk patient. The unit is closed to admissions if there is evidence of ongoing transmission. Bootsma and colleagues [78] have developed a mathematical model which proposes that effectively implementing isolation procedures for MRSA carriers and screening all patients when there is evidence of ongoing transmission will decrease the prevalence of MRSA to less than 1% in 8 years. Implementing the full search and destroy protocol will decrease the prevalence to less than 1% in 6 years. In this stochastic model, there are some major assumptions such as 100% effective isolation procedures, which may not be realistic. Nevertheless, this model is not just statistical theory. The Netherlands has had many years of enviably low rates of MRSA. Although Bootsma's model was created for an adult unit, it is a feasible protocol to be implemented in NICUs, especially with more NICUs incorporating single patient rooms into their design.

Candida in the neonatal intensive care unit

In the past 2 decades, understanding of the epidemiology, risk factors, management, and outcomes for *Candida* infections in the NICU population has substantially increased. Understanding of the pathogenesis, optimal therapy, and preventive strategies continues to evolve.

Epidemiology

Candida sp cause approximately 10% to 15% of cases of late-onset sepsis among VLBW infants less than 1500 g [21,79]. The overall rate of candidemia in the NICU is approximately 1.6% of all infants [35,80]. The rates among VLBW infants less than 1500 g and among extremely low birth weight (ELBW) infants less than 1000 g have been reported to be 5% to 10% and 7% to 20%, respectively [21,80]. The incidence of candidemia increased throughout the 1980s and 1990s as the number of VLBW infants who survived increased [81]. Nevertheless, in a study examining data accumulated by the Centers for Disease Control and Prevention National Nosocomial Infection Surveillance system, the incidence of candidemia among ELBW infants decreased from 3.51 cases per 1000 patient-days from 1995 to 1999 to 2.68 cases per 1000 patient-days from 2000 to 2004 [80], which may have reflected the increasing use of fluconazole prophylaxis. The incidence of candidemia may vary greatly from center to center as demonstrated in multicenter studies [21,80]. In addition, full-term infants with complex congenital anomalies and a prolonged length of stay are at high risk for *Candida* infections [82,83]. It is critical to perform active surveillance for candidemia in individual NICUs to document local epidemiologic trends.

Most cases of candidemia occur within the first 6 weeks of life (median, 21 days of age) [80], although a minority of cases occur at 3 months of age or older [9,81]. In most NICUs, *Candida albicans* is the most common species followed closely by *C parapsilosis* [21,35,79,80]. Fewer than 10% of *Candida* infections are caused by other species, including *C tropicalis, C lusitaniae, C guilliermondii, C glabrata,* and *C krusei.* This distribution of *Candida* sp has been relatively constant over 25 years [81].

Pathogenesis

Our understanding of the pathogenesis of candidemia is steadily evolving. Colonization generally precedes infection [84]. The most commonly colonized sites are the gastrointestinal tract [85], the skin, and, in some series, the respiratory tract [86]. Molecular typing has shown that strains colonizing the gastrointestinal tract subsequently cause blood stream infections [35], presumably as such strains translocate across the gastrointestinal tract epithelium. Overall, 23% to 37% of VLBW infants are colonized with *Candida* [35,87,88]. As expected, the rate of colonization has been shown to increase with increasing length of stay [35]. *Candida* strains may be acquired via vertical transmission from the maternal gastrointestinal/genitourinary tract [89] or, more commonly, via horizontal transmission from the hands of health care workers [35]. *C parapsilosis* is the most common species carried on the hands of health care workers; 19% of NICU staff were colonized with this organism [35,90].

The virulence factors of *Candida* sp are highly diverse. Various enzymes such as proteinases, lipases, phospholipases, and adhesins have been shown to have a role in virulence [91]. *Candida* can grow as budding yeast cells or as filamentous hyphae or pseudohyphae [92]. Coregulation of hyphal morphology and other virulence factors including adhesins has been described. Hyphae may mediate penetration into host tissues and facilitate escape from host cells [92]. As in numerous other health care–acquired infections, biofilms composed of matrix-enclosed *Candida* adhering to the catheter surface are thought to be a key step in catheter-related candidemia [93]. Microorganisms within a biofilm are resistant to antimicrobial agents due to several potential mechanisms, including poor penetration of drugs into the biofilm, a unique microbial phenotype characterized by slow growth due to limited nutrients, and the expression of resistance genes. Most recently, investigators have used genomics to assess differential gene expression in different environmental niches during the establishment of infection [91]. These gene patterns involve up-regulation of metabolic and stress responses postulated to reflect adaptation to environmental changes wrought by the transition from a commensal to pathogen.

Risk factors for infection

Numerous investigators have examined risk factors for *Candida* infections. As noted previously, premature and low birth weight infants are at much higher risk for candidemia. In addition to birth weight, central venous catheters are one of the most important risk factors for candidemia. Not surprisingly, the risk of candidemia increases with the duration of central catheter use [83]. Both hyperalimentation and intralipids are associated with an increased risk of candidemia, although these therapies are confounded by delays in enteral feeding. The precise contribution of the latter is difficult to measure, but candidal infections were less likely to develop in infants who received enteral feedings by the third day of life [9].

Several medications have been associated with an increased risk of candidemia. These include H_2 blockers [35], which have been shown in vitro to reduce neutrophil diapedesis, and the use of third- and fourth-generation cephalosporins and carbapenems [9], which presumably alter the gastrointestinal tract flora and increase the risk of *Candida* colonization or overgrowth of the gastrointestinal tract. Additional risk factors include a previous bacterial blood stream infection, which is obviously confounded by the duration of antibiotic use and the degree of prematurity, and gastrointestinal tract abnormalities such as necrotizing enterocolitis, congenital malformations (eg, intestinal atresias), or functional abnormalities (eg, Hirshsprung's disease) [83].

Clinical presentations and diagnosis

The two most common clinical manifestions of *Candida* in the NICU are catheter-related blood stream infections and disseminated candidiasis involving the central nervous system, kidneys, eyes, spleen, or bone. Signs and symptoms of candidemia are nonspecific and include temperature instability, apnea, bradycardia, glucose intolerance, and abdominal distension. Catheter-related blood stream infections present as late-onset sepsis and may be complicated by the formation of an intra-atrial thrombus and endocarditis [94]. It is likely that candidal meningitis is underdiagnosed. Infants with *Candida* meningitis may have negative blood cultures or normal CSF parameters [95]; therefore, all infants with candidemia should undergo a lumbar puncture. Due to the potential for disseminated candidiasis, infants with candidemia should have daily physical examinations for metastatic foci and should undergo evaluation including abdominal ultrasound, an echocardiogram, and eye examination.

If *Candida* infections are suspected, blood cultures with adequate blood volumes (at least one milliliter per culture) from both the central venous catheter and a peripheral vein should be obtained. Routine processing of blood cultures by the clinical microbiology laboratory will recover *Candida* sp. Approximately 10% of infants may have candidemia for 2 or more weeks [9].

There is increasing interest in developing alternative methods of diagnosing candidiasis, particularly because invasive disease may be associated with negative blood cultures, and cultures from sterile body fluids and deep tissues may be difficult to obtain in premature infants. Measuring the level of 1,3-β-D-glucan (a cell wall component of *Candida*) is being explored as an alternative diagnostic strategy [96], although, to date, there are no studies in infected children.

Management

Not surprisingly, because of the relative rarity of candidemia and the complexities of studying neonates, there are no randomized comparative treatment trials of *Candida* infections in neonates. Most management strategies are derived from studies in older patients and clinical experience.

Available antifungal agents include conventional amphotericin, lipid-associated amphotericin products, azoles such as fluconazole and voriconazole, and, most recently, the echinocandin agents such as caspofungin. Although amphotericin does not penetrate the central nervous system well, even in the setting of meningeal inflammation, case reports have demonstrated successful outcomes in preterm infants treated with either conventional or liposomal amphotericin [97]. Flucytosine, which must be given orally, does penetrate the central nervous system, but its use has been hampered by its formulation and the need to follow serum levels [98]. Flucytosine should never be used alone due to the rapid emergence of resistance. Fluconazole has been used with increased frequency among infants in the NICU due to its role in prophylaxis. There are several pharmacokinetic studies of this agent, which penetrates the central nervous system well [98]. Although resistance to antifungal agents in the NICU setting is rare, antifungal susceptibility testing should be performed if treatment with fluconazole is being considered. The use of newer agents such as voriconazole and caspofungin is hampered by the paucity of pharmacokinetic data and safety data in the newborn population.

In addition to prompt initiation of antifungal agents at appropriate doses, it is essential to remove the central venous catheter immediately in infants diagnosed with candidemia. Delayed removal or immediate replacement of central venous catheters in ELBW infants with candidemia was associated with a 2.7-fold increased risk of death or neurodevelopmental impairment in a comparison with ELBW infants without candidemia [9]. Documenting sterilization of the blood stream is recommended. Due to the frequency of false-negative blood cultures, two negative blood cultures at least 48 hours apart are needed to ensure that the blood stream has become negative.

Although fungal endocarditis in adults is managed by surgery and often requires valve replacement, surgical management may not be an option in a premature infant. There are several case reports describing successful treatment of infants with fungal endocarditis with prolonged medical management alone [99].

Outcomes

Crude mortality rates associated with candidemia are high and range from 26% to 32% of VLBW infants [23]. Candidemia is often associated with early mortality; most deaths occur within the first 7 days of the diagnosis [21,100]. The attributable mortality rate due to candidemia is estimated to be 13% [80]. In some studies, *C albicans* has been more virulent than *C parapsilosis*, because infection with the former has been associated with a higher mortality rate, 42% versus 20%, respectively [9]. This association has not been consistently observed [80].

A recent study from the NICHD Neonatal Research Network assessed neurodevelopmental outcomes among 320 ELBW infants who had been diagnosed with candidemia and *Candida* meningitis [9]. At 18 to 22 months of age, these infants had lower Bayley scores and higher rates of cerebral palsy, blindness, or deafness when compared with infants who did not experience infections due to *Candida*. A case-control study of hospital costs demonstrated that infants with candidemia, on average, incurred increased hospital costs of $28,500 due to increased costs per day and increased length of stay [101].

Prevention

Given the high rates of morbidity and mortality and the costs associated with candidemia, prevention of *Candida* infections would be highly desirable. One of the most intriguing developments in management of *Candida* in the NICU is the recent use of fluconazole prophylaxis in VLBW infants to prevent invasive candidiasis (Table 4). The rationale for this strategy is to prevent fungal colonization in these high-risk infants, with subsequent reduction of invasive disease [102,103]. Initially, single-center, placebo-controlled studies and studies using historic controls showed a reduction in *Candida* colonization, disease, or mortality [103–105]; however, reduced mortality was not demonstrated in a recent meta-analysis [106]. Most recently, a multicenter study conducted in Italy demonstrated a reduction in colonization and invasive disease among VLBW infants [102]. The incidence of invasive disease was 13.2% in infants treated with placebo compared with 3% in infants treated with fluconazole, but there was no difference in mortality. Fluconazole did not reduce the rate of invasive disease among the small number of infants colonized with *Candida* sp before the use of the study drug. Fluconazole was well tolerated, and there was no documentation of fluconazole-resistant strains, although the total duration of the study was only 15 months.

The neonatology and infectious disease communities have been concerned about widespread adaptation of fluconazole prophylaxis for several reasons [108]. Issues include (1) the emergence of resistance to fluconazole and of non-albicans *Candida* sp, particularly intrinsically resistant species such as *C glabrata* and *C krusei*; (2) the short- and long-term safety of prolonged use of fluconazole, especially in infants less than 750 g, because the pharmacokinetic properties of fluconazole are not well studied; and (3) the cost.

Many experts recommend focusing prevention efforts on implementing strategies that will minimize exposures to the risk factors cited previously rather than implementing fluconazole prophylaxis.

Infections in the NICU population due to *Candida* are associated with high rates of morbidity, particularly of the central nervous system, as well as high rates of crude and attributable mortality. Recent data suggest that the case rates of candidemia may be decreasing, perhaps owing to the increasing use of fluconazole prophylaxis and the implementation of quality improvement initiatives. It is critical to continue to monitor *Candida* infections in the NICU to detect potential changes in epidemiologic trends.

Table 4
Selected studies of fluconazole prophylaxis in preterm infants

Study	Design	Population and regimen	Findings
Kaufman, [103]	Single-center, placebo-controlled, RCT	Birth weight <1000 g 3 mg/kg × 42 days[a] Weeks 1–2: Dose administered every 3rd day Weeks 3–4: Dose administered every other day Weeks 5–6: Dose administered daily	↓ Colonization ↓ Invasive infections No impact on mortality
Kaufman, [104]	Single-center, RCT	Birth weight <1000 g 3 mg/kg × 42 days[a] Compared the dosing regimen of the Kaufman [103] study versus twice weekly	↓ Colonization ↓ Invasive infections No impact on mortality
Bertini, [107]	Single-center historic controls	Birth weight ≤1500 g 6 mg/kg × 28 days[b] Week 1: Dose administered every 3rd day Weeks 2–4: Dose administered daily	↓ Invasive infections No impact on mortality
Healy, [105]	Single-center historic controls	Birth weight <1000 g 3 mg/kg × 42 days[a] Followed the dosing regimen of Kaufman [103] Compared cohorts of infants <1000 grams (who received prophylaxis), and those ≥1000 grams for rates of invasive candidiasis	↓ Invasive infections ↓ Mortality
Manzoni, [102]	Multicenter, placebo-controlled, RCT	Birth weight <1500 g 3 versus 6 mg/kg administered every 3rd day for the first 2 weeks, and then every other day If 1000–1500 g, prophylaxis was for 28 days; and if <1000 g, prophylaxis was for 42 days	↓ Colonization ↓ Invasive infections No impact on mortality

Abbreviation: RCT, randomized clinical trial.
[a] If central venous catheter in place. Once CVC removed, prophylaxis was discontinued.
[b] If central venous catheter in place at time of enrollment. However, prophylaxis regimen continued using oral fluconazole if CVC was removed.

Summary

Bacterial and fungal blood stream, meningitis, and skin and soft tissue infections remain major causes of mortality and morbidity for infants hospitalized in the NICU. Newer strategies to reduce the frequency of fungal infections (ie, prophylactic fluconazole) appear to be effective and safe and may be appropriate for certain high-risk populations (eg, infants <750 g). Nasal mupirocin should be considered in infants colonized with MRSA, but this therapy has unproven efficacy at the present time. The following strategies to reduce the frequency of nosocomial infections are effective and relatively inexpensive:

- "Degerm" hands using an alcohol- based emollient.
- Avoid scrubbing the skin with brushes or harsh soaps.
- Gown and glove when inserting central lines or changing dressings.
- Develop antimicrobial stewardship programs to promote the use of the simplest and most effective antibiotic (avoid broad-spectrum antibiotics such as third- and fourth-generation cephalosporins).
- Avoid drugs associated with an increased risk of infection (H_2 blocking agents and systemic steroids).
- Minimize practices that bypass normal skin barrier defense mechanisms (eg, venipuncture and heel stick).
- Minimize central venous catheter days.
- Encourage the aggressive advancement of enteral feedings and the use of breast milk.
- Maximize space and staffing patterns.
- Isolate/cohort infants harboring virulent or resistant pathogens.

References

[1] Dunn PM. Ignac Semmelweis (1818–1865) of Budapest and the prevention of puerperal fever. Arch Dis Child Fetal Neonatal Ed 2005;90(4):F345–8.

[2] Wenzel RP, Edmond MB. Team-based prevention of catheter-related infections. N Engl J Med 2006;355(26):2781–3.

[3] Payne NR, Carpenter JH, Badger GJ, et al. Marginal increase in cost and excess length of stay associated with nosocomial bloodstream infections in surviving very low birth weight infants. Pediatrics 2004;114(2):348–55.

[4] Stoll BJ, Hansen NI, Adams-Chapman I, et al. Neurodevelopmental and growth impairment among extremely low-birth-weight infants with neonatal infection. JAMA 2004; 292(19):2357–65.

[5] Aly H, Herson V, Duncan A, et al. Is bloodstream infection preventable among premature infants? A tale of two cities. Pediatrics 2005;115(6):1513–8.

[6] Horbar JD, Rogowski J, Plsek PE, et al. Collaborative quality improvement for neonatal intensive care. NIC/Q Project Investigators of the Vermont Oxford Network. Pediatrics 2001;107(1):14–22.

[7] Klinger G, Chin CN, Beyene J, et al. Predicting the outcome of neonatal bacterial meningitis. Pediatrics 2000;106(3):477–82.

[8] Stoll BJ, Hansen N, Fanaroff AA, et al. To tap or not to tap: high likelihood of meningitis without sepsis among very low birth weight infants. Pediatrics 2004;113(5): 1181–6.

[9] Benjamin DK Jr, Stoll BJ, Fanaroff AA, et al. Neonatal candidiasis among extremely low birth weight infants: risk factors, mortality rates, and neurodevelopmental outcomes at 18 to 22 months. Pediatrics 2006;117(1):84–92.

[10] Sarff LD, Platt LH, McCracken GH Jr. Cerebrospinal fluid evaluation in neonates: comparison of high-risk infants with and without meningitis. J Pediatr 1976;88(3):473–7.

[11] Garges HP, Moody MA, Cotten CM, et al. Neonatal meningitis: what is the correlation among cerebrospinal fluid cultures, blood cultures, and cerebrospinal fluid parameters? Pediatrics 2006;117(4):1094–100.

[12] Krebs VL, Okay TS, Okay Y, et al. Tumor necrosis factor-alpha, interleukin-1beta and interleukin-6 in the cerebrospinal fluid of newborn with meningitis. Arq Neuropsiquiatr 2005; 63(1):7–13.

[13] Dulkerian SJ, Kilpatrick L, Costarino AT Jr, et al. Cytokine elevations in infants with bacterial and aseptic meningitis. J Pediatr 1995;126(6):872–6.

[14] Boyce JM. Increasing prevalence of methicillin-resistant *Staphylococcus aureus* in the United States. Infect Control Hosp Epidemiol 1990;11(12):639–42.

[15] Saiman L. Preventing infections in the neonatal intensive care unit. In: Wenzel R, editor. Prevention and control of nosocomial infections. 4th edition. Hagerstown (MD): Lippincott, Williams & Wilkins; 2003. p. 345.

[16] Stoll BJ, Hansen N. Infections in VLBW infants: studies from the NICHD Neonatal Research Network. Semin Perinatol 2003;27(4):293–301.

[17] Banerjee SN, Grohskopf LA, Sinkowitz-Cochran RL, et al. Incidence of pediatric and neonatal intensive care unit-acquired infections. Infect Control Hosp Epidemiol 2006;27(6): 561–70.

[18] Baltimore RS. Neonatal nosocomial infections. Semin Perinatol 1998;22(1):25–32.

[19] Tiemersma EW, Bronzwaer SL, Lyytikainen O, et al. Methicillin-resistant *Staphylococcus aureus* in Europe, 1999–2002. Emerg Infect Dis 2004;10(9):1627–34.

[20] Stoll BJ, Hansen N, Fanaroff AA, et al. Changes in pathogens causing early-onset sepsis in very-low-birth-weight infants. N Engl J Med 2002;347(4):240–7.

[21] Stoll BJ, Hansen N, Fanaroff AA, et al. Late-onset sepsis in very low birth weight neonates: the experience of the NICHD Neonatal Research Network. Pediatrics 2002;110(2 Pt 1): 285–91.

[22] Gonzalez BE, Martinez-Aguilar G, Hulten KG, et al. Severe staphylococcal sepsis in adolescents in the era of community-acquired methicillin-resistant *Staphylococcus aureus*. Pediatrics 2005;115(3):642–8.

[23] Miller LG, Perdreau-Remington F, Rieg G, et al. Necrotizing fasciitis caused by community-associated methicillin-resistant *Staphylococcus aureus* in Los Angeles. N Engl J Med 2005;352(14):1445–53.

[24] Mishaan AM, Mason EO Jr, Martinez-Aguilar G, et al. Emergence of a predominant clone of community-acquired *Staphylococcus aureus* among children in Houston, Texas. Pediatr Infect Dis J 2005;24(3):201–6.

[25] Lowy FD, Aiello AE, Bhat M, et al. *Staphylococcus aureus* colonization and infection in New York State prisons. J Infect Dis 2007;196(6):911–8.

[26] Lee NE, Taylor MM, Bancroft E, et al. Risk factors for community-associated methicillin-resistant *Staphylococcus aureus* skin infections among HIV-positive men who have sex with men. Clin Infect Dis 2005;40(10):1529–34.

[27] Zinderman CE, Conner B, Malakooti MA, et al. Community-acquired methicillin-resistant *Staphylococcus aureus* among military recruits. Emerg Infect Dis 2004;10(5): 941–4.

[28] James L, Gorwitz RJ, Jones RC, et al. Methicillin-resistant *Staphylococcus aureus* infections among healthy full-term newborns. Arch Dis Child Fetal Neonatal Ed 2008;93:40–4.

[29] Morel AS, Wu F, Della-Latta P, et al. Nosocomial transmission of methicillin-resistant *Staphylococcus aureus* from a mother to her preterm quadruplet infants. Am J Infect Control 2002;30(3):170–3.

[30] Saiman L, O'Keefe M, Graham PL 3rd, et al. Hospital transmission of community-acquired methicillin-resistant *Staphylococcus aureus* among postpartum women. Clin Infect Dis 2003;37(10):1313–9.

[31] Chen KT, Huard RC, Della-Latta P, et al. Prevalence of methicillin-sensitive and methicillin-resistant *Staphylococcus aureus* in pregnant women. Obstet Gynecol 2006;108(3 Pt 1): 482–7.

[32] Behari P, Englund J, Alcasid G, et al. Transmission of methicillin-resistant *Staphylococcus aureus* to preterm infants through breast milk. Infect Control Hosp Epidemiol 2004;25(9): 778–80.

[33] Gastelum DT, Dassey D, Mascola L, et al. Transmission of community-associated methicillin-resistant *Staphylococcus aureus* from breast milk in the neonatal intensive care unit. Pediatr Infect Dis J 2005;24(12):1122–4.

[34] von Eiff C, Becker K, Machka K, et al. Nasal carriage as a source of *Staphylococcus aureus* bacteremia: study group. N Engl J Med 2001;344(1):11–6.

[35] Saiman L, Ludington E, Dawson JD, et al. Risk factors for *Candida* species colonization of neonatal intensive care unit patients. Pediatr Infect Dis J 2001;20(12):1119–24.

[36] Waters V, Larson E, Wu F, et al. Molecular epidemiology of gram-negative bacilli from infected neonates and health care workers' hands in neonatal intensive care units. Clin Infect Dis 2004;38(12):1682–7.

[37] Saiman L, Cronquist A, Wu F, et al. An outbreak of methicillin-resistant *Staphylococcus aureus* in a neonatal intensive care unit. Infect Control Hosp Epidemiol 2003;24(5):317–21.

[38] Diederen BM, Kluytmans JA. The emergence of infections with community-associated methicillin resistant *Staphylococcus aureus*. J Infect 2006;52(3):157–68.

[39] Graham PL 3rd, Lin SX, Larson EL. A US population-based survey of *Staphylococcus aureus* colonization. Ann Intern Med 2006;144(5):318–25.

[40] Davis SL, Rybak MJ, Amjad M, et al. Characteristics of patients with healthcare-associated infection due to SCCmec type IV methicillin-resistant *Staphylococcus aureus*. Infect Control Hosp Epidemiol 2006;27(10):1025–31.

[41] Tsuji BT, Rybak MJ, Cheung CM, et al. Community- and health care-associated methicillin-resistant *Staphylococcus aureus*: a comparison of molecular epidemiology and antimicrobial activities of various agents. Diagn Microbiol Infect Dis 2007;58(1):41–7.

[42] Said-Salim B, Mathema B, Braughton K, et al. Differential distribution and expression of Panton-Valentine leucocidin among community-acquired methicillin-resistant *Staphylococcus aureus* strains. J Clin Microbiol 2005;43(7):3373–9.

[43] Steinkraus G, White R, Friedrich L. Vancomycin MIC creep in non-vancomycin-intermediate *Staphylococcus aureus* (VISA), vancomycin-susceptible clinical methicillin-resistant S aureus (MRSA) blood isolates from 2001–2005. J Antimicrob Chemother 2007;60(4): 788–94.

[44] Howden BP, Ward PB, Charles PGP, et al. Treatment outcomes for serious infections caused by methicillin-resistant *Staphylococcus aureus* with reduced vancomycin susceptibility. Clin Infect Dis 2004;38:521–8.

[45] Cunha BA. Methicillin-resistant *Staphylococcus aureus*: clinical manifestations and antimicrobial therapy. Clin Microbiol Infect 2005;11(Suppl 4):33–42.

[46] Tiwari HK, Sen MR. Emergence of vancomycin resistant *Staphylococcus aureus* (VRSA) from a tertiary care hospital from northern part of India. BMC Infect Dis 2006;6:156–61.

[47] Hanaki H, Hososaka Y, Yanagisawa C, et al. Occurrence of vancomycin-intermediate-resistant *Staphylococcus aureus* in Japan. J Infect Chemother 2007;13(2):118–21.

[48] Chuang YY, Huang YC, Lee CY, et al. Methicillin-resistant *Staphylococcus aureus* bacteraemia in neonatal intensive care units: an analysis of 90 episodes. Acta Paediatr 2004;93(6): 786–90.

[49] Frederiksen B, Christiansen P, Knudsen FU. Acute osteomyelitis and septic arthritis in the neonate, risk factors and outcome. Eur J Pediatr 1993;152(7):577–80.

[50] Korakaki E, Aligizakis A, Manoura A, et al. Methicillin-resistant *Staphylococcus aureus* osteomyelitis and septic arthritis in neonates: diagnosis and management. Jpn J Infect Dis 2007;60(2–3):129–31.

[51] Wang CL, Wang SM, Yang YJ, et al. Septic arthritis in children: relationship of causative pathogens, complications, and outcome. J Microbiol Immunol Infect 2003;36(1):41–6.

[52] Saiman L, Prince A, Gersony WM. Pediatric infective endocarditis in the modern era. J Pediatr 1993;122(6):847–53.

[53] Valente AM, Jain R, Scheurer M, et al. Frequency of infective endocarditis among infants and children with *Staphylococcus aureus* bacteremia. Pediatrics 2005;115(1):E15–9.

[54] Friedland IR, du Plessis J, Cilliers A. Cardiac complications in children with *Staphylococcus aureus* bacteremia. J Pediatr 1995;127(5):746–8.

[55] Kaufman D, Fairchild KD. Clinical microbiology of bacterial and fungal sepsis in very-low-birth-weight infants. Clin Microbiol Rev 2004;17(3):638–80, table of contents.

[56] Davenport M, Doig CM. Wound infection in pediatric surgery: a study in 1094 neonates. J Pediatr Surg 1993;28(1):26–30.

[57] Rodrigues MM, Patrocinio SJ, Rodrigues MG. *Staphylococcus aureus* meningitis in children: a review of 30 community-acquired cases. Arq Neuropsiquiatr 2000;58(3B):843–51.

[58] Krcmery V Jr, Filka J, Uher J, et al. Ciprofloxacin in treatment of nosocomial meningitis in neonates and in infants: report of 12 cases and review. Diagn Microbiol Infect Dis 1999; 35(1):75–80.

[59] Kluytmans JA, Mouton JW, VandenBergh MF, et al. Reduction of surgical-site infections in cardiothoracic surgery by elimination of nasal carriage of *Staphylococcus aureus*. Infect Control Hosp Epidemiol 1996;17(12):780–5.

[60] Nasal mupirocin prevents *Staphylococcus aureus* exit-site infection during peritoneal dialysis. Mupirocin Study Group. J Am Soc Nephrol 1996;7(11):2403–8.

[61] Sandri AM, Dalarosa MG, Ruschel de Alcantara L, et al. Reduction in incidence of nosocomial methicillin-resistant *Staphylococcus aureus* (MRSA) infection in an intensive care unit: role of treatment with mupirocin ointment and chlorhexidine baths for nasal carriers of MRSA. Infect Control Hosp Epidemiol 2006;27(2):185–7.

[62] Stein M, Navon-Venezia S, Chmelnitsky I, et al. An outbreak of new, nonmultidrug-resistant, methicillin-resistant *Staphylococcus aureus* strain (SCCmec type iiia variant-1) in the neonatal intensive care unit transmitted by a staff member. Pediatr Infect Dis J 2006;25(6): 557–9.

[63] Hitomi S, Kubota M, Mori N, et al. Control of a methicillin-resistant *Staphylococcus aureus* outbreak in a neonatal intensive care unit by unselective use of nasal mupirocin ointment. J Hosp Infect 2000;46(2):123–9.

[64] Simor AE, Stuart TL, Louie L, et al. Mupirocin-resistant, methicillin-resistant *Staphylococcus aureus* (MRSA) in Canadian hospitals. Antimicrob Agents Chemother 2007;51(11): 3880–6.

[65] Jones JC, Rogers TJ, Brookmeyer P, et al. Mupirocin resistance in patients colonized with methicillin-resistant *Staphylococcus aureus* in a surgical intensive care unit. Clin Infect Dis 2007;45(5):541–7.

[66] Machado JK, Feferbaum R, Kobayashi CE, et al. Vancomycin pharmacokinetics in preterm infants. Clinics 2007;62(4):405–10.

[67] Gabriel MH, Kildoo GC 3rd, Gennrich JL, et al. Prospective evaluation of a vancomycin dosage guideline for neonates. Clin Pharm 1991;10(2):129–32.

[68] Anderson BJ, Allegaert K, Van den Anker JN, et al. Vancomycin pharmacokinetics in preterm neonates and the prediction of adult clearance. Br J Clin Pharmacol 2007;63(1):75–84.

[69] Kearns GL, Jungbluth GL, Abdel-Rahman SM, et al. Impact of ontogeny on linezolid disposition in neonates and infants. Clin Pharmacol Ther 2003;74(5):413–22.

[70] Saiman L, Goldfarb J, Kaplan SA, et al. Safety and tolerability of linezolid in children. Pediatr Infect Dis J 2003;22(9 Suppl):S193–200.

[71] Tsuji BT, Rybak MJ. E-test synergy testing of clinical isolates of *Staphylococcus aureus* demonstrating heterogeneous resistance to vancomycin. Diagn Microbiol Infect Dis 2006;54(1):73–7.

[72] Abramson MA, Sexton DJ. Nosocomial methicillin-resistant and methicillin-susceptible *Staphylococcus aureus* primary bacteremia: at what costs? Infect Control Hosp Epidemiol 1999;20(6):408–11.

[73] Chaix C, Durand-Zaleski I, Alberti C, et al. Control of endemic methicillin-resistant *Staphylococcus aureus*: a cost-benefit analysis in an intensive care unit. JAMA 1999;282(18): 1745–51.

[74] Clancy M, Graepler A, Wilson M, et al. Active screening in high-risk units is an effective and cost-avoidant method to reduce the rate of methicillin-resistant *Staphylococcus aureus* infection in the hospital. Infect Control Hosp Epidemiol 2006;27(10):1009–17.

[75] Larson EL, Cimiotti J, Haas J, et al. Effect of antiseptic handwashing vs alcohol sanitizer on health care-associated infections in neonatal intensive care units. Arch Pediatr Adolesc Med 2005;159(4):377–83.

[76] Gerber SI, Jones RC, Scott MV, et al. Management of outbreaks of methicillin-resistant *Staphylococcus aureus* infection in the neonatal intensive care unit: a consensus statement. Infect Control Hosp Epidemiol 2006;27(2):139–45.

[77] Roberts RB, de Lencastre A, Eisner W, et al. Molecular epidemiology of methicillin-resistant *Staphylococcus aureus* in 12 New York hospitals: MRSA Collaborative Study Group. J Infect Dis 1998;178(1):164–71.

[78] Bootsma MC, Diekmann O, Bonten MJ. Controlling methicillin-resistant *Staphylococcus aureus*: quantifying the effects of interventions and rapid diagnostic testing. Proc Natl Acad Sci U S A 2006;103(14):5620–5.

[79] Stoll BJ, Gordon T, Korones SB, et al. Late-onset sepsis in very low birth weight neonates: a report from the National Institute of Child Health and Human Development Neonatal Research Network. J Pediatr 1996;129(1):63–71.

[80] Fridkin SK, Kaufman D, Edwards JR, et al. Changing incidence of *Candida* bloodstream infections among NICU patients in the United States: 1995–2004. Pediatrics 2006;117(5): 1680–7.

[81] Kossoff EH, Buescher ES, Karlowicz MG. Candidemia in a neonatal intensive care unit: trends during fifteen years and clinical features of 111 cases. Pediatr Infect Dis J 1998; 17(6):504–8.

[82] Rabalais GP, Samiec TD, Bryant KK, et al. Invasive candidiasis in infants weighing more than 2500 grams at birth admitted to a neonatal intensive care unit. Pediatr Infect Dis J 1996;15(4):348–52.

[83] Feja KN, Wu F, Roberts K, et al. Risk factors for candidemia in critically ill infants: a matched case-control study. J Pediatr 2005;147(2):156–61.

[84] Jarvis WR. The epidemiology of colonization. Infect Control Hosp Epidemiol 1996;17(1): 47–52.

[85] el-Mohandes AE, Johnson-Robbins L, Keiser JF, et al. Incidence of *Candida parapsilosis* colonization in an intensive care nursery population and its association with invasive fungal disease. Pediatr Infect Dis J 1994;13(6):520–4.

[86] Rowen JL, Rench MA, Kozinetz CA, et al. Endotracheal colonization with *Candida* enhances risk of systemic candidiasis in very low birth weight neonates. J Pediatr 1994; 124(5 Pt 1):789–94.

[87] Baley JE, Kliegman RM, Boxerbaum B, et al. Fungal colonization in the very low birth weight infant. Pediatrics 1986;78(2):225–32.

[88] Shattuck KE, Cochran CK, Zabransky RJ, et al. Colonization and infection associated with *Malassezia* and *Candida* species in a neonatal unit. J Hosp Infect 1996;34(2):123–9.

[89] Waggoner-Fountain LA, Walker MW, Hollis RJ, et al. Vertical and horizontal transmission of unique *Candida* species to premature newborns. Clin Infect Dis 1996;22(5):803–8.

[90] Strausbaugh LJ, Sewell DL, Ward TT, et al. High frequency of yeast carriage on hands of hospital personnel. J Clin Microbiol 1994;32(9):2299–300.

[91] Brown AJ, Odds FC, Gow NA. Infection-related gene expression in *Candida albicans*. Curr Opin Microbiol 2007;10(4):307–13.

[92] Kumamoto CA, Vinces MD. Contributions of hyphae and hypha-co-regulated genes to *Candida albicans* virulence. Cell Microbiol 2005;7(11):1546–54.

[93] Douglas LJ. *Candida* biofilms and their role in infection. Trends Microbiol 2003;11(1):30–6.

[94] Pearlman SA, Higgins S, Eppes S, et al. Infective endocarditis in the premature neonate. Clin Pediatr (Phila) 1998;37(12):741–6.

[95] Cohen-Wolkowiez M, Smith PB, Mangum B, et al. Neonatal *Candida* meningitis: significance of cerebrospinal fluid parameters and blood cultures. J Perinatol 2007;27(2):97–100.

[96] Smith PB, Benjamin DK Jr, Alexander BD, et al. Quantification of 1,3-beta-D-glucan levels in children: preliminary data for diagnostic use of the beta-glucan assay in a pediatric setting. Clin Vaccine Immunol 2007;14(7):924–5.

[97] Lopez Sastre JB, Coto Cotallo GD, Fernandez Colomer B. Neonatal invasive candidiasis: a prospective multicenter study of 118 cases. Am J Perinatol 2003;20(3):153–63.

[98] Frattarelli DA, Reed MD, Giacoia GP, et al. Antifungals in systemic neonatal candidiasis. Drugs 2004;64(9):949–68.

[99] Sanchez PJ, Siegel JD, Fishbein J. Candida endocarditis: successful medical management in three preterm infants and review of the literature. Pediatr Infect Dis J 1991;10(3):239–43.

[100] Benjamin DK, DeLong E, Cotten CM, et al. Mortality following blood culture in premature infants: increased with gram-negative bacteremia and candidemia, but not gram-positive bacteremia. J Perinatol 2004;24(3):175–80.

[101] Smith PB, Morgan J, Benjamin JD, et al. Excess costs of hospital care associated with neonatal candidemia. Pediatr Infect Dis J 2007;26(3):197–200.

[102] Manzoni P, Stolfi I, Pugni L, et al. A multicenter, randomized trial of prophylactic fluconazole in preterm neonates. N Engl J Med 2007;356(24):2483–95.

[103] Kaufman D, Boyle R, Hazen KC, et al. Fluconazole prophylaxis against fungal colonization and infection in preterm infants. N Engl J Med 2001;345(23):1660–6.

[104] Kaufman D, Boyle R, Hazen KC, et al. Twice weekly fluconazole prophylaxis for prevention of invasive *Candida* infection in high-risk infants of < 1000 grams birth weight. J Pediatr 2005;147(2):172–9.

[105] Healy CM, Baker CJ, Zaccaria E, et al. Impact of fluconazole prophylaxis on incidence and outcome of invasive candidiasis in a neonatal intensive care unit. J Pediatr 2005;147(2):166–71.

[106] Clerihew L, Austin N, McGuire W. Prophylactic systemic antifungal agents to prevent mortality and morbidity in very low birth weight infants. Cochrane Database Syst Rev 2007;4:CD003850.

[107] Bertini G, Perugi S, Dani C, et al. Fluconazole prophylaxis prevents invasive fungal infection in high-risk, very low birth weight infants. J Pediatr 2005;147:162–5.

[108] Long SS, Stevenson DK. Reducing *Candida* infections during neonatal intensive care: management choices, infection control, and fluconazole prophylaxis. J Pediatr 2005;147(2):135–41.

CLINICS IN
PERINATOLOGY

Clin Perinatol 35 (2008) 251–272

Necrotizing Enterocolitis

Pinchi S. Srinivasan, MD*, Michael D. Brandler, MD,
Antoni D'Souza, MD

*Division of Neonatology, Department of Pediatrics, New York Hospital Queens, Affiliate
Weill Medical College of Cornell University, 56-45, Main Street, Flushing, NY 11355, USA*

"Iatrogenesis" literally means "brought forth by a healer" ("iatros" means "healer" in Greek); as such, it can refer to good or bad effects, but it is used almost exclusively to refer to a state of ill health or adverse effect or complication caused by or resulting from medical treatment.

Necrotizing enterocolitis (NEC) is the most common acquired gastrointestinal disease that occurs predominantly in premature infants. In NEC the small (most often distal) and/or large bowel becomes injured, develops intramural air, and may progress to frank necrosis with perforation [1]. Even with early, aggressive treatment, the progression of necrosis, which is highly characteristic of NEC, can lead to sepsis and death.

When one considers common neonatal issues such as enteral feeding, bacterial infections, and clinical situations resulting in ischemic insults to bowels, one can see how NEC can be considered an unintentional iatrogenic disease associated with some of these factors. Several unresolved issues, such as an unproven pathogenesis, inadequate and often-difficult therapy, and the lack of an agreed-upon and effective prevention strategy, make this disease an enigmatic clinical entity that continues to occur in almost every neonatal ICU (NICU) caring for preterm babies, especially those weighing less than 1500 g. Approximately 12% of infants that have a birth weight less than 1500 g develop NEC, and about one third of those who develop NEC succumb to the disease. The possibly iatrogenic component of NEC relates to the epidemiologic nature of the disease, which occurs only in the postnatal period: the disease is never reported in stillborn infants and is rare in infants who have never been fed in NICU settings, even though clinical practices (eg, feeding regimens, fluid management) vary widely among NICUs.

---

* Corresponding author.
E-mail address: pns9001@nyp.org (P.S. Srinivasan).

0095-5108/08/$ - see front matter © 2008 Elsevier Inc. All rights reserved.
doi:10.1016/j.clp.2007.11.009 *perinatology.theclinics.com*

This article reviews the current scientific knowledge related to the etiology and pathogenesis of NEC and discusses some possible preventive measures.

Epidemiology and risk factors

NEC is a disease familiar to all practitioners who care for very low birth weight (VLBW) babies. It also can be considered a disease of medical progress, because the routine use of antenatal steroids and prophylactic surfactant has resulted in higher survival of preterm infants, and it is this group that is most susceptible to this potentially devastating disease [2]. There is a well-known inverse relationship between the incidence of NEC and gestational age at birth, with extremely premature and extremely low birth weight babies carrying the highest risk for developing NEC [3–6]. In selected series, the incidence of NEC has ranged from 1% to 5% of all NICU admissions [7].

Most recent population-based or multicentric epidemiologic studies have reported NEC rates that have remained stable for VLBW infants, ranging between 6% and 7% [6,8–11]. An exception is a study by New South Wales and Australian Capital Territory Neonatal Intensive Care Unit Study group (NSW ACT NICUS) reporting a reduction in the incidence of NEC from 12% in 1986–1987 and 1992–1993 to 6% in 1998–1999 for all infants born in New South Wales at 24 to 28 weeks' gestation [12]. This is the only large study to report a decline in the rate of the disease in VLBW preterm infants, although a smaller, single-center report from the United States also reported a decline in the incidence of NEC in infants with birth weights between 500 and 800 g [13].

The authors of the NSW CT NICUS speculate that reduced cardiorespiratory compromise secondary to patent ductus arteriosus (PDA), pneumothorax, and pulmonary morbidity and wider use of human-milk feeding may have played an indirect role in the reduced incidence of NEC [12]. In this study, however, the mortality rate from NEC remained unchanged, at 27% to 37%, as did the requirement for surgical intervention, at 41% to 57% [14]. During the decade of the 1990s, National Institute of Child Health and Human Development (NICHD) Neonatal Network centers saw no significant change in the incidence of NEC (≥ Bell stage 2), which remained at about 7% in infants with birth weights between 500 and 1500 g [15,16]. Within the NICHD Neonatal Network, between 1987 and 2000, several groups reported rates of the disease ranging from 1% to 22% of VLBW infants [15,17]. In a similar period, the Vermont Oxford Network reported an incidence of NEC 6% to 7.1% [11] despite the overall increased survival in infants with birth weights of less than 1000 g.

The risk of NEC seems to be increased in black infants, a finding often attributed to the high risk of prematurity in this group [5,18]. Although in the past no consistent association was identified between sex and rates of

NEC, recent studies have suggested an increased risk in males, with a slightly greater incidence [14,18] and higher mortality [19] among male VLBW infants.

Mortality rates from NEC range from 12% to 30% [7]. Higher fatality rates are associated with decreasing birth weight and gestational age [14,19]. Mortality associated with NEC has been shown to be higher for black infants than for other groups [18,19], and the racial disparity in deaths from the disease remains significant even after controlling for birth weight and other characteristics [19]. Fatality rates are relatively higher in infants requiring surgery than in those medically treated for NEC. The case fatality rate among patients who have NEC is as high as 50% in infants requiring surgical intervention, and an estimated 20% to 40% of all infants who have NEC undergo surgery [6,8,10]. Mortality for this group is related to underlying clinical status, especially the number of comorbidities [20] and surgical treatment [21,22].

Holman and colleagues [18] used the 2000 Kids' inpatient database to estimate the hospitalization rates and mortality associated with NEC in the United States. About 66% of these infants weighed less than 1500 g. An estimated 4463 (SE = 219) hospitalizations associated with NEC occurred among neonates in the United States during the year 2000. During 2000, there was one NEC hospitalization per 1000 live births, and approximately one in seven NEC hospitalizations ended in death. The incidence of NEC in infants delivered in level 3 hospitals was similar to that in infants delivered in community hospitals, so the nature of the birth hospital does not seem to affect the incidence of NEC [12,23].

The association of antenatal steroid administration and the incidence of NEC is unclear, with several studies reporting conflicting findings. The results from the Cochrane systematic review on treatment with antenatal corticosteroids show an overall reduction in NEC in addition to a reduction in neonatal deaths [24]. Two large, retrospective studies from a national database [6] and the multicenter NICHD network [25] have shown an increased risk of NEC with antenatal steroid exposure. Possible explanations for the increase in NEC after antenatal steroids include the increased survival of more immature infants who have decreased acute pulmonary morbidity. The improved pulmonary status of these infants may encourage caregivers to institute and advance feedings more rapidly than is prudent. Despite the possibility of an increased risk of NEC with the use of antenatal steroids, the continued use of a single course of antenatal corticosteroids to accelerate fetal lung maturation in women at risk of preterm birth is encouraged. Further studies may define more clearly the association between antenatal steroid administration and the incidence of NEC.

In a recent report of the Research Planning Workshop held on New Therapies and Preventive Approaches for Necrotizing Enterocolitis, PDA surgery and antenatal steroids were statistically significant predictors for increased risk of NEC for infants with birth weights between 400 and

1000 g. For infants with birth weights between 1001 and 1500 g, reaching full feeds by 14 days of age was associated with decreased risk of developing NEC [26].

The recent study by the NSW ACT NICUS Group found no effect of antenatal steroids on the incidence of NEC. These authors also reported NEC in the higher gestation group (28–31 weeks) to be associated with perinatal risk factors, including small for gestational age status, pneumothorax, younger maternal age, placental abruption, respiratory distress syndrome, and the use of surfactant [14]. In infants of less than 28 weeks' gestation, the significant factor associated with an increased risk of NEC was PDA requiring surgery [14].

Most cases of NEC are sporadic, although the observation of crops or epidemics of NEC cases has been reported widely. Many neonatal ICUs have had periods during which several infants have developed cases of NEC that seemingly were identical in presentation, clinical course, and causative agent. Outbreaks have been recorded more commonly in crowded nurseries and where there are high rates of gastrointestinal illness among care givers [27]. Boccia and colleagues [28] reviewed the characteristics of 17 NEC epidemics and found that although the outbreaks differed in the number of cases, the clinical presentations, and the management, there were some similarities. The authors concluded that, in general, a NEC epidemic is caused by the dissemination of a particular pathogen in a specific ward during a specific period of time, and that NICU staff may play a direct role in transmitting the infection. Observations made during these epidemics suggest that they are infectious outbreaks. No single infectious agent has been linked to epidemic NEC, but common infectious agents have been isolated from blood, stool, and peritoneal fluid during outbreaks. Still, many outbreaks of NEC have not been associated with any positive cultures.

Recent data suggest that the neonate's genetic background may contribute to the susceptibility for NEC. Because cytokines take the central role in tissue injury, cytokine genetics with exploration of cytokine polymorphism has been studied extensively. Attempts have been made to find the association between different polymorphisms and the incidence and severity of the disease. A carrier state of genetic polymorphisms may be associated with perinatal morbidity, including NEC. Vascular endothelial growth factor (VEGF) G+405C polymorphism is shown to be associated with a higher risk of preterm birth, and VEGF C-2578A polymorphism may participate in the development of perinatal complications such as NEC and acute renal failure [29,30]. The prevalence of the mutant variant of the interleukin (IL)-4 receptor α gene was lower in neonates who had NEC than in those who did not, suggesting that this mutation might protect against development of NEC in infants [31].

NEC rarely occurs in full-term infants [32–34]. Approximately 5% to 10% of NEC cases occur in infants at or above 37 weeks of gestation. In addition to occurring earlier in life, NEC almost always is associated with specific risk factors, such as peripartum asphyxia, intrauterine growth restriction, polycythemia or hyperviscosity, exchange transfusion, umbilical catheterization, congenital heart disease, or myelomeningocele [35–38]. When it does occur in full-term infants, NEC results in much the same morbidity and mortality as in preterm infants.

Etiology and pathogenesis

Although extensive research has investigated the pathophysiology of NEC, a complete understanding has not been elucidated fully. The most accepted epidemiologic precursors for NEC are prematurity [3,39] and gastrointestinal feeding [39].

Santulli and colleagues [40] described the classic triad of pathologic events in the pathogenesis of NEC: (1) intestinal ischemia (2) colonization by pathogenic bacteria, and (3) excess protein substrate in the intestinal lumen. Subsequently Kosloske [41] suggested that the coincidence of two of three classic pathologic events was sufficient to cause NEC. Kosloske's [41] model has been supported by the findings of pathologists reviewing specimens with NEC, which invariably showed coagulation (ischemic) necrosis, inflammation, and bacterial overgrowth, all present in varying degrees of severity [42]. Reparative tissue changes such as epithelial regeneration, granulation tissue formation, and fibrosis also were found in the majority of cases, suggesting ongoing tissue injury of at least several days' duration.

Kosloske [41] hypothesized that NEC is more likely to appear following quantitative extremes (ie, severe ischemia, highly pathogenic flora, or marked excess of substrate) and that NEC develops only if a threshold of injury, sufficient to initiate intestinal necrosis, is exceeded. This hypothesis may explain both typical occurrences of NEC among high-risk premature infants and the atypical occurrences among infants considered at low risk (eg, previously healthy term infants, infants fed breast milk exclusively, and infants never fed). Further, it may explain why NEC fails to develop in most high-risk infants in NICUs.

Kosloske's hypothesis may help identify possible iatrogenic situations that could contribute to the quantitative extremes of one of these three events. Inadequate pharmacologic stabilization of intestinal perfusion may result in ischemic injury to bowel. NICU practices (eg, delayed enteral feeding, a relatively sterile environment in incubators, and, frequently, administration of broad-spectrum antibiotics) may delay and impair natural intestinal bacterial colonization [43]. Certain feeding practices (eg, initiation of enteral feedings [44–46], duration of trophic feedings [47], advances in feeding volume [47–49], addition of fortifier, increases in caloric density [50,51], and use of breast milk versus formula [51]) have been implicated as having possible associations with the development of NEC.

Prematurity

Prematurity remains the most important and consistent risk factor for NEC. Although the specific underlying mechanisms responsible for the predilection of NEC in premature infants are not clearly known, certain factors are known to compromise intestinal host defense in premature infants. Among the factors known to place the premature infant at high risk of NEC are immaturity of gastrointestinal motility, digestive ability, circulatory regulation, and intestinal barrier function, abnormal colonization by pathologic bacteria [52], and underdeveloped intestinal defense mechanisms. Each of these factors is discussed in the following sections.

Intestinal motility and digestion

Immature intestinal motility and digestion probably predispose preterm infants to NEC. Fetal studies in both human [53] and animal models [54] suggest that development of gastrointestinal motility begins in the second trimester but matures in the third trimester. Intestinal motility studies have shown that premature infants can have less organized and immature motility patterns than full-term infants; enteral feeding can mature these responses [55–59]. An intrinsic immaturity of the enteric nervous system delays transit and may lead to poor clearance of bacteria and subsequent bacterial overgrowth. Peristalsis also serves as an important component of epithelial barrier integrity. Peristalsis limits the amount of time during which antigens are able to interact with the apical surface of the enterocytes and also speeds the process by which antigen–antibody complexes are eliminated [60]. Fetal hypoxia [61] or perinatal asphyxia associated with maternal or fetal disease states, including intrauterine growth restriction, in both preterm and full-term infants is known to reduce postnatal intestinal motility [62]. In addition to impaired intestinal motility, premature infants have poor digestive and absorptive ability [63]. Luminal digestion forms the first lines of defense against ingested pathogens and toxins. Lower hydrogen ion output in the stomach [64] and low proteolytic enzyme activity [65] related to gut immaturity impair this defense. Malabsorption coupled with poor gastrointestinal motility may have deleterious effects on mucosal integrity [59,66]. Immature luminal digestion can predispose the infant to the entry of pathogens from the environment and allow colonization by pathogens in the distal gastrointestinal tract.

Intestinal barrier

The intestinal barrier lies at the interface between microbes within the intestinal lumen and the immune system of the host and has both immunologic and mechanical components. Factors that impair the function of the intestinal barrier may predispose the host to the invasion of gut-derived microbes and to the development of systemic inflammatory disease. This process, termed "bacterial translocation," may be compounded when the mechanisms that regulate the repair of the intestinal barrier are disrupted. Preterm infants also have higher intestinal permeability than older children and adults because of various mechanical and nonmechanical factors including (1) the tight junctions that maintain the connections between adjacent cells (2) peristalsis of the intestinal lumen, and (3) components of the mucus coat including secretory IgA [67–69]. Disruption of the tight junctions by systemic stressors may lead to intestinal hyperpermeability (the "leaky gut"), predisposing the host to bacterial translocation and immune system activation in the pathogenesis of NEC.

Intestinal defense mechanisms

Three major categories of epithelial host defense include enhanced salt and water secretion, expression of antimicrobial proteins and peptides, and production of intestinal mucins [70]. Preterm infants have underdeveloped and immature intestinal secretion and absorption mechanisms, resulting in selective movement of small ions across the epithelial monolayer and, in the preterm infant, an inability to remove unwanted pathogens or toxins from the intestinal lumen [70].

The two main families of antimicrobial peptides produced by intestinal cells are the defensins (α and β) and cathelicidins [71,72] These antimicrobial peptides have bioactivity against a wide range of microbes, including bacteria, viruses, fungi, protozoa, and spirochetes, and the immature intestine may be vulnerable to such pathogens [73]. Reduced activity of these biochemical defenses may be caused by reduced defensin expression. Secretory IgA lines the intestinal lumen, serves to bind bacteria, and acts as an important part of the mucosal defense mechanism by neutralizing bacterial endotoxin, rotavirus, and influenza virus infection [74]. This activity underscores the immunologic benefits of breast-milk feeding.

A critical determinant of the integrity of the intestinal epithelial barrier is found in the mucus covering the enterocyte monolayer [75]. Mucin has many functions beneficial to the gastrointestinal tract, including lubrication, mechanical protection, and protection against the acidic environment provided by gastric and duodenal secretions. The degree of protection conferred to the gastrointestinal tract by mucins relates in part to the maturity of the mucins [76]. Mucin also aids in the fixation of pathogenic bacteria, viruses, and parasites.

Recent evidence suggests that platelet activating factor and human toll-like receptors contribute to the proinflammatory response that is characteristic of NEC pathology [77–80]. Inflammatory mediators implicated in the pathogenesis of NEC include platelet activating factor, tumor necrosis factor, and interleukins (IL-1, IL-6, IL-8, IL-10, IL-12, and IL-18) [78–82].

Intestinal circulatory regulation

Intestinal ischemia leading to mucosal damage is a critical predisposing factor in the development of NEC. Coagulation necrosis is the footprint of prior ischemia and is a hallmark of the pathologic findings of NEC. The increased incidence of NEC after perinatal asphyxia, indwelling umbilical catheters, PDA, and the use of indomethacin also supports the role of intestinal ischemia.

Lloyd [83] proposed redistribution of cardiac output away from the intestine during asphyxia as a cause of intestine ischemia and NEC. This phenomenon had been described earlier in a diving mammal model [84]. Although the laboratory studies by Alward and colleagues [85] and Touloukian and colleagues [86] seemed to confirm Lloyd's [83] hypothesis, the theory of the "diving reflex" as a cause of NEC has been questioned because of its inability to explain the epidemiologic pattern of NEC or the association of risk factors for NEC and because of recent physiologic information regarding sustained adrenergic stimulation. Sustained adrenergic stimulation, which is the physiologic basis for the diving reflex [84], does not cause sustained flow reduction or tissue hypoxia in newborn intestine [87,88]. In an excellent review on newborn intestinal circulation, Reber and colleagues [89] discuss how reperfusion injury may explain the mucosal damage noted by Alward and colleagues [85] and Touloukian and colleagues [86] in their experimental studies with restoration of normoxemia after a profound degree of asphyxia.

Fetal intestine is a relatively dormant organ engaged in minimal activity, so a relatively low level of blood flow and oxygen delivery is adequate to meet its limited tissue oxygen demand. Postnatally, however, the intestine is a site of intense metabolic activity; in most mammals it becomes the sole site for nutrient absorption, with a dramatic increase in growth during the first weeks after birth [90].

The basal vascular resistance within the newborn intestinal circulation significantly decreases in the first several days after birth. This decrease seems to be mediated by three vascular control systems: nitric oxide (NO) [91,92], which causes vasodilation; the myogenic response, a process in which an increase in intravascular pressure induces vasoconstriction in some blood vessels [93], and endothelin (ET-1) [92,94], which provides constrictor tone. The consequence of this reduction in resistance is a dramatic increase in the rate of intestinal blood flow and oxygen delivery, which is thought to be the normal transition in intestinal circulatory adaptation to meet the increased demands of a functional, rapidly growing intestine. Interruptions of this normal transition of the newborn intestinal circulation and its associated increased intestinal blood flow may result in intestinal ischemia.

As a novel hypothesis, Reber and colleagues [89] propose that disruption or loss of endothelial cell function within the newborn intestine circulation is the key antecedent of the intestinal ischemia relevant to the pathogenesis of NEC. The limitation of this hypothesis is based on gastrointestinal physiologic observations made in newborn swine.

Several factors or processes have the potential to disrupt endothelial function in a relatively specific manner, altering the ET-1–NO balance in favor of constriction. Ischemia-reperfusion sequence, platelet activating factor, a lipid proinflammatory mediator [80], bacterial translocation, and intestinal stasis consequent to dysmotility with subsequent short-chain fatty acids–related mucosal disruption are some of the potential factors that could lead to endothelial dysfunction. The best-studied of all these factors is the process of ischemia-reperfusion [87]. The unique ET-1–NO interaction then might facilitate rapid extension of this constriction, generating a viscous cascade wherein ischemia rapidly extends into larger portions of the intestine [95].

Abnormal bacterial colonization

Commensal bacteria interact symbiotically with the mammalian intestine to regulate the expression of genes important for barrier function, digestion, and angiogenesis [96]. Because NEC does not occur in utero, intestinal bacteria might have a role in its pathogenesis, especially if abnormal colonization occurs. Commensal bacteria can inhibit inflammatory pathways and perhaps contribute to the maintenance of homoeostasis [97]. Furthermore, reports indicate that pathogenic stimuli, including Salmonella and *Escherichia coli*, produce exaggerated proinflammatory responses in immature intestinal epithelial cells [98,99].

Although the fetal gut is sterile, colonization of the preterm gut occurs rapidly postnatally. In utero, a sterile fetal environment protects the intestine. The establishment of normal intestinal flora is the basis of a natural immunologic barrier against invasion by pathogenic bacteria. By convention, the natural microflora of healthy breast-fed term infants (ie, a bifidobacterial predominance) is considered the most normal condition [43].

The natural colonization process tends to be both delayed and impaired in preterm infants because of several factors, including delayed enteral feeding, a relatively sterile environment (incubators), and the frequent administration of broad-spectrum antibiotics [100]. Investigators have reported that duodenal colonization of Enterobacteriaceae is abnormal in VLBW infants and that early abnormal colonization of stools with *Clostridium perfringens* is correlated with the later development of NEC [101,102].

The intestinal bacterial colonization of preterm neonates differs from that of term infants both temporally and qualitatively. Preterm neonates are colonized by fewer bacterial strains and are more likely to be populated by pathogenic bacteria [100], predominantly Klebsiella, Enterobacter, and Clostridium organisms [103]. Even among infants receiving breast milk, bifidobacterial predominance is seen in very few VLBW infants in the first 3 to 4 weeks of life [104–106]. In a case-control study exploring the relationship of gut colonization and NEC, De la Cochetiere and colleagues [102] showed evidence for a temporal relationship between abnormal bacterial colonization and later development of NEC.

Natural resident gut microflora protect against invading bacteria by several different mechanisms: by competing for receptor sites on the gut wall and for available nutrients; by generating an environment hostile to pathogens (eg, via low pH); and by providing a physical barrier, decreasing the permeability of the gastrointestinal wall to protect against invasion and systemic dissemination of both pathogenic and commensal micro-organisms.

The abnormal colonization of premature neonates, together with the immaturity (increased absorptive capacity) of their intestinal epithelial barrier function predisposes these infants to pathogenic bacterial overgrowth. Bacterial translocation, the transmucosal passage of pathogenic bacteria across an intact intestinal barrier, is the process that enables the systemic spread of intestinal bacteria. To cause infection, however, bacteria first must colonize the intestine; only then can they translocate to extraintestinal sites. Although bacteria have long been suspected of playing a role in the development of NEC, only about 33% to 48% of infants who have NEC have a positive blood culture [25]. Although many pathogens are associated with NEC, their role in the causation of NEC is not clear. No particular species have been shown to be necessary for NEC to develop. Bacterial overgrowth in the intestine is one of the major factors that promote bacterial translocation [107]. Colonization must precede translocation, and colonization with more pathogenic bacteria renders the host even more susceptible to disease [108]. Musemeche and colleagues [109] developed an experimental model in germ-free rats to evaluate the comparative effects of ischemia, bacteria, and food substrate on induction of NEC. In this model the most important of the three factors in the pathogenesis of intestinal necrosis was the nature of colonizing bacteria.

Enteral feeding strategies and necrotizing enterocolitis

Although the fetus ingests as much as 500 mL of amniotic fluid daily at term, NEC does not occur in utero. At birth, the enteral nutrient ingested by the infant changes from amniotic fluid to breast milk or formula. Brown and Sweet [110] proposed that aggressive feeding protocols contribute to the pathogenesis of NEC. By instituting a very conservative feeding protocol with modest daily increments in enteral volume and stopping feedings with the slightest suggestion of feeding intolerance, they were able to reduce the incidence of NEC. Other studies have also suggested that infants who developed NEC were fed either too rapidly or with excessive daily increments [25,45,49,111].

Vascular responses to feeding in preterm infants

In a case-control analysis of early human milk feeding tolerance among infants given indomethacin, a drug known to reduce mesenteric vascular flow [112,113], the incidence of NEC was not significantly different compared to matched control infants who did not receive Indomethacin for symptomatic PDA. Bellander and colleagues [114] demonstrated that small feedings were well tolerated in preterm infants when indomethacin was used in the first week of life to treat symptomatic PDA. In a small, clinical trial, Huang and colleagues [115] assessed the effect of nonnutritive sucking and showed that vascular responses to feeding were significantly more intense among infants given a pacifier before feeding than in a control group fed without preprandial pacifiers. This study showed an additional potential benefit for nonnutritive sucking on gastrointestinal function.

Feeding volume increments and breast milk

The use of human milk seems to be highly advantageous, and the incidence of NEC is significantly lower among breast-fed infants than in those fed with commercial formulas [116–118]. There are a number of purported mechanisms to explain this protective effect, including the better tolerability of breast milk; earlier maturation of the mucosal barrier; the presence of constituents, such as glutamate, nucleotides, and growth factors; and the presence of inhibitors of proinflammatory cytokines, such as platelet activating factor acetylhydrolase. Although human milk clearly has been shown to reduce the risk of NEC, it has not eliminated the risk completely.

Two randomized, prospective trials have assessed infants with feeding volume increments of 30 mL/kg/d [119] and 35 mL/kg/d [48] compared with a control group whose feedings were increased by 15 mL/kg/d. Infants receiving the larger incremental volumes reached full feeding volumes earlier than the control infants ($P < .05$). Both studies showed no significant difference between the two groups in the incidence of NEC. The study by Salhotra and Ramji [119] was limited to infants with birth weights below 1250 g, and most were born with intrauterine growth retardation and gestational ages of 30 to 32 weeks. Thus, it is not clear whether these data are clinically applicable to appropriately sized VLBW infants. Also the results were conflict with those of Berseth and colleagues [47], who compared infants randomly assigned to daily increases in feeding volumes with infants whose feeds were held at a minimal volume (gut stimulation protocol or minimal enteral feeds) for the first 10 feeding days. This study demonstrated a significant increase in NEC in the group with advancing volumes, and the study was closed early because the incidence of NEC was 10% in the advancing volume group versus 1.4% in the minimal volume group [47]. The interpretation of this study, however, is complex, because enteral feedings were introduced only at 10 days of life, essentially providing a prolonged period of "bowel rest." This study also raises important questions: whether the gut-stimulation protocol is protective or advancing-volume protocols contribute to the development of NEC. Both may be correct [120]. A larger, multicenter, randomized, controlled trial may be required to answer these questions. Nonetheless, other randomized trials have not demonstrated that fast versus slow or early versus delayed feedings alter the incidence of NEC [48,121–123]. In a multicenter, case-control study looking at associations between enteral feeding practices and the development NEC in preterm infants,

Henderson, and colleagues [118] found significantly shorter duration of trophic feeding and significantly faster advancement of feeding volumes among
cases of NEC compared to a frequency-matched control infants who did not
develop NEC. Unblinded feeding trials have inherent sources of
bias—such as "surveillance bias"—a higher tendency to investigate and
diagnose NEC in infants that are considered to be at higher risk, and also
render interpretation of results difficult warranting caution in it's clinical application. Despite these data suggesting duration of trophic feeding and rate
of advancement of feed volumes as potential modifiable risk factors for
NEC, firm practice recommendation can only be made when sufficient
data from randomized controlled trials are available.

Other risk factors and associations

Recent interest has focused on several growth factors, including epidermal growth factor, as important trophic modulators of intestinal health in
premature infants [124]. Shin and colleagues [124] showed that saliva and
serum epidermal growth factor levels are diminished in premature patients
who have NEC compared with age-matched control subjects. In a study
looking at the ontogeny of salivary epidermal growth factor (sEGF) in premature infants Warner and colleagues [125] have reported patterns of sEGF
levels over the first 2 weeks of life that were significantly related to development of NEC in VLBW infants.

An increased risk of NEC associated with maternal cocaine abuse has
been observed in both animal models [126,127] and human neonates
[128,129].

H2-blocker therapy was associated with higher rates of NEC, as reported
in the large case-control study from the NICHD data registry, supporting
the hypothesis that gastric pH level may be a factor in the pathogenesis of
NEC [10].

Development of a fulminant form of NEC in a subset of stable, growing,
premature neonates who were transfused electively for symptomatic anemia
of prematurity has been described by Mally and others [130]. The authors
speculate a combination of host-specific and transfusion storage issues contributed to the onset of NEC.

Prevention

Because the onset of NEC often is abrupt and overwhelming, with rapid
progression, it seems unlikely that intervention strategies to halt the progression will succeed after the presentation of clinical signs and symptoms. In
contrast, preventive approaches have had some success, and clinical trials
have reported reduction of disease with the use of breast-milk feeding
[34,116,117,131,132], enteral antibiotic prophylaxis [133], probiotics
[134,136], and arginine supplements [137]. Evidence suggests that oral

antibiotics reduce the incidence of NEC in low birth weight infants, but concerns about adverse outcomes persist, particularly related to the development of resistant bacteria [138].

Probiotics are nonpathogenic, beneficial species of bacteria that colonize and replicate within the human intestinal tract and, when ingested in sufficient quantities, exert a positive influence on host health or physiology [43]. Probiotic micro-organisms consist primarily of strains of Lactobacillus, Bifidobacterium, and Streptococcus. Lactobacilli are bacterial strains originating from human microflora. Ingested probiotic bacteria act essentially as exogenous lactobacteria. Attempts to normalize abnormal bowel colonization with lactobacteria supplementation have shown a reduction in the incidence of NEC-like intestinal lesions in several animal models [139,140].

Schanler [141] reviewed three large, randomized trials of use of probiotics [134–136] and concluded that 43 infants would need treatment to prevent one case of NEC. Deshpande and colleagues [142] systematically reviewed randomized, controlled trials evaluating efficacy and safety of any probiotic supplementation (started within first 10 days, duration > 7 days) in preventing stage 2 or greater NEC in VLBW preterm neonates (gestation < 33 weeks). Meta-analysis of seven randomized, controlled trials (n = 1393) using a fixed effects model estimated a lower risk of NEC (relative risk, 0.36; 95% CI, 0.20–0.65) in the probiotic group than in controls. The reviewers conclude that probiotics might reduce the risk of NEC in preterm neonates of less than 33 weeks' gestation.

The short-term and long-term safety of probiotics still needs to be assessed in large trials [142,143]. Other unanswered questions pertaining to probiotic use relate to the selection of the optimal probiotic mixture (species, strain, single or combined), the dose and frequency of dosing, the rates of colonization, the duration of colonization, the role or efficacy of killed bacteria or their DNA in preventing NEC, adverse effects (especially systemic infection as a result of exposure to probiotics), and long-term effects on immune and gastrointestinal functions.

Swallowing amniotic fluid in utero is believed to be necessary for proper intestinal maturation. In a phase I trial, infants receiving simulated amniotic fluid (a sterile, noncaloric, growth factor–containing solution named "SAFEstart" [Simulated Amniotic Fluid for Enteral administration]), when compared to a control group consisting of neonates who met study criteria but were cared for during the period immediately preceding the study without the test fluid (SAFEstart), had higher caloric intakes over a period of first 21 day of life [144]. Subsequently a small randomized, controlled, masked trial has been completed with the findings of a trend towards better tolerance of milk feedings among infants who received test solution compared to control group who were given sham solution [145]. This finding suggests that supplementing at-risk infants with appropriate growth factors may help protect infants from developing NEC. SAFEstart contains erythropoietin and granulocyte-colony stimulating factor.

Receptors for these growth factors are found on luminal villus surfaces in the neonatal intestine; the binding of granulocyte-colony stimulating factor and erythropoietin to their receptors induces an antiapoptotic effect.

Another strategy proposed for the prevention of NEC involves the administration of enteral administration of a combination of IgG and IgA. There are no randomized, controlled trials of the use of oral IgA alone for the prevention of NEC. A Cochrane Neonatal Collaborative Review Group [146] concluded that the available evidence does not support the administration of oral immunoglobulin for the prevention of NEC.

Pentoxifylline has a significant role in inhibiting tumor necrosis factor-alpha and in reducing mucosal injury and improving healing in ischemia–reperfusion experiments. Experimental animal models using pentoxifyllin to prevent NEC have found mixed results [147,148].

Preoccupation with preventing NEC has contributed to the chronic undernourishment of stable, growing VLBW infants. Inadequate nutrient intakes can affect neurocognitive development adversely. Furthermore, delayed feeding and/or starvation is associated with fewer mucosal antibody cells, reduction in the local immune response, decreased enzyme levels, damage to mucosal barriers, increased susceptibility to infections, morphologic injury, bacterial overgrowth, and decreased secretion of IgA.

There is a substantial lack of uniformity in practice in the nutritional management of VLBW infants. This variability in practice includes practices such as initiation of enteral feeding, duration of trophic feeding, advances in feeding volume, addition of fortifiers, and increases in caloric density. The diversity of practice often exists even within institutions and among individual neonatologists working in a single group [149]. This diversity results from the poor understanding of the mechanisms involved in the pathophysiology of NEC and especially its relationship with feeding. Because NEC seldom occurs in infants who are not being fed, feedings have come to be seen as a major contributor to the onset of NEC. The notion that food is noxious has dominated the thinking; that notion continues to some extent today and is responsible for the major emphasis being placed on how to make feedings safe. Several aspects of feeding practices aimed at assessing measures of feeding tolerance and neonatal outcome have focused on the time of introduction of feedings, on the volume of feedings volumes, on the type of milk, and on the rate of increase in feeding volumes [46,121,123,150–152]. Despite the suggested advantages of advancing feedings more rapidly in premature low-birth-weight infants (ie, shorter time to regain birth weight and shorter time to achieve full feedings), the ideal rate of advancement remains unclear, particularly for extremely low birth weight infants (<1000 g) [121,122]. For high-risk neonates a universally tolerable safe limit of enteral feeding volume (daily total or increments per kg/d) may never be defined because of difficulties in interpreting "feeding intolerance" and the presence of other comorbid conditions that could alter the normal feeding tolerance. The use of dilute feedings has little rationale and should be avoided, because there is clear evidence that diluted feedings and water do not promote maturation of gastroduodenal motility as well as full-strength formula [153,154].

Summary

The incidence of neonatal NEC and the mortality stemming from this disease have not improved significantly during the last 40 years. Still, many animal and human studies have emerged to help clinicians unfold numerous pathophysiologic abnormalities at the cellular level. A better understanding of this basic information may improve significantly the outcomes of patients who have this potentially devastating disease. One of the more promising of the various strategies proposed for the prevention of NEC is the use of probiotics. Directions for future research to prevent NEC include investigation of (1) NO modulation of mucosal and vascular protective mechanisms in the developing intestine, in particular the role of arginine supplementation of the diet of preterm infants; (2) the use of platelet activating factor receptor antagonists or recombinant platelet activating factor-acetylhydrolase in preterm infants; (3) altering the nutrient composition of preterm infant formula, in particular as it relates to the lipid composition; (4) dietary supplementation with growth factors such as endothelial growth factor, insulin-like growth factor, and glutamine; and (5) further understanding of probiotics in terms of selection, dosing, duration, and short- and long-term effects.

Acknowledgments

The authors thank Rita Maier, Director, Health Education Library, New York Hospital Queens, and her staff for their timely help in providing the necessary resources related to literature search.

References

[1] Kliegman RM, Fanaroff AA. Necrotizing enterocolitis. N Engl J Med 1984;310(17): 1093–103.
[2] Srinivasan P, Burdjalov V. Necrotizing Enterocolitis. In: Spitzer AR. Intensive care of the Fetus and Neonate. 2nd edition. Philadelphia: Elsevier Mosby; 2005. p. 1027–45.
[3] Stoll BJ, Kanto WP Jr, Glass RI, et al. Epidemiology of necrotizing enterocolitis: a case control study. J Pediatr 1980;96(3 Pt 1):447–51.
[4] Hsueh W, Caplan MS, Qu XW, et al. Neonatal necrotizing enterocolitis: clinical considerations and pathogenetic concepts. Pediatr Dev Pathol 2003;6(1):6–23.
[5] Llanos AR, Moss ME, Pinzon MC, et al. Epidemiology of neonatal necrotising enterocolitis: a population-based study. Paediatr Perinat Epidemiol 2002;16(4):342–9.
[6] Guthrie SO, Gordon PV, Thomas V, et al. Necrotizing enterocolitis among neonates in the United States. J Perinatol 2003;23(4):278–85.
[7] Lin PW, Stoll BJ. Necrotising enterocolitis. Lancet 2006;368(9543):1271–83.
[8] Sankaran K, Puckett B, Lee DS, et al. Variations in incidence of necrotizing enterocolitis in Canadian neonatal intensive care units. J Pediatr Gastroenterol Nutr 2004;39(4):366–72.

[9] Lee SK, McMillan DD, Ohlsson A, et al. Variations in practice and outcomes in the Canadian NICU network: 1996–1997. Pediatrics 2000;106(5):1070–9.

[10] Guillet R, Stoll BJ, Cotten CM, et al. Association of H2-blocker therapy and higher incidence of necrotizing enterocolitis in very low birth weight infants. Pediatrics 2006;117(2): E137–42.

[11] Horbar JD, Badger GJ, Carpenter JH, et al. Trends in mortality and morbidity for very low birth weight infants, 1991–1999. Pediatrics 2002;110(1 Pt 1):143–51.

[12] Luig M, Lui K. Epidemiology of necrotizing enterocolitis–part I: changing regional trends in extremely preterm infants over 14 years. J Paediatr Child Health 2005;41(4):169–73.

[13] Harper RG, Rehman KU, Sia C, et al. Neonatal outcome of infants born at 500 to 800 grams from 1990 through 1998 in a tertiary care center. J Perinatol 2002;22(7):555–62.

[14] Luig M, Lui K. Epidemiology of necrotizing enterocolitis–part II: risks and susceptibility of premature infants during the surfactant era: a regional study. J Paediatr Child Health 2005; 41(4):174–9.

[15] Fanaroff AA, Hack M, Walsh MC. The NICHD Neonatal Research Network: changes in practice and outcomes during the first 15 years. Semin Perinatol 2003;27(4):281–7.

[16] Fanaroff AA, Stoll BJ, Wright LL, et al. Trends in neonatal morbidity and mortality for very low birthweight infants. Am J Obstet Gynecol 2007;196(2)(147):E141–8.

[17] Lemons JA, Bauer CR, Oh W, et al. Very low birth weight outcomes of the National Institute of Child Health and Human Development Neonatal Research Network, January 1995 through December 1996. NICHD Neonatal Research Network. Pediatrics 2001; 107(1):E1.

[18] Holman RC, Stoll BJ, Curns AT, et al. Necrotising enterocolitis hospitalisations among neonates in the United States. Paediatr Perinat Epidemiol 2006;20(6):498–506.

[19] Holman RC, Stoll BJ, Clarke MJ, et al. The epidemiology of necrotizing enterocolitis infant mortality in the United States. Am J Public Health 1997;87(12):2026–31.

[20] Ehrlich PF, Sato TT, Short BL, et al. Outcome of perforated necrotizing enterocolitis in the very low-birth weight neonate may be independent of the type of surgical treatment. Am Surg 2001;67(8):752–6.

[21] Henry MC, Lawrence Moss R. Surgical therapy for necrotizing enterocolitis: bringing evidence to the bedside. Semin Pediatr Surg 2005;14(3):181–90.

[22] Blakely ML, Lally KP, McDonald S, et al. Postoperative outcomes of extremely low birth-weight infants with necrotizing enterocolitis or isolated intestinal perforation: a prospective cohort study by the NICHD Neonatal Research Network. Ann Surg 2005;241(6):984–9 [discussion: 989–94].

[23] Warner B, Musial MJ, Chenier T, et al. The effect of birth hospital type on the outcome of very low birth weight infants. Pediatrics 2004;113(1 Pt 1):35–41.

[24] Roberts D, Dalziel S. Antenatal corticosteroids for accelerating fetal lung maturation for women at risk of preterm birth. Cochrane Database Syst Rev 2006;(3):CD004454.

[25] Uauy RD, Fanaroff AA, Korones SB, et al. Necrotizing enterocolitis in very low birth weight infants: biodemographic and clinical correlates. National Institute of Child Health and Human Development Neonatal Research Network. J Pediatr 1991;119(4):630–8.

[26] Grave GD, Nelson SA, Walker WA, et al. New therapies and preventive approaches for necrotizing enterocolitis: report of a research planning workshop. Pediatr Res 2007; 62(4):510–4.

[27] Gerber AR, Hopkins RS, Lauer BA, et al. Increased risk of illness among nursery staff caring for neonates with necrotizing enterocolitis. Pediatr Infect Dis 1985;4(3):246–9.

[28] Boccia D, Stolfi I, Lana S, et al. Nosocomial necrotising enterocolitis outbreaks: epidemiology and control measures. Eur J Pediatr 2001;160(6):385–91.

[29] Banyasz I, Bokodi G, Vasarhelyi B, et al. Genetic polymorphisms for vascular endothelial growth factor in perinatal complications. Eur Cytokine Netw 2006;17(4):266–70.

[30] Treszl A, Tulassay T, Vasarhelyi B. Genetic basis for necrotizing enterocolitis—risk factors and their relations to genetic polymorphisms. Front Biosci 2006;11:570–80.

[31] Treszl A, Heninger E, Kalman A, et al. Lower prevalence of IL-4 receptor alpha-chain gene G variant in very-low-birth-weight infants with necrotizing enterocolitis. J Pediatr Surg 2003;38(9):1374–8.

[32] Ostlie DJ, Spilde TL, St Peter SD, et al. Necrotizing enterocolitis in full-term infants. J Pediatr Surg 2003;38(7):1039–42.

[33] Ng S. Necrotizing enterocolitis in the full-term neonate. J Paediatr Child Health 2001;37(1): 1–4.

[34] Lambert DK, Christensen RD, Henry E, et al. Necrotizing enterocolitis in term neonates: data from a multihospital health-care system. J Perinatol 2007;27(7):437–43.

[35] McElhinney DB, Hedrick HL, Bush DM, et al. Necrotizing enterocolitis in neonates with congenital heart disease: risk factors and outcomes. Pediatrics 2000;106(5):1080–7.

[36] Maayan-Metzger A, Itzchak A, Mazkereth R, et al. Necrotizing enterocolitis in full-term infants: case-control study and review of the literature. J Perinatol 2004;24(8):494–9.

[37] Wiswell TE, Robertson CF, Jones TA, et al. Necrotizing enterocolitis in full-term infants. A case-control study. Am J Dis Child 1988;142(5):532–5.

[38] Bolisetty S, Lui K, Oei J, et al. A regional study of underlying congenital diseases in term neonates with necrotizing enterocolitis. Acta Paediatr 2000;89(10):1226–30.

[39] Kliegman RM, Walker WA, Yolken RH. Necrotizing enterocolitis: research agenda for a disease of unknown etiology and pathogenesis. Pediatr Res 1993;34(6):701–8.

[40] Santulli TV, Schullinger JN, Heird WC, et al. Acute necrotizing enterocolitis in infancy: a review of 64 cases. Pediatrics 1975;55(3):376–87.

[41] Kosloske AM. Pathogenesis and prevention of necrotizing enterocolitis: a hypothesis based on personal observation and a review of the literature. Pediatrics 1984;74(6):1086–92.

[42] Ballance WA, Dahms BB, Shenker N, et al. Pathology of neonatal necrotizing enterocolitis: a ten-year experience. J Pediatr 1990;117(1 Pt 2):S6–13.

[43] Hammerman C, Kaplan M. Probiotics and neonatal intestinal infection. Curr Opin Infect Dis 2006;19(3):277–82.

[44] Dunn L, Hulman S, Weiner J, et al. Beneficial effects of early hypocaloric enteral feeding on neonatal gastrointestinal function: preliminary report of a randomized trial. J Pediatr Apr 1988;112(4):622–9.

[45] McKeown RE, Marsh TD, Amarnath U, et al. Role of delayed feeding and of feeding increments in necrotizing enterocolitis. J Pediatr 1992;121(5 Pt 1):764–70.

[46] LaGamma EF, Ostertag SG, Birenbaum H. Failure of delayed oral feedings to prevent necrotizing enterocolitis. Results of study in very-low-birth-weight neonates. Am J Dis Child 1985;139(4):385–9.

[47] Berseth CL, Bisquera JA, Paje VU. Prolonging small feeding volumes early in life decreases the incidence of necrotizing enterocolitis in very low birth weight infants. Pediatrics 2003; 111(3):529–34.

[48] Rayyis SF, Ambalavanan N, Wright L, et al. Randomized trial of "slow" versus "fast" feed advancements on the incidence of necrotizing enterocolitis in very low birth weight infants. J Pediatr 1999;134(3):293–7.

[49] Anderson DM, Kliegman RM. The relationship of neonatal alimentation practices to the occurrence of endemic necrotizing enterocolitis. Am J Perinatol 1991;8(1):62–7.

[50] Bhat BA, Gupta B. Effects of human milk fortification on morbidity factors in very low birth weights infants. Ann Saudi Med 2001;21(5–6):292–5.

[51] Lucas A, Fewtrell MS, Morley R, et al. Randomized outcome trial of human milk fortification and developmental outcome in preterm infants. Am J Clin Nutr 1996;64(2):142–51.

[52] Claud EC, Walker WA. Hypothesis: inappropriate colonization of the premature intestine can cause neonatal necrotizing enterocolitis. Faseb J 2001;15(8):1398–403.

[53] Sase M, Miwa I, Sumie M, et al. Ontogeny of gastric emptying patterns in the human fetus. J Matern Fetal Neonatal Med 2005;17(3):213–7.

[54] Sase M, Lee JJ, Park JY, et al. Ontogeny of fetal rabbit upper gastrointestinal motility. J Surg Res 2001;101(1):68–72.

[55] Berseth CL. Neonatal small intestinal motility: motor responses to feeding in term and preterm infants. J Pediatr 1990;117(5):777–82.

[56] Berseth CL. Gestational evolution of small intestine motility in preterm and term infants. J Pediatr 1989;115(4):646–51.

[57] Berseth CL, Ittmann PI. Antral and duodenal motor responses to duodenal feeding in preterm and term infants. J Pediatr Gastroenterol Nutr 1992;14(2):182–6.

[58] Ittmann PI, Amarnath R, Berseth CL. Maturation of antroduodenal motor activity in preterm and term infants. Dig Dis Sci 1992;37(1):14–9.

[59] Di Lorenzo M, Bass J, Krantis A. An intraluminal model of necrotizing enterocolitis in the developing neonatal piglet. J Pediatr Surg 1995;30(8):1138–42.

[60] Sarna SK. Cyclic motor activity; migrating motor complex: 1985. Gastroenterology 1985; 89(4):894–913.

[61] Sase M, Lee JJ, Ross MG, et al. Effect of hypoxia on fetal rabbit gastrointestinal motility. J Surg Res 2001;99(2):347–51.

[62] Berseth CL, McCoy HH. Birth asphyxia alters neonatal intestinal motility in term neonates. Pediatrics 1992;90(5):669–73.

[63] Lebenthal A, Lebenthal E. The ontogeny of the small intestinal epithelium. JPEN J Parenter Enteral Nutr 1999;23(Suppl 5):S3–6.

[64] Hyman PE, Clarke DD, Everett SL, et al. Gastric acid secretory function in preterm infants. J Pediatr 1985;106(3):467–71.

[65] Antonowicz I, Lebenthal E. Developmental pattern of small intestinal enterokinase and disaccharidase activities in the human fetus. Gastroenterology 1977;72(6):1299–303.

[66] Lin J. Too much short chain fatty acids cause neonatal necrotizing enterocolitis. Med Hypotheses 2004;62(2):291–3.

[67] Muller CA, Autenrieth IB, Peschel A. Innate defenses of the intestinal epithelial barrier. Cell Mol Life Sci 2005;62(12):1297–307.

[68] Neu J, Chen M, Beierle E. Intestinal innate immunity: how does it relate to the pathogenesis of necrotizing enterocolitis. Semin Pediatr Surg 2005;14(3):137–44.

[69] Han X, Fink MP, Delude RL. Proinflammatory cytokines cause NO*-dependent and independent changes in expression and localization of tight junction proteins in intestinal epithelial cells. Shock 2003;19(3):229–37.

[70] Hecht G. Innate mechanisms of epithelial host defense: spotlight on intestine. Am J Physiol 1999;277(3 Pt 1):C351–8.

[71] Otte JM, Kiehne K, Herzig KH. Antimicrobial peptides in innate immunity of the human intestine. J Gastroenterol 2003;38(8):717–26.

[72] Ganz T. Defensins: antimicrobial peptides of innate immunity. Nat Rev Immunol 2003; 3(9):710–20.

[73] Chen H, Xu Z, Peng L, et al. Recent advances in the research and development of human defensins. Peptides 2006;27(4):931–40.

[74] van der Waaij LA, Mesander G, Limburg PC, et al. Direct flow cytometry of anaerobic bacteria in human feces. Cytometry 1994;16(3):270–9.

[75] Corfield AP, Myerscough N, Longman R, et al. Mucins and mucosal protection in the gastrointestinal tract: new prospects for mucins in the pathology of gastrointestinal disease. Gut 2000;47(4):589–94.

[76] Allen A, Bell A, Mantle M, et al. The structure and physiology of gastrointestinal mucus. Adv Exp Med Biol 1982;144:115–33.

[77] Caplan MS, Simon D, Jilling T. The role of PAF, TLR, and the inflammatory response in neonatal necrotizing enterocolitis. Semin Pediatr Surg 2005;14(3):145–51.

[78] Kliegman RM. Models of the pathogenesis of necrotizing enterocolitis. J Pediatr 1990; 117(1 Pt 2):S2–5.

[79] Edelson MB, Bagwell CE, Rozycki HJ. Circulating pro- and counterinflammatory cytokine levels and severity in necrotizing enterocolitis. Pediatrics 1999;103(4 Pt 1):766–71.

[80] Caplan MS, Sun XM, Hseuh W, et al. Role of platelet activating factor and tumor necrosis factor-alpha in neonatal necrotizing enterocolitis. J Pediatr 1990;116(6):960–4.

[81] Harris MC, D'Angio CT, Gallagher PR, et al. Cytokine elaboration in critically ill infants with bacterial sepsis, necrotizing enterocolitis, or sepsis syndrome: correlation with clinical parameters of inflammation and mortality. J Pediatr 2005;147(4):462–8.

[82] Harris MC, Costarino AT Jr, Sullivan JS, et al. Cytokine elevations in critically ill infants with sepsis and necrotizing enterocolitis. J Pediatr 1994;124(1):105–11.

[83] Lloyd JR. The etiology of gastrointestinal perforations in the newborn. J Pediatr Surg 1969; 4(1):77–84.

[84] Scholander PF. The master switch of life. Sci Am 1963;209:92–106.

[85] Alward CT, Hook JB, Helmrath TA, et al. Effects of asphyxia on cardiac output and organ blood flow in the newborn piglet. Pediatr Res 1978;12(8):824–7.

[86] Touloukian RJ, Posch JN, Spencer R. The pathogenesis of ischemic gastroenterocolitis of the neonate: selective gut mucosal ischemia in asphyxiated neonatal piglets. J Pediatr Surg 1972;7(2):194–205.

[87] Nowicki PT. The effects of ischemia-reperfusion on endothelial cell function in postnatal intestine. Pediatr Res 1996;39(2):267–74.

[88] Buckley NM, Jarenwattananon M, Gootman PM, et al. Autoregulatory escape from vaso-constriction of intestinal circulation in developing swine. Am J Physiol 1987;252(1 Pt 2): H118–24.

[89] Reber KM, Nankervis CA, Nowicki PT. Newborn intestinal circulation. Physiology and pathophysiology. Clin Perinatol 2002;29(1):23–39.

[90] Stoddart RW, Widdowson EM. Changes in the organs of pigs in response to feeding for the first 24 h after birth. III. Fluorescence histochemistry of the carbohydrates of the intestine. Biol Neonate 1976;29(1–2):18–27.

[91] Nankervis CA, Nowicki PT. Role of nitric oxide in regulation of vascular resistance in post-natal intestine. Am J Physiol 1995;268(6 Pt 1):G949–58.

[92] Nankervis CA, Dunaway DJ, Miller CE. Endothelin ET(A) and ET(B) receptors in post-natal intestine. Am J Physiol Gastrointest Liver Physiol 2001;280(4):G555–62.

[93] Su BY, Reber KM, Nankervis CA, et al. Development of the myogenic response in postnatal intestine: role of PKC. Am J Physiol Gastrointest Liver Physiol 2003;284(3): G445–52.

[94] Nankervis CA, Schauer GM, Miller CE. Endothelin-mediated vasoconstriction in postis-chemic newborn intestine. Am J Physiol Gastrointest Liver Physiol 2000;279(4):G683–91.

[95] Nowicki PT, Dunaway DJ, Nankervis CA, et al. Endothelin-1 in human intestine resected for necrotizing enterocolitis. J Pediatr 2005;146(6):805–10.

[96] Hooper LV, Wong MH, Thelin A, et al. Molecular analysis of commensal host-microbial relationships in the intestine. Science 2001;291(5505):881–4.

[97] Collier-Hyams LS, Neish AS. Innate immune relationship between commensal flora and the mammalian intestinal epithelium. Cell Mol Life Sci 2005;62(12):1339–48.

[98] Nanthakumar NN, Fusunyan RD, Sanderson I, et al. Inflammation in the developing hu-man intestine: a possible pathophysiologic contribution to necrotizing enterocolitis. Proc Natl Acad Sci U S A 2000;97(11):6043–8.

[99] Claud EC, Lu L, Anton PM, et al. Developmentally regulated IkappaB expression in intes-tinal epithelium and susceptibility to flagellin-induced inflammation. Proc Natl Acad Sci U S A 2004;101(19):7404–8.

[100] Stoll BJ, Gordon T, Korones SB, et al. Late-onset sepsis in very low birth weight neonates: a report from the National Institute of Child Health and Human Development Neonatal Research Network. J Pediatr 1996;129(1):63–71.

[101] Hoy CM, Wood CM, Hawkey PM, et al. Duodenal microflora in very-low-birth-weight neonates and relation to necrotizing enterocolitis. J Clin Microbiol 2000;38(12): 4539–47.

[102] de la Cochetiere MF, Piloquet H, des Robert C, et al. Early intestinal bacterial colonization and necrotizing enterocolitis in premature infants: the putative role of Clostridium. Pediatr Res 2004;56(3):366–70.

[103] Fanaro S, Chierici R, Guerrini P, et al. Intestinal microflora in early infancy: composition and development. Acta Paediatr Suppl 2003;91(441):48–55.

[104] Sakata H, Yoshioka H, Fujita K. Development of the intestinal flora in very low birth weight infants compared to normal full-term newborns. Eur J Pediatr 1985;144(2):186–90.

[105] Blakey JL, Lubitz L, Barnes GL, et al. Development of gut colonisation in pre-term neo-nates. J Med Microbiol 1982;15(4):519–29.

[106] Gewolb IH, Schwalbe RS, Taciak VL, et al. Stool microflora in extremely low birthweight infants. Arch Dis Child Fetal Neonatal Ed 1999;80(3):F167–73.

[107] Deitch EA. Role of bacterial translocation in necrotizing enterocolitis. Acta Paediatr Suppl 1994;396:33–6.

[108] Van Camp JM, Drongowski R, Gorman R, et al. Colonization of intestinal bacteria in the normal neonate: comparison between mouth and rectal swabs and small and large bowel specimens. J Pediatr Surg 1994;29(10):1348–51.

[109] Musemeche CA, Kosloske AM, Bartow SA, et al. Comparative effects of ischemia, bacteria, and substrate on the pathogenesis of intestinal necrosis. J Pediatr Surg 1986;21(6):536–8.

[110] Brown EG, Sweet AY. Preventing necrotizing enterocolitis in neonates. JAMA 1978; 240(22):2452–4.

[111] La Gamma EF, Browne LE. Feeding practices for infants weighing less than 1500 g at birth and the pathogenesis of necrotizing enterocolitis. Clin Perinatol 1994;21(2):271–306.

[112] Yanowitz TD, Yao AC, Werner JC, et al. Effects of prophylactic low-dose indomethacin on hemodynamics in very low birth weight infants. J Pediatr 1998;132(1):28–34.

[113] Pezzati M, Vangi V, Biagiotti R, et al. Effects of indomethacin and ibuprofen on mesenteric and renal blood flow in preterm infants with patent ductus arteriosus. J Pediatr 1999;135(6): 733–8.

[114] Bellander M, Ley D, Polberger S, et al. Tolerance to early human milk feeding is not com-promised by indomethacin in preterm infants with persistent ductus arteriosus. Acta Pae-diatr 2003;92(9):1074–8.

[115] Huang CF, Tsai MC, Chu CH, et al. The influence of pacifier sucking on mesenteric blood flow in infants. Clin Pediatr (Phila) 2003;42(6):543–6.

[116] Lucas A, Cole TJ. Breast milk and neonatal necrotising enterocolitis. Lancet 1990; 336(8730):1519–23.

[117] McGuire W, Anthony MY. Donor human milk versus formula for preventing necrotising enterocolitis in preterm infants: systematic review. Arch Dis Child Fetal Neonatal Ed 2003; 88(1):F11–4.

[118] Henderson G, Craig S, Brocklehurst P, et al. Enteral feeding regimens and necrotising en-terocolitis in preterm infants: multi-centre case-control study. Arch Dis Child Fetal Neona-tal Ed, Epub ahead of print.

[119] Salhotra A, Ramji S. Slow versus fast enteral feed advancement in very low birth weight infants: a randomized control trial. Indian Pediatr 2004;41(5):435–41.

[120] Kliegman RM. The relationship of neonatal feeding practices and the pathogenesis and prevention of necrotizing enterocolitis. Pediatrics 2003;111(3):671–2.

[121] Kennedy KA, Tyson JE, Chamnanvanakij S. Rapid versus slow rate of advancement of feedings for promoting growth and preventing necrotizing enterocolitis in parenterally fed low-birth-weight infants. Cochrane Database Syst Rev 2000;(2):CD001241.

[122] Kennedy KA, Tyson JE, Chamnanvanikij S. Early versus delayed initiation of progressive enteral feedings for parenterally fed low birth weight or preterm infants. Cochrane Data-base Syst Rev 2000;(2):CD001970.

[123] Schanler RJ, Lau C, Hurst NM, et al. Randomized trial of donor human milk versus pre-term formula as substitutes for mothers' own milk in the feeding of extremely premature infants. Pediatrics 2005;116(2):400–6.

[124] Shin CE, Falcone RA Jr, Stuart L, et al. Diminished epidermal growth factor levels in infants with necrotizing enterocolitis. J Pediatr Surg 2000;35(2):173–6 [discussion: 177].

[125] Warner BB, Ryan AL, Seeger K, et al. Ontogeny of salivary epidermal growth factor and necrotizing enterocolitis [see comment]. J Pediatr 2007;150(4):358–63.

[126] Buyukunal C, Kilic N, Dervisoglu S, et al. Maternal cocaine abuse resulting in necrotizing enterocolitis–an experimental study in a rat model. Acta Paediatr Suppl 1994;396:91–3.

[127] Kilic N, Buyukunal C, Dervisoglu S, et al. Maternal cocaine abuse resulting in necrotizing enterocolitis. An experimental study in a rat model. II. Results of perfusion studies. Pediatr Surg Int 2000;16(3):176–8.

[128] Lopez SL, Taeusch HW, Findlay RD, et al. Time of onset of necrotizing enterocolitis in newborn infants with known prenatal cocaine exposure. Clin Pediatr (Phila) 1995;34(8): 424–9.

[129] Czyrko C, Del Pin CA, O'Neill JA Jr, et al. Maternal cocaine abuse and necrotizing enterocolitis: outcome and survival. J Pediatr Surg 1991;26(4):414–8 [discussion: 419–21].

[130] Mally P, Golombek SG, Mishra R, et al. Association of necrotizing enterocolitis with elective packed red blood cell transfusions in stable, growing, premature neonates. Am J Perinatol 2006;23(8):451–8.

[131] Schanler RJ. Evaluation of the evidence to support current recommendations to meet the needs of premature infants: the role of human milk. Am J Clin Nutr 2007;85(2):625S–8S.

[132] Schanler RJ, Shulman RJ, Lau C. Feeding strategies for premature infants: beneficial outcomes of feeding fortified human milk versus preterm formula. Pediatrics 1999;103(6 Pt 1): 1150–7.

[133] Siu YK, Ng PC, Fung SC, et al. Double blind, randomised, placebo controlled study of oral vancomycin in prevention of necrotising enterocolitis in preterm, very low birthweight infants. Arch Dis Child Fetal Neonatal Ed 1998;79(2):F105–9.

[134] Lin HC, Su BH, Chen AC, et al. Oral probiotics reduce the incidence and severity of necrotizing enterocolitis in very low birth weight infants. Pediatrics 2005;115(1):1–4.

[135] Bin-Nun A, Bromiker R, Wilschanski M, et al. Oral probiotics prevent necrotizing enterocolitis in very low birth weight neonates. J Pediatr 2005;147(2):192–6.

[136] Dani C, Biadaioli R, Bertini G, et al. Probiotics feeding in prevention of urinary tract infection, bacterial sepsis and necrotizing enterocolitis in preterm infants. A prospective double-blind study. Biol Neonate 2002;82(2):103–8.

[137] Shah P, Shah V. Arginine supplementation for prevention of necrotising enterocolitis in preterm infants. Cochrane Database Syst Rev 2007;(3):CD004339.

[138] Bury RG, Tudehope D. Enteral antibiotics for preventing necrotizing enterocolitis in low birthweight or preterm infants. Cochrane Database Syst Rev 2001;(1):CD000405.

[139] Caplan MS, Miller-Catchpole R, Kaup S, et al. Bifidobacterial supplementation reduces the incidence of necrotizing enterocolitis in a neonatal rat model. Gastroenterology 1999; 117(3):577–83.

[140] Barlow B, Santulli TV, Heird WC, et al. An experimental study of acute neonatal enterocolitis—the importance of breast milk. J Pediatr Surg 1974;9(5):587–95.

[141] Schanler RJ. Probiotics and necrotising enterocolitis in premature infants. Arch Dis Child Fetal Neonatal Ed 2006;91(6):F395–7.

[142] Deshpande G, Rao S, Patole S. Probiotics for prevention of necrotising enterocolitis in preterm neonates with very low birthweight: a systematic review of randomised controlled trials. Lancet 2007;369(9573):1614–20.

[143] Bell EF. Preventing necrotizing enterocolitis: what works and how safe? Pediatrics 2005; 115(1):173–4.

[144] Christensen RD, Havranek T, Gerstmann DR, et al. Enteral administration of a simulated amniotic fluid to very low birth weight neonates. J Perinatol 2005 Jun;25(6):380–5.

[145] Barney CK, Lambert DK, Alder SC, et al. Treating feeding intolerance with an enteral solution patterned after human amniotic fluid: a randomized, controlled, masked trial. J Perinatol 2007 Jan;27(1):28–31.

[146] Foster J, Cole M. Oral immunoglobulin for preventing necrotizing enterocolitis in preterm and low birth-weight neonates. Cochrane Database Syst Rev 2004;(1):CD001816.

[147] Travadi J, Patole S, Charles A, et al. Pentoxifylline reduces the incidence and severity of necrotizing enterocolitis in a neonatal rat model. Pediatr Res 2006;60(2):185–9.

[148] Erdener D, Bakirtas F, Alkanat M, et al. Pentoxifylline does not prevent hypoxia/reoxygenation-induced necrotizing enterocolitis. An experimental study. Biol Neonate 2004;86(1): 29–33.

[149] Ziegler EE, Thureen PJ, Carlson SJ. Aggressive nutrition of the very low birthweight infant. Clin Perinatol 2002;29(2):225–44.

[150] Ostertag SG, LaGamma EF, Reisen CE, et al. Early enteral feeding does not affect the incidence of necrotizing enterocolitis. Pediatrics 1986;77(3):275–80.

[151] Tyson JE, Kennedy KA. Minimal enteral nutrition for promoting feeding tolerance and preventing morbidity in parenterally fed infants. Cochrane Database Syst Rev 2000;(2): CD000504.

[152] Tyson JE, Kennedy KA. Trophic feedings for parenterally fed infants. Cochrane Database Syst Rev 2005;(3):CD000504.

[153] Baker JH, Berseth CL. Duodenal motor responses in preterm infants fed formula with varying concentrations and rates of infusion. Pediatr Res 1997;42(5):618–22.

[154] Berseth CL, Nordyke C. Enteral nutrients promote postnatal maturation of intestinal motor activity in preterm infants. Am J Physiol 1993;264(6 Pt 1):G1046–51.

ELSEVIER
SAUNDERS

CLINICS IN
PERINATOLOGY

Clin Perinatol 35 (2008) 273–281

Pulmonary Complications of Mechanical Ventilation in Neonates

J. Davin Miller, MD, Waldemar A. Carlo, MD*

*Division of Neonatology, Department of Pediatrics, University of Alabama at Birmingham,
525 New Hillman Building, 619 19th Street South, Birmingham, AL 35233-7335, USA*

Mechanical ventilation is a common therapy to treat infants with respiratory insufficiency. Advances in pulmonary care such as surfactant replacement therapy and improved mechanical ventilation have reduced the mortality of infants, but important respiratory morbidities continue to affect preterm and term infants [1,2]. Lung and airway injury can be attributed to natural causes, such as pulmonary or systemic infection, or to complications of mechanical ventilation. Complications of mechanical ventilation include volutrauma, extrapulmonary air leak syndromes, traumatic injury to large airways, and endotracheal tube complications.

Volutrauma

Experimental data demonstrate that mechanical ventilation using both high tidal volumes and high peak pressures can cause lung injury [3–6]; however, data from various investigators consistently demonstrate that, regardless of the peak pressure, markers of lung injury in animals are increased with high tidal volume ventilation but not with low tidal volume ventilation [7–10]. Only a few breaths of large tidal volume ventilation immediately after birth can reduce subsequent lung compliance and diminish the response to exogenous surfactant in surfactant-deficient lambs [11]. Furthermore, most experimental animal studies investigating ventilator-associated lung injury use high tidal volumes, not low tidal volumes, to induce the injury.

At the microscopic and molecular level, volutrauma caused by mechanical overdistention leads to a diverse array of abnormalities. Alveolar

---

* Corresponding author.
E-mail address: wcarlo@peds.uab.edu (W.A. Carlo).

0095-5108/08/$ - see front matter © 2008 Elsevier Inc. All rights reserved.
doi:10.1016/j.clp.2007.11.004   *perinatology.theclinics.com*

epithelial cell damage, alveolar protein leakage, altered lymphatic flow, hyaline membrane formation, and inflammatory cell influx can be seen in the lungs of animals after high tidal volume ventilation [12–15]. Volutrauma can also decrease lung compliance and alter surfactant structure and function [11,15–18]. The expression of genes involved in inflammatory signaling is up-regulated after mechanical ventilation with high tidal volumes [14,15,19,20]. These data suggest that changes at the microscopic and molecular level due to injurious mechanical ventilation could adversely affect the structure and function of the lung.

Because lung injury contributes to bronchopulmonary dysplasia (BPD), efforts to decrease volutrauma in preterm infants should decrease the risk of this disorder [21]. Most published randomized controlled trials in neonates testing "lung protective" strategies with conventional mechanical ventilation have compared volume-targeted modes with pressure-limited modes and have not used different predetermined tidal volumes in each treatment arm [22–25]. The assumption while using volume-targeted modes of conventional mechanical ventilation is that lower tidal volumes are delivered as compliance improves when compared with the volumes associated with pressure-limited ventilation. Over time, these lower volumes may translate into decreased volutrauma and decrease the risk of BPD. Various investigators have compared these two modes of ventilation to test the hypothesis that volume-targeted ventilation decreases the incidence of BPD. A meta-analysis of four such trials demonstrated a significant decrease in pneumothorax (2% versus 13%; relative risk [RR], 0.23; CI, 0.07–0.76; number needed to treat [NNT], 9) and trends toward decreased death and BPD [26]. The combined outcome of death or BPD was not reported in any trial included in the analysis. Other protective ventilatory strategies such as permissive hypercapnia have been tested using randomized controlled trials in preterm infants. Even though all three permissive hypercapnia trials aimed to decrease volutrauma, respiratory frequency, not tidal volume, was changed the most to achieve different PCO_2 targets [27–29].

Only one recent prospective randomized controlled trial has evaluated the effects of using different predetermined tidal volumes to ventilate preterm infants. Lista and colleagues [30] used volume-guarantee ventilation and compared tracheal aspirate cytokine levels in 30 preterm infants ventilated with 3 mL/kg versus 5 mL/kg of tidal volume. The primary hypothesis was that, when compared with a tidal volume of 5 mL/kg, using low tidal volumes (3 mL/kg) would induce less inflammation, reduce ventilation time, and reduce the incidence of BPD. Interestingly, reduction of the tidal volume from 5 mL/kg to 3 mL/kg actually increased the markers of lung injury, prolonged the total time of mechanical ventilation, and did not change the incidence of BPD [30]. Another mechanism of lung injury is repeated collapse and re-opening of alveoli, but there are insufficient data in immature lungs [5]. The best ventilator strategy may consist of using adequate positive end-expiratory pressure (PEEP) to maintain functional residual capacity (FRC) to avoid atelectrauma and using an optimal tidal volume to avoid volutrauma (Fig. 1) [31].

A single respiratory intervention (ie, using a particular ventilator mode or a specific tidal volume) may minimize lung injury from volutrauma but is unlikely to substantially decrease the incidence of a multifactorial disease such as BPD. To improve long-term respiratory outcomes, clinicians must focus on many aspects of neonatal care. Walsh and colleagues [32] designed a randomized controlled trial to test the hypothesis that care practices at hospitals with a low incidence of BPD (benchmark centers) could be emulated and to determine whether those practices would decrease the incidence of BPD. The respiratory practices at benchmark centers thought to be effective in reducing BPD were using lower tidal volumes and peak pressures, aggressively weaning infants from the ventilator to nasal continuous positive airway pressure, avoiding routine suction procedures, avoiding hand-bagging ventilated infants, accepting higher PCO_2 values, and using surfactant early once an infant was intubated. Interestingly, the trial reported that successfully changing respiratory care practices did not reduce the incidence of BPD. A multifactorial benchmarking approach to neonatal respiratory care and ventilator management may help minimize lung injury from pulmonary complications such as volutrauma, but more data are needed to identify potential better care practices.

Few clinical trials have investigated pulmonary and long-term outcomes using low versus high tidal volume ventilation in preterm infants. Current evidence from experimental studies suggests that volutrauma from high tidal volume ventilation or from inadequate maintenance of the FRC with PEEP is injurious to the preterm lung and should be avoided [5,7–10]. Although the

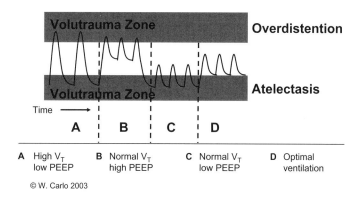

© W. Carlo 2003

Fig. 1. Which volumes cause lung injury? (A) A large tidal volume (V_T) with inadequate PEEP may cause lung injury due to overdistention and atelectasis. (B) A normal tidal volume with high PEEP may also cause volutrauma. (A and C) A low PEEP may cause lung injury secondary to collapse and reopening of alveoli. (D) Optimal ventilation with a tidal volume and PEEP that avoids both injury zones. (Courtesy of W. Carlo, MD, Birmingham, AL.)

pathogenesis of BPD is multifactorial, volutrauma caused by mechanical ventilation may be an important factor to minimize with ventilator strategies that avoid overdistention and atelectasis. The precise tidal volume required to minimize volutrauma is not known; however, efforts to limit tidal volume may be a beneficial practice in the neonatal intensive care unit [32].

Air leak syndromes

Complications of mechanical ventilation related to volutrauma include various types of extrapulmonary air leakage, such as pneumothorax and pulmonary interstitial emphysema. Air leak syndromes are important causes of morbidity and mortality in neonates [33,34]. In fact, Powers and colleagues reported that infants weighing less than 1500 g and diagnosed with pneumothorax during the first 24 hours of life were 13 times more likely to die or have BPD [34]. Pneumothorax is associated with respiratory distress syndrome, meconium aspiration syndrome, and pulmonary hypoplasia but can also occur in non-ventilated neonates. The incidence of pneumothorax in infants weighing less than 1500 g during 1991 to 1999 in the Vermont Oxford Neonatal Network Database ranged from 8.6% in 1991 to 5.1% in 1996 [35]. Recent retrospective data from the National Institute of Child Health and Development (NICHD) Neonatal Research Network suggest that pneumothorax is more common in extremely low birth weight infants, but this is confounded by the higher need for mechanical ventilation and severity of lung disease in these infants [1]. The incidence of pneumothorax in the NICHD Neonatal Research Network from 1990 to 2002 was 13% in infants weighing 501 to 750 g and 2% in infants weighing 1251 to 1500 g [1].

Clinical data identifying risk factors associated with pneumothorax can be obtained from randomized controlled trials comparing different ventilator modes or strategies for preterm infants. Analysis of three randomized controlled trials comparing high rate positive-pressure ventilation (rate > 60 breaths per minute) with conventional mechanical ventilation in neonates showed that using rates greater than 60 breaths per minute was associated with a decreased risk of air leakage (RR, 0.69; CI, 0.51–0.93; NNT, 11) [36]. Another analysis of four randomized controlled trials evaluating long versus short inspiratory times using conventional mechanical ventilation in intubated infants with respiratory distress syndrome showed that a long inspiratory time (> 0.5 seconds) was associated with an increased risk of pneumothorax (36% versus 24%; RR, 1.56; CI, 1.24–1.97; NNH, 8) [37]. Elective high-frequency oscillatory ventilation has also been evaluated in multiple randomized controlled trials to determine whether this therapy is beneficial in preterm infants. An analysis of 16 trials comparing elective high-frequency ventilation with conventional ventilation showed a significant increase in air leakage in the high-frequency group (29% versus 24%; RR, 1.23; CI, 1.06–1.44; NNH, 28) [38]. This association was consistent in the fixed effect model and random effects model in this analysis. One randomized controlled trial investigated the role of high-frequency oscillatory ventilation in preventing new air leaks in high-risk infants versus conventional mechanical ventilation [39]. This study reported a significant decrease in new air leaks (42% versus 63%; $P < .005$; NNT, 5), although the incidence of air leaks in the control group with conventional mechanical ventilation was high (63%), and the majority of patients were not treated with surfactant [39]. High-frequency jet ventilation has also been studied as a means to decrease chronic lung disease. Two trials demonstrated a nonsignificant decrease in the risk for air leaks in favor of elective high-frequency jet ventilation (39% versus 32%; RR, 0.82; CI, 0.55–1.22) [40].

Retrospective data can also help define care practices or risk factors associated with extrapulmonary air leakage. In a case-control study of very low birth weight infants from 1997 to 2002, pneumothorax developed in 10.9% of infants. Multivariate analysis showed that maximal peak inspiratory pressures during the 24 hours before diagnosis (odds ratio [OR], 2.84; CI, 1.6–5.4) and the number of suction procedures during the 8 hours before diagnosis (OR, 1.56; CI 1.09–2.23) were both independently associated with pneumothorax [41]. Other studies that included both ventilated preterm and term infants in the analysis identified low birth weight (OR, 19.3; CI 2.3–160.2), the administration of bag and mask ventilation (OR, 29; CI 3.6–233.5), endotracheal tube displacement (64% in infants with air leaks versus 18.5% in controls, $P < .05$), and an increase in clinical interventions including suction procedures, chest radiography, reintubation, and chest compressions as variables associated with pneumothorax [42–44]. Watkinson and Tiron [42] analyzed data from 606 ventilated neonates and reported that overventilation (defined as a $PaCO_2$ <30 mm Hg) was not associated with pneumothorax. Regardless of whether associated variables are causative or merely a result of an undiagnosed air leak, identifying those infants at highest risk is important and may improve long-term outcome if subsequent air leak is prevented.

Pulmonary interstitial emphysema is another form of air leak that is associated with increases in mortality and morbidity in preterm infants [34,45]. It is characterized by leakage of gas from the alveoli that becomes trapped inside the interstitial spaces of the lung. Pulmonary interstitial emphysema is diagnosed based on the presence of coarse, non-branching, radiolucencies on chest radiography that project toward the periphery of the lung in a disorganized fashion [46]. This appearance must not be confused with an air bronchogram, a classic radiographic sign of respiratory distress syndrome. Air bronchograms show long, smooth, branching radiolucencies that follow normal anatomic distributions similar to the bronchial tree [46]. The incidence of pulmonary interstitial emphysema in the randomized controlled trials evaluating prophylactic versus rescue surfactant therapy was about 3% to 5% [47]. In one recent retrospective study, risk factors for pulmonary interstitial emphysema included a higher maximum inspired oxygen concentration and higher mean airway pressures when compared with that in control subjects, and these factors were associated with an increased risk of death in infants weighing less than 1000 g [34].

Tracheal injury and endotracheal tube complications

Subglottic stenosis is a complication that occurs in approximately 1% to 2% of intubated neonates [48,49]. In one study, the incidence of subglottic stenosis was greater if the ratio of the external diameter of the endotracheal tube divided by the gestational age of the infant in weeks was more than 0.1 [50]. A recent case series described subglottic cysts as an abnormality often seen in conjunction with subglottic stenosis. Subglottic cysts are a recognized complication of intubation in preterm infants and may develop many months after extubation [51]. Tracheal perforation is a rare complication of endotracheal intubation. The data identifying risk factors and the incidence of tracheal perforation are limited to case reports. The mortality associated with this complication is high (75% in one study) and is likely due to vascular, cardiac, and respiratory compromise secondary to air leak [52]. Palatal deformities such as palatal grooves, asymmetry, and a high-arched palate also occur after long-term mechanical ventilation [53]. Despite subsequent palatal growth and remodeling after extubation, abnormalities can persist for many years [53,54]. Tracheal trauma and endotracheal tube complications may be minimized by using smaller endotracheal tubes, by minimizing reintubation attempts, and by aggressively weaning preterm infants off of mechanical ventilator support.

Summary

Mechanical ventilation is necessary and life saving in many neonates. Most complications are inherent to this intervention and cannot be confused with iatrogenic errors in judgment or care practices by clinicians. Clinical data suggest that complications such as volutrauma and air leak syndromes can negatively affect long-term pulmonary and non-pulmonary outcomes. One specific intervention or strategy is unlikely to decrease complications of mechanical ventilation. Careful attention to many aspects of neonatal care, such as delivery room resuscitation, ventilatory support, and routine care practices, is needed to decrease pulmonary complications of mechanical ventilation. Clinical research is needed to improve mechanical ventilator strategies to reduce pulmonary complications and improve long-term outcomes.

References

[1] Fanaroff AA, Stoll BJ, Wright LL, et al. Trends in neonatal morbidity and mortality for very low birth weight infants. Am J Obstet Gynecol 2007;147:e1–147.

[2] Lemons JA, Bauer CR, Oh W, et al. Very low birth weight outcomes of the National Institute of Child Health and Human Development Neonatal Research Network, January 1995 through December 1996. Pediatrics 2001;107:1–8.

[3] Attar MA, Donn SM. Mechanisms of ventilator-induced lung injury in premature infants. Semin Neonatol 2002;7:353–60.

[4] Dreyfuss D, Saumon G. Role of tidal volume, FRC and end-inspiratory volume in the development of pulmonary edema following mechanical ventilation. Am Rev Respir Dis 1993;48:1194–203.

[5] Muscedere JG, Mullen JB, Gan K, et al. Tidal ventilation at low airway pressures can augment lung injury. Am J Respir Crit Care Med 1994;149:1327–34.

[6] Auten RL, Vozzelli M, Clark RH. Volutrauma: what is it, and how do we avoid it? Clin Perinatol 2001;28:505–15.

[7] Peevy KJ, Hernandez LA, Moise AA, et al. Barotrauma and microvascular injury in lungs of nonadult rabbits: effect of ventilation pattern. Crit Care Med 1990;18:634–7.

[8] Carlton DP, Cummings JJ, Scheerer RG, et al. Lung overexpansion increases pulmonary microvascular protein permeability in young lambs. J Appl Physiol 1990;9:577–83.

[9] Hernandez LA, Peevy KJ, Moise AA, et al. Chest wall restriction limits high airway pressure-induced lung injury in young rabbits. J Appl Physiol 1999;66:2364–8.

[10] Parker JC, Hernandez LA, Peevy KJ. Mechanisms of ventilator-induced lung injury. Crit Care Med 1993;21:131–43.

[11] Ingimarsson J, Björklund LJ, Curstedt T, et al. Incomplete protection by prophylactic surfactant against the adverse effects of large lung inflations at birth in immature lambs. Intensive Care Med 2004;30(7):1446–53.

[12] Björklund LJ, Ingimarsson J, Curstedt T, et al. Manual ventilation with a few large breaths at birth compromises the therapeutic effect of subsequent surfactant replacement in immature lambs. Pediatr Res 1997;42(3):348–55.

[13] Wada K, Jobe AH, Ikegami M. Tidal volume effects on surfactant treatment responses with the initiation of ventilation in preterm lambs. J Appl Physiol 1997;83(4):1054–61.

[14] Hillman NH, Moss TJM, Kallapur SG, et al. Brief, large tidal volume ventilation initiates lung injury and a systemic response in fetal sheep. Am J Respir Crit Care Med 2007;176:575–81.

[15] Copland IB, Kavanagh BP, Engelberts D, et al. Early changes in lung gene expression due to high tidal volume. Am J Respir Crit Care Med 2003;168:1051–9.

[16] Simbruner G, Mittal RA, Smith J, et al. Effects of duration and amount of lung stretch at biophysical, biochemical, histological, and transcriptional levels in an in vivo rabbit model of mild lung injury. Am J Perinatol 2007;24(3):149–59.

[17] Veldhuizen RAW, Welk B, Harbottle R, et al. Mechanical ventilation of isolated rat lungs changes the structure and biophysical properties of surfactant. J Appl Physiol 2002;92:1169–75.

[18] Panda AK, Nag K, Harbottle RR, et al. Effect of acute lung injury on structure and function of pulmonary surfactant films. Am J Respir Cell Mol Biol 2004;30:641–50.

[19] Copland IB, Martinez F, Kavanagh BP, et al. High tidal volume ventilation causes different inflammatory responses in newborn versus adult lung. Am J Respir Crit Care Med 2004;169:739–48.

[20] Copland IB, Post M. Stretch-activated signaling pathways responsible for early response gene expression in fetal lung epithelial cells. J Cell Physiol 2007;210:133–43.

[21] Jobe AH, Ikegami M. Mechanisms initiating lung injury in the preterm. Early Hum Dev 1998;53:81–94.

[22] Keszler M, Abubakar K. Volume guarantee: stability of tidal volume and incidence of hypocarbia. Pediatr Pulmonol 2004;38:240–5.

[23] Lista G, Colnaghi M, Castoldi F, et al. Impact of targeted-volume ventilation on lung inflammatory response in preterm infants with respiratory distress syndrome (RDS). Pediatr Pulmonol 2004;37:510–4.

[24] Piotrowski A, Sobala W, Kawczynski P. Patient-initiated, pressure-regulated, volume-controlled ventilation compared with intermittent mandatory ventilation in neonates: a prospective, randomised study. Intensive Care Med 1997;23:975–81.

[25] Sinha S, Donn S, Gavey J, et al. Randomised trial of volume controlled versus time cycled, pressure limited ventilation in preterm infants with respiratory distress syndrome. Arch Dis Child Fetal Neonatal Ed 1997;77:F202–5.

[26] McCallion N, Davis PG, Morley CJ. Volume-targeted versus pressure-limited ventilation in the neonate. Cochrane Database Syst Rev 2005;(3):20:CD003666.

[27] Mariani G, Cifuentes J, Carlo WA. Randomized trial of permissive hypercapnia in preterm infants. Pediatrics 1999;104:1082–8.

[28] Carlo WA, Stark AR, Wright LL, et al. Minimal ventilation to prevent bronchopulmonary dysplasia in extremely-low-birth-weight infants. J Pediatr 2002;141:370–4.

[29] Thome UH, Carroll W, Wu TJ, et al. Outcome of extremely preterm infants randomized at birth to different PaCO$_2$ targets during the first seven days of life. Biol Neonate 2006;90: 218–25.

[30] Lista G, Castoldi F, Fontana P, et al. Lung inflammation in preterm infants with respiratory distress syndrome: effects of ventilation with different tidal volumes. Pediatr Pulmonol 2006; 41:357–63.

[31] Carlo WA. Permissive hypercapnia and permissive hypoxemia in neonates. J Perinatol 2007; 27(Suppl):S64–70.

[32] Walsh M, Laptook A, Kazzi SN, et al. A cluster-randomized trial of benchmarking and multimodal quality improvement to improve rates of survival free of bronchopulmonary dysplasia for infants with birth weights of less than 1250 grams. Pediatrics 2007;119:876–90.

[33] Powers WF, Clemens JD. Prognostic implications of age at detection of air leak in very low birth weight infants requiring ventilatory support. J Pediatr 1993;123(4):611–7.

[34] Verma RP, Chandra S, Niwas R, et al. Risk factors and clinical outcomes of pulmonary interstitial emphysema in extremely low birth weight infants. J Perinatol 2006;26(3):197–200.

[35] Horbar JD, Badger GJ, Carpenter JH, et al. Trends in mortality and morbidity for very low birth weight infants 1991–1999. Pediatrics 2002;110:143–51.

[36] Greenough A, Milner AD, Dimitriou G. Synchronized mechanical ventilation for respiratory support in newborn infants. Cochrane Database Syst Rev 2004;(4):18:CD000456.

[37] Kamlin CO, Davis PG. Long versus short inspiratory times in neonates receiving mechanical ventilation. Cochrane Database Syst Rev 2004;(4):CD004503.

[38] Thome UH, Carlo WA, Pohlandt F. Ventilation strategies and outcome in randomised trials of high frequency ventilation. Arch Dis Child Fetal Neonatal Ed 2005;90(6):F466–73.

[39] HiFO Study Group. Randomized study of high-frequency oscillatory ventilation in infants with severe respiratory distress syndrome. J Pediatr 1993;122(4):609–19.

[40] Bhuta T, Henderson-Smart DJ. Elective high frequency jet ventilation versus conventional ventilation for respiratory distress syndrome in preterm infants. Cochrane Database Syst Rev 2000;(2):CD000328.

[41] Klinger G, Ish-Hurwitz S, Sirota L, et al. Risk factors for pneumothorax in very low birth weight infants. Presented at the Pediatric Academic Societies' 2006 Annual Meeting. San Francisco, April 29–May 2, 2006.

[42] Watkinson M, Tiron I. Events before the diagnosis of a pneumothorax in ventilated neonates. Arch Dis Child Fetal Neonatal Ed 2001;85:F201–3.

[43] Niwas R, Nadroo AM, Sutija VG, et al. Malposition of endotracheal tube: association with pneumothorax in ventilated neonates. Arch Dis Child Fetal Neonatal Ed 2007;92:F233–4.

[44] Ngerncham S, Kittiratsatcha P, Pacharn P. Risk factors of pneumothorax during the first 24 hours of life. J Med Assoc Thai 2005;88(8):S135–41.

[45] Kraybill EN, Rynan DK, Bose CL, et al. Risk factors for chronic lung disease in infants with birth weight of 751–1000 gms. J Pediatr 1989;155:115–20.

[46] Sivit CJ. Diagnostic imaging. In: Martin RJ, Fanaroff AA, Walsh MC, editors. Neonatal-perinatal medicine: diseases of the fetus and newborn, vol. 1. 8th edition. Philadelphia: Mosby; 2007. p. 713–31.

[47] Morley CJ. Systematic review of prophylactic vs. rescue surfactant. Arch Dis Child Fetal Neonatal Ed 1997;77(1):F70–4.

[48] Walner DL, Loewen MS, Kimura RE. Neonatal subglottic stenosis: incidence and trends. Laryngoscope 2001;111(1):48–51.

[49] Choi SS, Zalzal GH. Changing trends in neonatal subglottic stenosis. Otolaryngol Head Neck Surg 2000;122(1):61–3.

[50] Sherman JM, Nelson H. Decreased incidence of subglottic stenosis using an "appropriate-sized" endotracheal tube in neonates. Pediatr Pulmonol 1989;6(3):183–5.

[51] Johnson LB, Rutter MJ, Shott SR, et al. Acquired subglottic cysts in preterm infants. J Otolaryngol 2005;34(2):75–8.

[52] Doherty KM, Tabaee A, Castillo M, et al. Neonatal tracheal rupture complicating endotracheal intubation: a case report and indications for conservative management. Int J Pediatr Otorhinolaryngol 2005;69(1):111–6.

[53] Macey-Dare LV, Moles DR, Evans RD, et al. Long-term effect of neonatal endotracheal intubation on palatal form and symmetry in 8–11-year-old children. Eur J Orthod 1999; 21(6):703–10.

[54] Fadavi S, Adeni S, Dziedzic K, et al. The oral effects of orotracheal intubation in prematurely born preschoolers. ASDC J Dent Child 1992;59(6):420–4.

ELSEVIER
SAUNDERS

CLINICS IN
PERINATOLOGY

Clin Perinatol 35 (2008) 283–291

Index

Note: Page numbers of article titles are in **boldface** type.

A

Abruption, placental, medically indicated preterm birth and, 58–61

Abscess, after neuraxial block, 44–45

Adverse events, definition of, 6

Age, maternal, uterine rupture risk and, 90–91

Agency for Healthcare Research and Quality, 27

Air leak syndromes, in mechanical ventilation, 24, 276–278

Allergy, drug, monitoring of, 148–149

Alveolar injury, in mechanical ventilation, 273–274

Amino acid preparations, complications of, 19–20

Aminoglycosides, hearing loss due to, 167

Ammonium compounds, hazards of, 176

Amniotic fluid, simulated, for necrotizing enterocolitis, 263–264

Amphotericin, for candidiasis, 240–241

Anesthesia
errors with, 105, 107
malignant hyperthermia of, 192–193
neuraxial. *See* Neuraxial block.

Angiogenic factors, in ischemic placental disease, 59–60

Antibiotics
errors with, 112, 152–153
for necrotizing enterocolitis, 263

Anticoagulants, for thrombosis, 210

Antidepressants, in pregnancy, 104–105

Antimicrobial peptides, necrotizing enterocolitis and, 257

Aorta, thrombosis of, in umbilical catheter use, 213–214

Arterial catheters, complications of, 211–212, 216

Arthritis, septic, MRSA, 233

Asphyxia, necrotizing enterocolitis in, 256, 258

Assisted ventilation. *See* Mechanical ventilation.

Atrium, right, central venous catheter in, 203, 205

Auditory system, noise effects on, 166–168

Autonomic nervous system, noise effects on, 167

B

Backache, postpartum, 40–41

Bacteremia, MRSA, 233–235

Bacterial translocation, necrotizing enterocolitis in, 256–257, 260

Barotrauma, in mechanical ventilation, 24

Benzethonium chloride, hazards of, 176–177

Benzyl alcohol, toxicity of, 174

Bifidobacterium, for necrotizing enterocolitis, 263

Bleach, hazards of, 176

Bleeding. *See* Hemorrhage.

Blindness, from oxygen exposure, 26–27, 164–165

Blood patch, epidural, for post–dural puncture headache, 39–40

Blood stream infections
Candida, 240–242
MRSA, 233–235

Blood transfusions, hazards of, 175

Bradycardia, fetal, in uterine rupture, 87–88

doi:10.1016/S0095-5108(08)00010-9